300 Single Best Answers
in Clinical Medicine

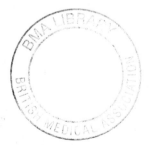
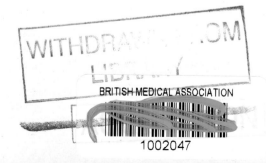

300 Single Best Answers in Clinical Medicine

George Collins BSc MBBS
Foundation Year 1 Doctor
Addenbrooke's Hospital
Cambridge University Hospitals NHS Foundation Trust

James Davis BSc MBBS
Foundation Year 1 Doctor
King's College Hospital
King's College Hospital NHS Foundation Trust

Oscar Swift BSc MBBS
Foundation Year 1 Doctor
Lister Hospital
East and North Hertfordshire NHS Trust

Edited by **Huw Beynon** BSc MD FRCP
Consultant in Rheumatology and General Medicine
Royal Free Hospital
Royal Free London NHS Foundation Trust

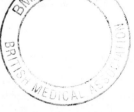

Imperial College Press

ICP

Published by

Imperial College Press
57 Shelton Street
Covent Garden
London WC2H 9HE

Distributed by

World Scientific Publishing Co. Pte. Ltd.
5 Toh Tuck Link, Singapore 596224
USA office: 27 Warren Street, Suite 401-402, Hackensack, NJ 07601
UK office: 57 Shelton Street, Covent Garden, London WC2H 9HE

Library of Congress Cataloging-in-Publication Data
Collins, George (George Benjamin), 1989–   , author.
    300 single best answers in clinical medicine / George Collins, James Davis, Oscar Swift ;
[editor] Huw Beynon.
    p. ; cm.
    Includes bibliographical references and index.
    ISBN 978-1-78326-436-0 (hardcover : alk. paper) --
    ISBN 978-1-78326-437-7 (paperback : alk. paper)
    I. Davis, James (James Stephen), 1989–   , author. II. Swift, Oscar, 1988–   , author.
III. Beynon, H. L. C., editor. IV. Title.
    [DNLM: 1. Clinical Medicine--methods--Examination Questions. WB 18.2]
    RC58
    616.0076--dc23

                                    2014025833

British Library Cataloguing-in-Publication Data
A catalogue record for this book is available from the British Library.

Typeset by Stallion Press
Email: enquiries@stallionpress.com

Printed in Singapore by B & Jo Enterprise Pte Ltd

Preface

Under the auspices of Dr Huw Beynon, renowned medical educator, we wrote this collection of 300 single best answer questions during our final year at medical school. We have drawn on our experiences of medical education to produce a book we wish we could have read as students ourselves. We were keen near-peer educators at medical school and have taken this forward to our junior doctor years.

Like the challenges set by our patients, those set by these best of five questions are far-reaching, complex and multi-dimensional. Many of the questions are difficult and span various aspects of general medicine. They aim to translate basic science, pathology and clinical practice into real-life clinical scenarios, mirroring the thought processes physicians require in the diagnosis, investigation and management of their patients' medical problems. Although they are no substitute for real-life clinical encounters, books like this are a valuable addition to a student's repertoire of learning and revision aids.

In contrast to many revision books and online question banks, our answers are comprehensive and, in most cases, include thorough justification of both the correct and incorrect answers. The learning points apply not only to the case in point but also to other clinical scenarios. It is this understanding-based approach to learning clinical medicine that we find most rewarding and hope we can impart to our readers as they transition from medical students to foundation year doctors and beyond. The book is divided into five mock exam papers of 60 questions each. We would suggest a time limit of 75 minutes per paper. Alternatively, topics can be covered by keyword or specialty. We have tried to replicate the layout of questions delivered in formal examinations by avoiding, as much as possible, negatively phrased questions and by ordering options in alphabetical order.

In addition to Dr Huw Beynon, our educators at University College London and our respective families and friends, we would like to thank Catharina Weijman, Jacqueline Downs and Alice Oven at Imperial College Press for their patience and guidance during the production of this book. Finally, we are grateful to the patients we have learned from, without whom a book like this would not be possible.

GC, JD, OS
April 2014

Contents

Laboratory Reference Ranges

Haematology	Normal value
Haemoglobin (male)	13.5–17.5 g/dL
Haemoglobin (female)	11.5–15.5 g/dL
Haemoglobin A	96–98%
Haemoglobin A2	1.5–3.2%
Foetal haemoglobin	0.5–0.8%
Mean corpuscular volume	76–96 fL
Haematocrit (male)	0.4–0.54
Haematocrit (female)	0.37–0.47
Erythropoietin	5–25 U/L
White cell count	$4\text{--}11 \times 10^9/L$
Neutrophils	$2\text{--}7.5 \times 10^9/L$
Lymphocytes	$1.3\text{--}3.5 \times 10^9/L$
Eosinophils	$0.0\text{--}0.4 \times 10^9/L$
Basophils	$0\text{--}0.1 \times 10^9/L$
Platelets	$150\text{--}400 \times 10^9/L$
Reticulocyte count	0.8–2.0%
Erythrocyte sedimentation rate (ESR) (male)	(~(age in years) ÷ 2) mm per hour
Erythrocyte sedimentation rate (ESR) (female)	(~(age in years + 10) ÷ 2) mm per hour
Prothrombin time	10–14 seconds
Activated partial thromboplastin time	35–45 seconds
Thrombin time	15–19 seconds
Fibrinogen	1.5–3 g/L
International normalised ratio	0.9–1.2

Biochemistry

Alanine aminotransferase (ALT)	5–35 IU/L
Albumin	35–50 g/L
Alkaline phosphatase (ALP)	30–300 IU/L
Amylase	0–180 Somogyi U/dL
Aspartate transaminase (AST)	5–35 IU/L
Bicarbonate	24–30 mmol/L
Bilirubin	3–17 µmol/L
Calcium	2.12–2.65 mmol/L
Chloride	95–105 mmol/L
Cholesterol	3.9–5.5 mmol/L
Low-density lipoprotein cholesterol	1.55–4.4 mmol/L
High-density lipoprotein cholesterol	0.9–1.93 mmol/L
Cortisol (9 am)	450–700 nmol/L
Creatine kinase (male)	25–195 IU/L
Creatine kinase (female)	25–170 IU/L
Creatinine	70–130 µmol/L
C-reactive protein	0–10
Ferritin	12–200 µg/L
Folate	5–6.3 nmol/L (2.1–2.8 µg/L)
Gamma-glutamyl transpeptidase (male)	11–51 IU/L
Gamma-glutamyl transpeptidase (female)	7–33 IU/L
Gastrin (fasting)	<100 ng/L
Glucose (fasting)	3.5–5.5 mmol/L
Glycosylated haemoglobin (HbA$_1$C)	5–8%
Growth hormone	<20 mU/L
Iron	12–30 µmol/L
Lactate dehydrogenase	70–250 IU/L
Magnesium	0.75–1.05 mmol/L

Osmolality	278–305 mOsmol/kg
Parathyroid hormone	<0.8–8.5 pmol/L
Phosphate	0.8–1.45 mmol/L
Potassium	3.5–5.0 mmol/L
Prolactin (male)	<450 U/L
Prolactin (female)	<600 U/L
Prostate specific antigen	0–4 ng/ml
Protein (total)	60–80 g/L
Red cell folate	0.36–1.44 µmol/L (160–640 µg/L)
Sodium	135–145 mmol/L
Thyroid-stimulating hormone	0.3–3.8 mU/L
Thyroxine (T_4)	70–140 nmol/L
Thyroxine (free)	10.0–26.0 nmol/L
Total iron-binding capacity	45–72 µmol/L
Triglyceride (fasting)	0.55–1.90 mmol/L
Triiodothyronine (T_3)	1.2–3.0 nmol/L
Troponin T	<0.1 µg/L
Urea	2.5–6.7 mmol/L
Urate (male)	0.21–0.48 mmol/L
Urate (female)	0.15–0.39 mmol/L
Vitamin B_{12}	0.13–0.68 nmol/L (>150 ng/L)
Vitamin D	>50 nmol/L = adequate, 25–50 nmol/L = insufficiency, <25 nmol/L = deficiency

Immunology

C3	0.70–1.65 g/L
C4	0.16–0.54 g/L
CD4 lymphocyte absolute count	404–1612 cells/ml
Immunoglobulin G concentration	6.34–18.11 g/L
Immunoglobulin A concentration	0.87–4.12 g/L
Immunoglobulin M concentration	0.53–2.23 g/L

Immunoglobulin E concentration	0–81 kU/L
Serum free light chains – kappa	3.3–19.4 mg/L
Serum free light chains – lambda	5.71–26.3 mg/L

Urine

Cortisol (free)	<280 nmol/24h
Hydroxyindole acetic acid	16–73 µmol/24h
Hydroxymethylmandelic acid	16–48 µmol/24h
Osmolality	350–1000 mOsmol/kg
Phosphate	15–50 mmol/24h
Potassium	14–120 mmol/24h
Sodium	100–250 mmol/24h

Arterial blood gas

pH	7.35–7.45
PaO_2	>10 kPa on air
$PaCO_2$	4.7–6.0 kPa
Lactate	0.5–2.2 mmol/L
Base excess	+/−2 mmol/L

CSF analysis

	Bacterial	**Viral**	**TB meningitis**
Appearance	Turbid	Clear	Clear/slightly cloudy
Cells (ml)	5–2000	5–500	5–1000
Predominant cell type	Neutrophils	Lymphocytes	Lymphocytes
Glucose	Very low	Normal	Low
Protein (mg/dL)	Often >1.0	0.5–0.9	Often 0.5–0.9
Other tests	Gram stain Bacterial antigen	PCR	Ziehl–Neelsen PCR

Abbreviations

5HT	Serotonin
50S	50 Svedberg units
AA	Serum amyloid protein A amyloidosis
ACE	Angiotensin-converting enzyme
AchR	Acetylcholine receptor
ADH	Antidiuretic hormone
AIDS	Acquired immunodeficiency syndrome
AL	Light chain amyloidosis
ANCA	Anti-neutrophil cytoplasmic antigen
Anti-HbcAg IgG	Immunoglobulin G antibodies against hepatitis B core antigen
Anti-HbcAg IgM	Immunoglobulin M antibodies against hepatitis B core antigen
Anti-HbeAg	Antibodies against hepatitis Be antigen
APC	Adenomatous polyposis coli gene
ATP	Adenosine triphosphate
aVF	Augmented vector foot
aVL	Augmented vector left
aVR	Augmented vector right
β-HCG	Beta human chorionic gonadotrophin
BCR-ABL	Breakpoint cluster-Abelson gene
BRCA1	Breast cancer 1, early-onset gene
BRCA2	Breast cancer 2, early-onset gene
C7	Cervical spine root seven
C8	Cervical spine root eight
CD	Cluster of differentiation
Creatine kinase MB	Creatine kinase muscle-brain
CMV	Cytomegalovirus
CO	Carbon monoxide
COPD	Chronic obstructive pulmonary disease

CT	Computed tomography
CYP450	Cytochrome P450
DC cardioversion	Direct current cardioversion
DNA	Deoxyribonucleic acid
dsDNA	Double-stranded deoxyribonucleic acid
ECG	Electrocardiogram
ESR	Erythrocyte sedimentation rate
EBV	Epstein–Barr virus
Fc	Fragment, crystallisable
FEV_1	Forced expiratory volume over 1 second
F_iO_2	Inspiratory concentration of oxygen
FVC	Forced vital capacity
GD1	Ganglioside GD1
GQ1B	Ganglioside GQ1B
GM1	Ganglioside GM1
GMP	Guanosine monophosphate
HACEK	*Haemophilus*, *Actinobacillus*, *Cardiobacterium*, *Eikenella* and *Kingella*
HBeAg	Hepatitis B e antigen
HBsAg	Hepatitis B surface antigen
HER2	Human epidermal growth factor receptor 2
HFE	Human haemochromatosis protein
HHV	Human herpes virus
HMG-CoA	3-Hydroxy-3-methylglutaryl-coenzyme A
HIV	Human immunodeficiency virus
IgA	Immunoglobulin A
IgE	Immunoglobulin E
IgG	Immunoglobulin G
IgM	Immunoglobulin M
JAK2	Janus kinase 2
kCO	Carbon monoxide transfer coefficient
L2	Lumbar spine root two
L4	Lumbar spine root four
L5	Lumbar spine root five

LASER	Light amplification by stimulated emission of radiation
MEN1	Menin gene
mGluR1	Metabotropic glutamate receptor 1
MRI	Magnetic resonance imaging
MSH2	MutS protein homologue 2
MST	Morphine sulphate
MuSK	Muscle-specific tyrosine kinase
NAPQI	N-acetyl-p-benzoquinone imine
NSAID	Non-steroidal anti-inflammatory drug
NSTEMI	Non-ST elevation myocardial infarction
$PaCO_2$	Partial pressure of carbon dioxide in the blood
PaO_2	Partial pressure of oxygen in the blood
PEFR	Peak expiratory flow rate
PiMZ	Protease inhibitor type MZ
PiSS	Protease inhibitor type SS
PiSZ	Protease inhibitor type SZ
PiZZ	Protease inhibitor type ZZ
PKD	Polycystic kidney disease gene
PML	Promyelocytic leukaemia gene
RARA	Retinoic acid receptor alpha gene
Rb	Retinoblastoma gene
REM	Rapid eye movement
RET	Rearranged during transfection gene
RNA	Ribonucleic acid
SCN4A	Sodium channel, voltage-gated type IV, alpha subunit
SOD1	Super-oxide dismutase one
STEMI	ST elevation myocardial infarction
T1	Thoracic spine root one
T4	Thoracic spine root four
TDP-43	TAR DNA-binding protein 43
TNF	Tumour necrosis factor
TP53	Tumour protein p53 gene

S1	Sacral nerve root one
S2	Sacral nerve root two
SSA	Sjögren's syndrome A antigen
SSB	Sjögren's syndrome B antigen
VHL	Von Hippel–Lindau gene
VZV	Varicella zoster virus

Paper 1

Paper 1

Paper 1: Questions

1.1 A 46-year-old male who is started on treatment for hypercholesterolaemia complains of the foul taste of his medication.

Which one of the following medications is he most likely to be taking?

A Benecol
B Cholestyramine
C Nicotinic acid
D Simvastatin
E Verapamil

1.2 An 83-year-old female with atrial fibrillation is reviewed in clinic. The patient and her relatives are discussing whether or not she should be started on warfarin.

In which one of the following situations can warfarin still be used?

A Frequent falls
B Mitral regurgitation
C Platelets less than $50 \times 10^9/L$
D Potential compliance issues
E Previous intracranial bleeds

1.3 A 36-year-old pregnant female presents with sudden-onset shortness of breath and pleuritic chest pain. Her observations are as follows:

Heart rate	110 beats per minute
Respiratory rate	30 breaths per minute
Blood pressure	100/60 mmHg
Oxygen saturations on room air	93%
Temperature	37.3 °C

Which one of the following is the most likely diagnosis?

A Deep vein thrombosis
B Myocardial infarction
C Pericarditis
D Pneumothorax
E Pulmonary embolus

1.4 A 46-year-old male presents with cough and general malaise. 'Target' lesions are present on his arms and legs. Chest X-ray shows bilateral alveolar shadowing and *Mycoplasma* serology is positive for IgM antibodies.

Which one of the following is the most appropriate treatment?

A Amoxicillin
B Ceftriaxone
C Erythromycin
D Meropenem
E Vancomycin

1.5 A 28-year-old male with a history of asthma presents with chest-tightness, shortness of breath, wheeze and cough.

Which one of the following is the best indicator that this asthma attack is life threatening?

A Heart rate of 115 beats per minute
B Oxygen saturations of 94%
C PEFR 35% of predicted
D Respiratory rate of 35 breaths per minute
E Silent chest

1.6 A 78-year-old female presents to the Emergency Department for the third time in one month with nausea, headache, weakness and unsteadiness on her feet. On examination coarse crackles are heard bibasally. Her observations are as follows:

Heart rate   110 beats per minute
Respiratory rate   28 breaths per minute
Oxygen saturations (pulse oximetry)   99%
  on room air

Arterial blood gas sampling reveals a PaO_2 of 12 kPa and oxygen saturations of 80% on room air.

Which one of the following is the most likely explanation in this patient?

A Acute pulmonary haemorrhage
B Acute pulmonary oedema
C Carbon monoxide poisoning
D Community-acquired pneumonia
E Pulmonary fibrosis

1.7 A 66-year-old male is diagnosed with COPD. The post-bronchodilator FEV_1:FVC is 0.58 and the FEV_1 is 37% that of predicted. He is a smoker with a 50-pack year history. He wants to give up smoking and has been referred for smoking cessation therapy.

Which one of the following subsequent management options is most likely to prolong survival in this patient?

A Corticosteroids
B Influenza vaccination
C Ipratropium bromide
D Long-term oxygen therapy
E Salmeterol inhalers

1.8 A 53-year-old male is being treated for aspiration pneumonia. Twenty-four hours after admission to hospital he develops worsening shortness of breath and cough. The patient is subsequently placed on high-flow oxygen using a non-rebreather mask with a reservoir bag. There are coarse crackles bilaterally and a chest X-ray shows the presence of extensive bilateral lung infiltrates. The arterial blood gas result is as follows:

PaO_2 10.8 kPa
$PaCO_2$ 4.3 kPa
F_iO_2 65%

Which one of the following pathological changes is most likely to explain this patient's clinical presentation?

A Alveolar hyaline membrane formation
B Alveolar wall destruction
C Diffuse pulmonary haemorrhage
D Granulomatous inflammation
E Mucous gland hypertrophy

1.9 A 32-year-old female with known ulcerative colitis presents with bloody diarrhoea and abdominal pain. Her observations are as follows:

Blood pressure   90/55 mmHg
Heart rate   120 beats per minute

Abdominal X-ray shows 'thumb-printing'.

Which one of the following medications is contraindicated?

A Aminosalicylate
B Ciclosporin
C Ciprofloxacin
D Morphine sulphate
E Prednisolone

1.10 A 46-year-old male presents with upper epigastric pain, anorexia and a three-month history of weight loss. On endoscopy a malignant ulcer is visualised. Subsequent biopsy reveals a low-grade gastric mucosal-associated lymphoid tissue lymphoma. *Helicobacter pylori* infection is also shown to be present.

Which one of the following is the most appropriate initial treatment of this patient?

A Band ligation
B Chemotherapy
C Injection sclerotherapy
D Proton pump inhibitor and antibiotics
E Radiotherapy

1.11 A 47-year-old male presents with fatigue, renal colic and depression. His corrected serum calcium is found to be 3.12 mmol/L.

Which one of the following is the most likely cause of his hypercalcaemia?

A Loop diuretic administration
B Osteomalacia
C Osteoporosis
D Sarcoidosis
E Secondary hyperparathyroidism

1.12 A 63-year-old female presents with lethargy, blurred vision and weight loss. Clinical examination reveals splenomegaly and blood tests reveal pancytopaenia with a raised ESR.

Which one of the following is the most likely diagnosis?

A Acute lymphoblastic leukaemia
B Chronic myeloid leukaemia
C Monoclonal gammopathy of uncertain significance
D Multiple myeloma
E Waldenström's macroglobulinaemia

1.13 A 36-year-old female with sickle cell disease presents with shortness of breath, joint pains and a maculopapular rash on the face, arms and legs. Blood tests are as follows:

Haemoglobin	6.9 g/dL
Reticulocyte count	0.2%

Which one of the following is the most likely aetiological agent in this patient?

A *Escherichia coli* O157
B Measles virus
C *Mycoplasma pneumoniae*
D Parvovirus B19
E *Salmonella* species

1.14 A 79-year-old female is admitted to the Intensive Care Unit with severe community-acquired pneumonia. Blood cultures grow *Streptococcus pneumoniae*. Bloods for urea and electrolytes and urine biochemistry tests are also taken and show evidence of pre-renal acute kidney injury.

Which one of the following profiles is most likely to be found in this patient?

A Increased urea:creatinine ratio, high urinary sodium
B Increased urea:creatinine ratio, low urinary sodium
C Normal urea:creatinine ratio, high urinary sodium
D Normal urea:creatinine ratio, low urinary sodium
E Reduced urea:creatinine ratio, high urinary sodium

1.15 A 66-year-old male is seen in the Emergency Department with generalised malaise, arthralgia and haematuria. On examination there is significant peripheral oedema. He also complains that his fingers become white, cold and numb when exposed to cold temperatures. On taking his past medical history, it is revealed that he is under the care of the hepatology department at the hospital for chronic liver disease. Urine dipstick reveals +++ blood and ++++ protein. Selected blood tests are as follows:

Albumin	21 g/L
Low-density lipoprotein cholesterol	5.2 mmol/L
C3	0.72 g/L
C4	0.11 g/L

A renal biopsy is performed and examined under the light microscope. Which one of the following is the most likely histological abnormality to be identified?

A Crescentic glomerulonephritis
B Focal segmental glomerulosclerosis
C Membranous nephropathy
D Mesangiocapillary glomerulonephritis
E Minimal change nephropathy

1.16 A 37-year-old previously healthy male presents to the Emergency Department after an episode of 'pricking' sensation on the tip of his left index finger that progressed to involve his left hand and arm over the course of two minutes. He reports that he has had four similar episodes over the past six weeks and they all resolved spontaneously after about three minutes. There is no associated motor weakness or loss of consciousness.

Which one of the following is the most likely diagnosis in this patient?

A C7 radiculopathy
B Complex partial seizure
C Diabetic neuropathy
D Jacksonian seizure
E Transient ischaemic attack

1.17 A 72-year-old female undergoes a dual-energy X-ray absorptiometry bone scan that reveals a T-score of −2.8. She has a 50-pack year smoking history and underwent the menopause aged 39. She subsequently commences treatment on risedronate but soon after stops taking it due to intolerable odynophagia.

Which one of the following treatment options is now the most appropriate for this patient?

A Alendronate
B Hormone replacement therapy
C Omeprazole
D Ranitidine
E Zoledronate

1.18 A 38-year-old male with Raynaud's syndrome presents to the Emergency Department. Clinical examination reveals the presence of tight skin over his hands, face and chest and 'red spots' that blanch when pressure is applied to them on his chest, face and arms. His blood pressure is 201/138 mmHg. Blood tests are as follows:

Serum creatinine   389 µmol/L
Serum urea   24.3 mmol/L

Which one of the following antibodies is most associated with this clinical scenario?

A Anti-centromere
B Anti-Jo1
C Anti-liver kidney microsomal
D Anti-RNA polymerase III
E Anti-SSA

1.19 A 38-year-old intravenous drug user presents with an acutely painful swollen left knee and a temperature of 38.3 °C. Joint aspiration reveals a turbid, yellow fluid that is sent for culture.

Which one of the following is the most appropriate initial empirical treatment?

A Intravenous cefotaxime and intravenous gentamicin
B Intravenous flucloxacillin and intravenous benzylpenicillin
C Oral amoxicillin and oral erythromycin
D Oral flucloxacillin and oral penicillin V
E Oral metronidazole

1.20 A 73-year-old male presents with lethargy, weight loss, scalp tenderness and shoulder and hip girdle pain. On examination the temporal arteries are tender to palpation, power is 5/5 throughout and vision is normal. The ESR is 114 mm per hour. The patient is immediately commenced on high-dose oral prednisolone following a clinical diagnosis of giant cell arteritis. However, upon review six weeks later, the patient's symptoms have not improved and the ESR is now 136 mm per hour.

Which one of the following is most appropriate in the management of this patient?

A Add azathioprine
B Add methotrexate
C Administer high-dose intravenous methylprednisolone
D CT chest, abdomen and pelvis
E Temporal artery ultrasound

1.21 A 37-year-old female presents with bloody nasal crusting and haemoptysis. Urine dipstick demonstrates 2+ protein and 3+ blood. On examination there is collapse of the nasal bridge and a palpable purpuric rash over both legs. A chest X-ray identifies a cavitating lesion in the left upper zone.

Which one of the following is the most likely diagnosis?

A Eosinophilic granulomatosis with polyangiitis (Churg–Strauss syndrome)
B Granulomatosis with polyangiitis (Wegener's granulomatosis)
C Histoplasmosis
D Sarcoidosis
E Tuberculosis

1.22 A 32-year-old pregnant female with a history of malar rash, photosensitivity and joint pain in her hands is seen in the antenatal clinic. An appropriate autoantibody screen is performed.

Which one of the following autoantibodies is most associated with poor foetal cardiac function with respect to this patient?

A Anti-dsDNA
B Anti-La
C Anti-nuclear
D Anti-phospholipid
E Anti-Ro

1.23 A 59-year-old male develops increasing pain in his right hip two years after a right total hip replacement. A right hip X-ray reveals marked periosteal reaction around the prosthesis. Joint aspiration of the hip yields straw-coloured fluid. Gram stain identifies Gram-positive bacilli.

Which one of the following is the most likely causative organism?

A *Neisseria gonorrhoeae*
B *Propionibacterium acnes*
C *Pseudomonas aeruginosa*

D *Staphylococcus aureus*
E *Streptococcus pneumoniae*

1.24 A 45-year-old male presents one month after a renal transplant with fever, cough and dyspnoea. A chest X-ray is performed and shows 'hazy shadowing'. Lung biopsy reveals the presence of 'owl's eye' inclusion bodies.

Which one of the following is the most likely causative organism?

A *Aspergillus fumigatus*
B CMV
C EBV
D *Pneumocystis jiroveci*
E VZV

1.25 A 65-year-old female on treatment for ovarian cancer presents with deafness and parasthesiae in her hands and feet.

Which one of the following medications is most likely to be responsible for her symptoms?

A Cisplatin
B Doxorubicin
C Paclitaxel
D Tobramycin
E Topotecan

1.26 A 78-year-old male develops sudden, painless loss of vision in his left eye. Examination of the fundus reveals a pale, oedematous retina. At the fovea the underlying vascular choroidal layer is well visualised.

Which one of the following is the most likely diagnosis?

A Central retinal artery occlusion
B Central retinal vein occlusion
C Giant cell arteritis
D Optic neuritis
E Vitreous haemorrhage

1.27 A 28-year-old female presents to the Emergency Department with nausea and severe abdominal pain.

Which one of the following is the most appropriate initial investigation?

A β-HCG
B Abdominal CT
C Abdominal ultrasound
D Abdominal X-ray
E Full blood count, urea and electrolytes, liver function tests and C-reactive protein

1.28 A 75-year-old male with New York Heart Association stage III heart failure has developed gynaecomastia after recently starting a new medication.

Which one of the following is the most likely cause of his symptoms?

A Bisoprolol
B Bumetanide
C Enalapril
D Furosemide
E Spironolactone

1.29 A 65-year-old male presents to the Emergency Department with fever, pleuritic chest pain and shortness of breath. He reports having suffered a myocardial infarction two weeks previously. On examination there is an audible rub in the left parasternal region. An initial chest X-ray is unremarkable and subsequent CT pulmonary angiogram does not reveal any filling defects.

Which one of the following is the most likely diagnosis in this patient?

A Acute mitral regurgitation
B Dressler's syndrome
C Pleural effusion
D Pneumonia
E Pulmonary embolism

1.30 A 20-year-old female with primary amenorrhoea presents to her General Practitioner complaining of dizziness, shortness of breath and leg pains, which are all brought on by exercise. On examination she is noticed to have an ejection systolic murmur heard loudest on the back in between the scapulae. The blood pressure in both arms is 150/95 mmHg.

Which one of the following is the most likely underlying diagnosis in this patient?

A Down's syndrome
B Ebstein's anomaly
C Kallmann's syndrome
D Primary hyperparathyroidism
E Turner syndrome

1.31 A 77-year-old female is admitted to hospital with severe shortness of breath. She has a productive cough with pink, frothy sputum and bibasal inspiratory crackles. Her observations are as follows:

Respiratory rate   20 breaths per minute
Temperature   36.7 °C
Blood pressure   135/80 mmHg

A chest X-ray shows interstitial and alveolar shadowing throughout both lung fields with engorgement of the pulmonary vasculature.

Which one of the following medications is most appropriate in this patient?

A Intravenous bumetanide
B Intravenous ceftriaxone
C Intravenous co-amoxiclav
D Oral sildenafil
E Oral spironolactone

1.32 A 32-year-old intravenous drug user has a hepatitis B serology screen. It reveals the following:

HBsAg	Positive
Anti-HbcAg IgM	Negative
Anti-HbcAg IgG	Positive
HBeAg	Negative
Anti-I IbeAg	Negative

Which one of the following best describes his clinical state?

A Acute hepatitis B infection
B Hepatitis B carrier of high infectivity
C Hepatitis B carrier of low infectivity
D Immunisation with hepatitis B vaccine
E Previous infection with hepatitis B

1.33 A 41-year-old female presents with indigestion, bloating and diarrhoca. On further questioning her stools are foul smelling and more than one flush of the toilet is required to dispose of them. She also has an itchy, blistering rash on her elbows. On further investigation, she is found to have iron deficiency anaemia; jejunal biopsy reveals the presence of subtotal villous atrophy and absence of periodic acid-Schiff-positive macrophages. Anti-tissue transglutaminase antibodies are negative. There is no significant past medical history or recent history of foreign travel.

Which one of the following is the most likely explanation for these test results?

A Selective IgA deficiency
B Systemic scleroderma
C Tropical sprue
D Ulcerative colitis
E Whipple's disease

1.34 A 40-year-old male with galactorrhoea has a serum prolactin level of 1260 U/L. He subsequently undergoes an MRI scan which reveals a small suprasellar mass. A preliminary diagnosis of a microprolactinoma is made.

Which one of the following treatment options is most suitable in this patient?

A Initiate treatment with cabergoline
B Refer for radiation therapy
C Refer for transsphenoidal adenectomy
D Repeat prolactin levels in 12 months
E Start the patient on low-dose clozapine

1.35 A 65-year-old male presents with difficulty standing from his chair, muscular cramps, rigidity and painful muscles. On examination there is a sinus bradycardia, slow relaxing reflexes and enlarged calf muscles.

Which one of the following is the most likely diagnosis?

A Amiodarone-induced hyperthyroidism
B De Quervain's thyroiditis
C Graves' disease
D Hoffman's syndrome
E Hyperparathyroidism

1.36 A 43-year-old male presents with tiredness and lethargy. The patient has the following investigation results:

Haemoglobin	9.6 g/dL
Reticulocyte count	7%
Direct Coombs test	Positive
Serum bilirubin	59 μmol/L
Serum unconjugated bilirubin	54 μmol/L
Serum conjugated bilirubin	5 μmol/L

Which one of the following is the most likely cause of this clinical scenario?

A Epstein–Barr virus infection
B Glucose-6-phosphate disease
C *Mycoplasma* virus infection
D Sickle cell disease
E Systemic lupus erythematosus

1.37 A 65-year-old female presented to her General Practitioner complaining of pruritus after a hot bath. Her full blood count revealed a haemoglobin of 19.6 g/dL.

Which one of the following is she most at risk of developing?

A Acute myeloid leukaemia
B Chronic lymphocytic leukaemia
C Chronic myeloid leukaemia
D Multiple sclerosis
E Systemic lupus erythematosus

1.38 A 19-year-old female with known sickle cell disease presents with a two-week history of worsening pain in her right hip. She also complains of feeling lethargic and was noted to have a temperature of 38.5 °C. An MRI scan revealed localised bone marrow abnormalities in the right femoral head.

Which of the following would be the most likely organism cultured from a bone biopsy in this patient?

A *Escherichia coli*
B *Pseudomonas aeruginosa*
C *Salmonella typhi*
D *Staphylococcus epidermidis*
E *Streptococcus viridans*

1.39 A 70-year-old female with postural hypotension is noted to have microalbuminuria on three occasions over a one-year period. Her estimated glomerular filtration rate is 65 mL/min/1.73 m^2 and a renal biopsy reveals nodular glomerulosclerosis.

Which of the following is the most likely diagnosis?

A Diabetic nephropathy
B Idiopathic nephropathy
C HIV nephropathy
D Hypertensive nephropathy
E Multiple myeloma

1.40 A 22-year-old male presents with a two-month history of nausea and vomiting. He also complains of frontal headaches that are worse at night and relieved by an episode of vomiting. Which one of the following investigations is it most important to perform in this patient?

A Abdominal ultrasound
B CT abdomen
C CT head
D Lumbar puncture
E T2-weighted MRI brain

1.41 A 78-year-old female presents with a six-month history of increasing difficulties with speech fluency. Her close relative states that this was preceded by marked personality changes including impulsivity and severe mood swings. She has also been recently diagnosed with the early stages of motor neuron disease. Which one of the following is the most likely diagnosis in this patient?

A Alzheimer's disease
B Frontotemporal lobe dementia
C Hypothyroidism
D Lewy body dementia
E Vascular dementia

1.42 A 35-year-old female presents with worsening double vision and an unsteady gait. Three weeks prior she suffered an episode of severe bloody diarrhoea. A full neurological examination reveals generalised areflexia.

Which one of the following antibodies is most associated with this patient's condition?

A Anti-GD1a
B Anti-GD3
C Anti-GM1
D Anti-GQ1B
E Anti-MuSK

1.43 A 66-year-old female with advanced metastatic breast cancer presents to the Emergency Department with pain in her lumbar spine and complains of difficulty walking for the last 12 hours. Neurological examination reveals marked sensory loss in dermatomes L4, L5 and S1.

Which one of the following is the single most appropriate imaging modality in this patient?

A MRI cervical spine
B MRI cervical, thoracic and lumbar spine
C MRI lumbar spine
D MRI thoracic spine
E X-ray cervical, thoracic and lumbar spine

1.44 A 62-year-old female with type II diabetes mellitus recently started long-term anticoagulant therapy with warfarin for permanent atrial fibrillation. She subsequently presented to her General Practitioner with fever, shortness of breath and pleuritic chest pain and was treated for a chest infection. Following this, she returns to her General Practitioner complaining that during her regular glucose finger prick monitoring she is bleeding much more than usual. Clotting investigations reveal that her international normalised ratio is eight.

Which one of the following antibiotics is most likely to have been prescribed?

A Amoxicillin
B Ampicillin
C Erythromycin
D Penicillin V
E Rifampicin

1.45 A 39-year-old female attends her General Practitioner complaining of shortness of breath that has been worsening over the previous few months. On examination there is a pansystolic murmur that obscures the second heart sound.

Which one of the following additional findings most supports the likely diagnosis?

A The murmur radiates to the carotids
B The murmur gets quieter on squatting
C The murmur is loudest at the apex
D The patient has pale conjunctiva
E The patient is in her third trimester of pregnancy

1.46 A four-year-old girl is admitted to hospital with a chest infection, her fourth admission since birth. She has been producing thick, yellow-green sputum and her mother also says that her stools are 'oily, foul-smelling and float in the pan'.

Which one of the following is the most likely diagnosis?

A Asthma
B Cystic fibrosis
C Gastroesophageal reflux
D Kartagener's syndrome
E Sarcoidosis

1.47 A 13-year-old female with a known nut allergy is brought into the Emergency Department by her father. She has severe stridor and swollen lips and tongue after accidentally consuming nuts at a restaurant.

Which one of the following is not advocated in the management of this patient?

A   0.5 ml 1:1000 intramuscular adrenaline
B   5 mg nebulised salbutamol
C   10 ml 1:10000 intravenous adrenaline
D   10 mg intravenous chlorphenamine
E   Tracheal intubation

1.48 A 63-year-old male is suffering from weight loss and generalised itching and books in to see his local General Practitioner. The remainder of the history is unremarkable and there are no further symptoms. On examination he is clearly icteric and has a painless, palpable mass in the right upper quadrant. What is the single most appropriate test to confirm your clinical diagnosis?

A   Abdominal CT scan
B   Alpha fetoprotein
C   Endoscopic retrograde cholangiopancreatography
D   Full blood count and peripheral blood film
E   Ultrasound scan of the biliary system

1.49 A six-week-old boy with a one-week history of projectile vomiting is brought to the Emergency Department by his mother. A capillary blood gas measurement is performed.

Which one of the following metabolic disturbances would be the most likely finding?

A   Hyperglycaemic hyperketotic metabolic acidosis
B   Hypernatraemic hypokalaemic metabolic alkalosis
C   Hypochloraemic hyperkalaemic metabolic alkalosis
D   Hypochloraemic hypokalaemic metabolic alkalosis
E   Hyponatraemic hyperkalaemic metabolic acidosis

1.50 A 37-year-old female presents to the Emergency Department with jaundice and acute epigastric pain that radiates to the back and has built up over about an hour. After receiving the results for her blood tests, a diagnosis of acute pancreatitis secondary to cholelithiasis is made.

In the assessment of acute pancreatitis, which one of the following investigations is of diagnostic, but not prognostic, value?

A Serum amylase
B Serum calcium
C Serum glucose
D Serum lactate dehydrogenase
E White blood cell count

1.51 A patient with type I diabetes mellitus is having convulsions in the Emergency Department. Finger prick capillary glucose is 1.3 mmol/L. At present there is no intravenous access.

Which one of the following is the most appropriate immediate management?

A Intramuscular adrenaline
B Intramuscular glucagon
C Oral glucose
D Subcutaneous 10% dextrose solution
E Subcutaneous insulin

1.52 A 45-year-old man is complaining to his General Practitioner that his rings, gloves and hat no longer fit. Which one of the following is the most appropriate initial screening test to support the diagnosis?

A An oral glucose tolerance test
B MRI of the pituitary fossa
C Serum growth hormone levels
D Serum insulin-like growth factor 1 levels
E Serum prolactin levels

1.53 A 24-year-old female presents to her General Practitioner complaining that over the past 12 months she has felt increasingly tired all of the time. She reports having to regularly change heavily soaked sanitary wear during her menstrual period. Her General Practitioner sends off some blood tests and she is found to be anaemic. Other tests include vitamin B_{12} and folate, iron studies and a blood film.

Which one of the following is the most likely set of findings?

A High transferrin saturation, nucleated red blood cells and target cells

B Low ferritin, spherocytes and thrombocythaemia

C Low serum iron, anisocytosis and a dimorphic picture

D Normal serum iron, macrocytosis and poikilocytosis

E Raised total iron-binding capacity, pencil cells and anisocytosis

1.54 A 14-year-old boy presents with periorbital oedema, scrotal swelling and generalised pitting oedema, which has developed gradually since a viral upper respiratory tract infection one week ago. The urine dipstick shows 4+ protein and no trace of blood.

Which one of the following is the most likely diagnosis?

A Focal glomerular sclerosis

B Henoch–Schönlein purpura

C Membranous glomerulonephritis

D Mesangiocapillary glomerulonephritis

E Minimal change glomerulonephritis

1.55 A 35-year-old male recently visited his General Practitioner complaining of a painless left-sided scrotal swelling which had developed over many weeks and seemed to disappear at night. On examination the swelling felt soft like a bag of worms and did not transilluminate. The General Practitioner reassured the man that surgical treatment was not needed unless it caused problems, and asked him to return if the symptoms worsened. The man has now returned with frank painless haematuria.

Which one of the following is the most likely cause of his symptoms?

A Bladder transitional cell carcinoma
B Idiopathic varicocoele
C Renal cell carcinoma
D Testicular hydrocoele
E Urinary tract infection

1.56 A 58-year-old hypertensive male presented to his General Practitioner with urinary symptoms. After a careful history, the patient's complaints were difficulty initiating micturition, urinary frequency, terminal dribbling and nocturia. A urine dipstick showed microscopic haematuria. The patient was then counselled before a PSA test was sent off and a digital rectal examination performed. The prostate gland was non-tender, hard, enlarged and irregularly nodular, with loss of the midline sulcus.

Which one of the following is the next most appropriate course of action?

A Abdominal and pelvic CT scan
B Abdominal ultrasound
C Prescribe tamsulosin
D Start ciprofloxacin
E Transrectal ultrasound

1.57 A 19-year-old male presents to the Emergency Department one week after returning from his gap year in sub-Saharan Africa. He is noted to be pyrexial, clinically jaundiced and has palpable splenomegaly.

Which one of the following is the most likely diagnosis?

A Loa loa
B Malaria
C Schistosomiasis
D Toxoplasmosis
E Trypanosomiasis

1.58 A previously healthy 16-year-old male is brought into the Emergency Department by his mother, who informs the doctor that her son has become very unwell over the last 24 hours with nausea, vomiting and loss of appetite. His mother also says that he started acting very strangely and has developed a sunburn-like rash all over his body. Dermatological examination reveals a widespread erythematous, macular rash, marked inflammation of the oral mucosa and a small, slightly inflamed abrasion on the skin overlying the left tibial tuberosity. Initial investigations demonstrate a high fever, marked hypotension, tachycardia, tachypnoea, deranged liver and kidney function tests and thrombocytopaenia. He is admitted to the Intensive Care Unit and after initial resuscitation and shock management is started on antibiotics.

Which one of the following is the most appropriate option?

A Benzylpenicillin
B Ceftriaxone and metronidazole
C Ciprofloxacin
D Flucloxacillin and clindamycin
E Gentamicin

1.59 A 40-year-old male presents with a three-month history of increasing lethargy. A full blood count shows iron deficiency anaec mia. Colonoscopy reveals the presence of a tumour situated in the caecum. His father died of colorectal cancer aged 38 and his sister was recently diagnosed with ovarian cancer aged 36.

Which one of the following genes is most likely to be mutated in this patient?

A *APC*
B *BRCA1*
C *BRCA2*
D *MSH2*
E *VHL*

1.60 A 32-year-old female on long-term treatment for severe acne presents with a three-week history of headaches that are worse in the morning. On examination there is impaired abduction of the left eye. Fundoscopy reveals bilateral papilloedema.

Which of the following are the most appropriate set of initial investigations to perform in this patient?

A Blood cultures and lumbar puncture
B CT scan of head and blood cultures
C CT scan of head and visual evoked potentials
D Electroencephalogram and lumbar puncture
E MRI venography and lumbar puncture

Paper 1: Answers

1.1

B – Cholestyramine

Cholestyramine is a second-line agent used to treat hypercholesterol-aemia. It is unpopular with some patients due to its gritty, metallic taste. It acts as an anion exchange resin that prevents the reabsorption of bile acids in the gastrointestinal tract. Cholesterol is subsequently utilised to replenish the levels of bile acids. Benecol (a fatty acid ester of plant stanols) and nicotinic acid (vitamin B_3) are dietary supplements that can play an important role in the management of patients with hypercholesterolaemia. Simvastatin is an HMG-CoA reductase inhibitor and is the first-line therapy in the management of hypercholesterolaemia. The side effects of simvastatin include myositis and raised liver function tests. Verapamil is a calcium channel blocker and is not used as a treatment for hypercholesterolaemia.

1.2

B – Mitral regurgitation

A patient who has mitral regurgitation and is in atrial fibrillation requires anticoagulation with warfarin in order to prevent thrombi formation. These thrombi typically form in the left atrial appendage, which is a blind-ended trabeculated sac in the lateral wall of the left atrium. These features make the left atrial appendage highly thrombogenic, especially in the presence of haemostasis as occurs inside the fibrillating atria. Thrombi can subsequently embolise throughout the systemic arterial circulation and cause downstream ischaemic complications (e.g. stroke, myocardial infarction, mesenteric ischaemia, ischaemic limb).

However, in patients taking warfarin the reduced risk of emboli formation must be balanced against the increased risk of bleeding. It is therefore not advised that patients who are already at an increased risk of bleeding be commenced on warfarin (e.g. frequent falls, thrombocytopaenia or previous intracranial bleeds).

In patients taking warfarin the international normalised ratio needs to be maintained within strict boundaries (between two and three for atrial fibrillation).

1.3

E – Pulmonary embolus

This patient is in a prothrombotic state (pregnancy), has experienced a sudden onset of symptoms and is tachycardic, tachypnoeic, hypotensive and hypoxic. Sinus tachycardia is the ECG finding most commonly associated with pulmonary embolus. The patient experiences chest pain when they inhale because the embolus in the pulmonary vasculature irritates the nerve endings of the parietal (outer) pleura. Pulmonary emboli usually arise from thrombi migrating from the deep veins of the legs or pelvis.

Pneumothorax can present in a similar fashion; however, it is less likely given this patient's risk factor for pulmonary embolism. Myocardial infarction is unlikely to present with pleuritic chest pain.

1.4

C – Erythromycin

Mycoplasma pneumoniae is a member of the Mollicute class of bacteria. It is a cause of atypical pneumonia and can result in erythema multiforme (characterised by 'target' lesions). All members of the Mollicute class of bacteria lack a peptidoglycan cell wall, and hence will be unaffected by antibiotics whose mechanism of action occurs at this site (e.g. penicillins, carbapenems, cephalosporins and glycopeptides). Erythromycin is a macrolide antibiotic that binds to the 50S subunit of the bacterial ribosome and inhibits bacterial protein synthesis. This makes it an ideal choice for the treatment of *Mycoplasma pneumoniae* infection.

Amoxicillin (a penicillin), meropenem (a carbapenem) and ceftriaxone (a cephalosporin) are all members of the beta-lactam group of antibiotics. Beta-lactams inhibit penicillin-binding proteins, a group of proteins that are involved in the final stage of cell wall transpeptidation. Vancomycin is a glycopeptide antibiotic that also inhibits cell wall synthesis, but at an earlier stage than beta-lactams. Glycopeptide antibiotics inhibit polymerisation of the peptides *N*-acetylmuramic acid and *N*-acetylglucosamine, which are important in forming the backbone strands of the bacterial cell wall.

1.5

E – Silent chest

A silent chest implies that the upper airways have become so narrow that air is no longer able to move into and out of their lungs. This is an important sign as it means that the asthma attack is life threatening. Other clinical signs of a life-threatening asthma attack are altered level of consciousness, exhaustion, arrhythmia, hypotension, cyanosis and poor respiratory effort. Measurements that indicate a life-threatening attack are a PEFR of less than 33% of predicted, oxygen saturations of less than 92%, PaO_2 of less than 8 kPa and a 'normal' $PaCO_2$ of 4.6–6 kPa. A heart rate greater than 110 beats per minute, a PEFR of 33–50% of predicted and a respiratory rate of greater than 25 breaths per minute and an inability to complete sentences in one breath all indicate a severe asthma attack.

1.6

C – Carbon monoxide poisoning

This patient has carbon monoxide poisoning and needs her carboxyhaemoglobin levels measured using a carbon monoxide oximeter. Accidental carbon monoxide poisoning occurs in homes with poorly maintained heating mechanisms and is therefore more common in the winter months. The strength with which carbon monoxide binds to haemoglobin is 250 times that for oxygen, and carbon monoxide also distorts haemoglobin in such a way that any oxygen bound is less likely to dissociate. These two mechanisms result in a reduction in oxygen delivery to the tissues and contribute to the clinical features found in this patient. Importantly, carboxyhaemoglobin has similar absorption spectra to oxyhaemoglobin, which means that pulse oximetry results will be normal and cannot be used to assess for hypoxia. Arterial blood gas will yield the PaO_2, which is usually normal, and a low oxygen saturation. PaO_2 levels are usually normal as they reflect oxygen levels dissolved in the blood. This process is not affected by carbon monoxide. Management involves removing carbon monoxide from the body via displacement with oxygen. Oxygen at the highest possible concentration is required. Intubation and 100% oxygen may be necessary, and where facilities exist, hyperbaric oxygen may also help to further expediate recovery.

Old textbooks describe a cherry red appearance of the lips and a cherry red spot at the macula in carbon monoxide poisoning but these are insensitive signs.

1.7

D – Long-term oxygen therapy

Long-term oxygen therapy is the only treatment proven to prolong survival in COPD. It is also associated with the additional benefits of reducing secondary polycythaemia, improving sleep quality by reducing hypoxia-induced brain arousals, and reducing cardiac arrhythmias. Long-term oxygen therapy is considered in patients with severe or very severe airflow obstruction (FEV_1 of less than 49% of predicted). For long-term oxygen therapy to be effective patients must breathe supplemental oxygen for at least 15 hours per day and it is essential to warn them about the risks of fire and explosion if they continue to smoke.

Corticosteroids have an important role in patients who have frequent exacerbations; however, they do not prolong survival. Bronchodilators, such as ipratropium (an anti-cholinergic) and salmeterol (a long-acting beta-adrenoreceptor agonist), act to reduce airway resistance but provide symptomatic improvement only and do not alter the forced expiratory volume in 1 second in the long term. All patients with COPD should be offered the influenza vaccine annually in order to reduce acute exacerbations.

1.8

A – Alveolar hyaline membrane formation

This patient has developed acute respiratory distress syndrome as a complication of aspiration pneumonia. Acute respiratory distress syndrome is characterised pathologically by the formation of an alveolar hyaline membrane, which occurs as a result of acute, persistent inflammation in the lung. Patients with acute respiratory distress syndrome have extensive, bilateral infiltrates on chest X-ray and very poor oxygenation despite being given high amounts of inspired oxygen.

Alveolar wall destruction is found in emphysema. This is most commonly due to smoking as cigarette smoke inhibits the enzyme alpha 1-antitrypsin (more rarely, emphysema occurs as a result of alpha 1-antitrypsin deficiency). The function of alpha 1-antitrypsin is to inhibit neutrophil elastase; therefore when its levels decrease there is increased breakdown of alveolar walls.

Diffuse pulmonary haemorrhage is characteristic of anti-glomerular basement membrane disease, granulomatosis with polyangiitis (Wegener's granulomatosis) and systemic lupus erythematosus. The kCO is increased in these diseases because the erythrocytes that line the alveoli take up carbon monoxide readily and 'falsely' increase the measurement.

Granulomatous inflammation in the lung is seen as a result of infections (usually mycobacterial or fungal), sarcoidosis, extrinsic allergic

pneumonitis, granulomatosis with polyangiitis, eosinophilic granulomatosis with polyangiitis and a variety of other conditions.

Mucous gland hypertrophy is seen in patients with COPD.

1.9
D – Morphine sulphate

This patient's abdominal X-ray is suggestive of a toxic megacolon.
Bowel wall inflammation causes thickened mucosa; thickened
haustral folds give the abdominal X-ray a 'thumb-printed' appearance. Toxic megacolon is a serious complication of ulcerative colitis
and patients are at a high risk of perforation. Morphine should be
avoided in these patients as it causes constipation and so further
increases the risk of perforation.

Patients are often dehydrated and so require fluid replacement.
Aminosalicylates (e.g. sulphasalazine), ciclosporin, a calcineurin
inhibitor, and predisolone are all immunosuppressive medications
and have been shown to reduce inflammation and improve outcomes in ulcerative colitis.

1.10
D – Proton pump inhibitor and antibiotics

Gastric mucosal-associated lymphoid tissue lymphomas are
indolent B-cell lymphomas that comprise approximately 10% of
all types of non-Hodgkin's lymphoma. Ninety percent of gastric
mucosal-associated lymphoid tissue lymphomas are caused by
Helicobacter pylori infection. Therefore eradication therapy with a
proton pump inhibitor (omeprazole) and antibiotics (clarithromycin with either metronidazole or amoxicillin) are appropriate
first-line management options. In 50% of cases eradication therapy is successful and the mucosal-associated lymphoid tissue
lymphoma resolves. If these measures do not work, then chemotherapy, with or without radiotherapy, is required. Band ligation

and injection sclerotherapy are reserved for the treatment of oesophageal varices.

1.11

D – Sarcoidosis

This patient has significantly raised serum calcium and the only cause of hypercalcaemia from the options listed above is sarcoidosis. The presenting complaint of patients with hypercalcaemia is usually one or more of 'stones (renal or biliary colic), bones (bone pain), groans (abdominal pain, nausea and vomiting) and moans (fatigue, confusion and depression)'. Sarcoidosis, multiple myeloma, primary hyperparathyroidism and malignancy are the four major causes of hypercalcaemia. In sarcoidosis, granulomatous lesions convert 1-alpha hydroxylate 25-hydroxycholecalciferol (calcidiol) to its active form, 1,25-dihydroxycholecalciferol (calcitriol). Increased levels of calcitriol and parathyroid hormone lead to a rise in serum calcium levels through increased renal reabsorption of calcium and increased bone turnover. Calcitriol also increases calcium absorption from the gastrointestinal tract. In primary hyperparathyroidism and certain malignancies (both solid organ and haematological) there are increased levels of parathyroid hormone and parathyroid hormone-related peptide.

Loop diuretics are associated with hypocalcaemia; thiazide diuretics may cause hypercalcaemia. Osteoporosis is usually associated with a normal serum calcium level (along with normal phosphate and alkaline phosphatase) and so should not be considered as a cause in this situation. Osteomalacia is characterised by defective bone and cartilage mineralisation and accumulation of unmineralised bone matrix. Reduced calcium and phosphate with a raised alkaline phosphatase is associated with osteomalacia. Secondary hyperparathyroidism occurs in response to hypocalcaemia and is associated with normal calcium levels. It is most commonly seen in chronic kidney disease due to failure of the kidney to convert

1-alpha hydroxylate 25-hydroxycholecalciferol (calcidiol) to its active form, 1,25-dihydroxycholecalciferol (calcitriol).

1.12

E – Waldenström's macroglobulinaemia

Waldenström's macroglobulinaemia is a monoclonal B-cell disorder characterised by secretion of an IgM paraprotein. The B-cells in this disorder have an appearance halfway between small lymphocytes and plasma cells; hence this disease can also be described as a lymphoplasmacytoid proliferative disorder. IgM is a pentameric antibody that polymerises easily, causing plasma hyperviscosity, which can manifest as blurred vision. Waldenström's macroglobulinaemia can present in a similar fashion to multiple myeloma except for a few differences. Unlike myeloma, bone pain, hypercalcaemia and renal failure are not seen. In Waldenström's macroglobulinaemia, organomegaly, particularly splenomegaly, is common.

Chronic myeloid leukaemia and acute lymphoblastic leukaemia can cause splenomegaly; however, they are less likely to produce symptoms of hyperviscosity. Monoclonal gammopathy of uncertain significance refers to the presence of a serum paraprotein in patients who have no clinical evidence of multiple myeloma or Waldenström's macroglobulinaemia. This patient's pancytopaenia rules out this diagnosis.

1.13

D – Parvovirus B19

Parvovirus infects erythrocyte precursors, such as reticulocytes, via the P antigen on their cell surface and causes a transient red cell aplasia that lasts for five to ten days. In patients who have preexisting conditions that shorten red cell survival, such as sickle cell disease, there is a rapid onset of severe anaemia. Parvovirus B19 is an erythrovirus that also classically causes an erythematous rash on the face and limbs, and arthralgia.

Mycoplasma pneumoniae is a bacterium that causes an atypical pneumonia associated with cold agglutinins and erythema multiforme. *Escherichia coli* O157 is an enterohaemorrhagic bacterium associated with production of the Shiga-like toxin that can lead to development of the haemolytic uraemic syndrome. The measles virus is an RNA paramyxovirus associated with the onset of the 'three Cs': cough, coryza and conjunctivitis, and subsequent development of a diffuse maculopapular rash. White spots present on the buccal mucosa (Koplik's spots) are pathognomonic for measles. *Salmonella* species are mostly associated with gastrointestinal infections but are of particular interest in the context of patients with sickle cell disease as they are the most common cause of osteomyelitis in this group of patients.

1.14

B – Increased urea:creatinine ratio, low urinary sodium

This patient is septic and has developed pre-renal acute kidney injury as a result. Patients with pre-renal acute kidney injury have an increased urea:creatinine ratio and low urinary sodium.

In pre-renal acute kidney injury the urea:creatinine ratio is increased and the urinary sodium is decreased (less than 20 mmol/L). This is because urea and sodium, both of which are highly osmotic, are actively reabsorbed into the bloodstream to try and maintain an effective circulating volume and reperfuse the kidneys. For this reason, the urine osmolality is increased (more than 500 mOsm/L) in pre-renal acute kidney injury as water is being reabsorbed. In contrast, patients who develop acute tubular necrosis will have a normal urea:creatinine ratio, a high urinary sodium level (greater than 40 mmol/L) and a low urine osmolality (less than 350 mOsm/L) because the ability of the kidney to concentrate the urine and reabsorb sodium and urea is lost.

1.15

D – Mesangiocapillary glomerulonephritis

Mesangiocapillary glomerulonephritis, also known as membrano-proliferative glomerulonephritis, is associated with the presence of cryoglobulins in the setting of chronic hepatitis C infection. Cryoglobulins are proteins that precipitate at reduced temperatures and dissolve on re-warming. In hepatitis C infection, the cryoglobulins are rheumatoid factors (either monoclonal or poly-clonal IgM antibodies that bind the Fc portion of polyclonal IgG antibodies). Cryoglobulins are deposited in small- and medium-sized vessels in the skin, joints and glomeruli, activating the classical complement pathway (with a typical complement picture of a low C4 and a normal C3) and causing local inflammation and tissue damage. This gives rise to Raynaud's phenomenon, arthralgia and mesangiocapillary glomerulonephritis respectively. Patients can present with nephrotic syndrome (as in this patient), an acute nephritis, asymptomatic urinary abnormalities or rapidly progressive renal failure. Hypertension is also a common finding in these patients. Histologically, sub-endothelial immune complex deposition and mesangial hypercellularity is seen.

Crescentic glomerulonephritis is a rapidly progressive glomerulonephritis that is either idiopathic or associated with anti-glomerular basement membrane disease, systemic lupus erythematosus or granulomatosis with polyangiitis. There is glomerular basement membrane rupture and leakage of plasma proteins, including fibrin, into Bowman's capsule. The epithelial cells lining Bowman's capsule proliferate in response to the leaked fibrin and form a scar that is visible on light microscopy of a renal biopsy in a crescent shape. Focal segmental glomerulosclerosis involves sclerosis of the glomeruli that is both focal (less than 50% of all glomeruli are affected) and segmental (only part of affected glomeruli are sclerotic). It is either idiopathic, or secondary to diseases where there is a reduced nephron number, such as reflux nephropathy, or glomerular disease, such as diabetes mellitus, HIV nephropathy and Alport's syndrome.

Membranous nephropathy occurs as a result of IgG deposition on the outer aspect of the glomerular basement membrane. Activation of the classical pathway of the complement cascade leads to podocyte damage and thickening of the glomerular basement membrane (hence 'membranous'). Membranous nephropathy can be either idiopathic or secondary to infections (hepatitis B and C, malaria and streptococcus), malignancy (lymphoma, lung and colon cancer), multisystem disease (systemic lupus erythematosus and sarcoidosis) or drugs (captopril, gold and D-penicillamine).

Minimal change nephropathy is the most common cause of nephrotic syndrome in children and accounts for approximately 25% of cases in adults. Examination of the renal biopsy under the light microscope is normal; however, when viewed under the electron microscope there is diffuse effacement of the podocyte foot processes. This is due to damage to the glomerular protein nephrin, which allows albumin to leak into the tubules. In children with nephrotic syndrome, renal biopsy is not indicated as it is unlikely to show any evidence of glomerular disease when viewed under the light microscope.

1.16

D – Jacksonian seizure

A simple partial (focal) seizure originating within the somatosensory cortex that has spread to involve the left hand and arm is the most likely diagnosis. The spread of a seizure in this manner is known as the Jacksonian march. Seizures in the somatosensory cortex produce contralateral paraesthesia; following the seizure there may be reduced sensation in the region affected.

It is unlikely to be a sensory migranous aura as the symptoms are not followed by a headache. There is no evidence of impaired consciousness in this patient; this rules out a complex partial seizure.

A C7 radiculopathy would present with symptoms of pain in the C7 myotome and sensory loss over the C7 dermatome. There may also be wasting of the triceps, wrist and finger extensors and loss of the triceps jerk if the lesion had been present for a significant period of time. This would also be unlikely in this patient due to the transient nature of the symptoms.

In diabetic neuropathy the longest nerves are affected first and therefore distal sensation is affected prior to proximal sensation. It would therefore be unusual to experience symptoms in the arms but not the legs, and they would not be transient in nature.

Transient ischaemic attacks do not present with positive sensory symptoms.

1.17

E – Zoledronate

This patient has developed odynophagia as a result of oesophageal ulceration due to oral bisphosphonate use. She should therefore be switched to an intravenous bisphosphonate such as zoledronate. Bisphosphonates are the first-line medication in treating osteoporosis and act by inhibiting bone reabsorption. They have been shown to reduce the rate of both vertebral and non-vertebral fractures in patients with osteoporosis. Another important side effect of bisphosphonates is osteonecrosis.

This patient's T-score is less than −2.5, which means that she already has osteoporosis; hormone replacement therapy only plays a role in the prevention of osteoporosis. Recent reports suggest that proton pump inhibitors, such as omeprazole, may cause osteoporosis.

1.18

D – Anti-RNA polymerase III

This patient has scleroderma renal crisis, a rheumatological emergency that presents with acute renal failure and severe hypertension. This manifestation occurs more commonly in diffuse cutaneous systemic sclerosis, and patients who are positive for anti-RNA polymerase III antibodies are 11–16 times more likely to develop scleroderma renal crisis.

Anti-topoisomerase-I (scl-70) antibodies are most commonly found in diffuse cutaneous systemic sclerosis, whereas anti-centromere antibodies are more associated with the limited form of the disease.

Anti-SSA (Ro) antibodies are more commonly seen in Sjögren's syndrome and systemic lupus erythematosus and can cross the placenta and cause congenital heart block in 1 in 20 children born to mothers with these antibodies. Anti-liver kidney microsomal antibodies are associated with autoimmune hepatitis type II and anti-Jo1 antibodies are found in polymyositis and dermatomyositis.

1.19

B – Intravenous flucloxacillin and intravenous benzylpenicillin

This patient is systemically unwell with septic arthritis and requires urgent intravenous antibiotics. Treatment is with intravenous flucloxacillin and intravenous benzylpenicillin. These antibiotics are penicillin based, have good tissue penetration and are used to treat staphylococcal and streptococcal infections respectively. These are the most likely causative organisms in this scenario. *Staphylococcus aureus* is a particularly likely culprit given the fact that this patient is an intravenous drug user. Antibiotics should not be given orally in septic arthritis because a high concentration in the blood must be achieved as quickly as possible.

Metronidazole is used to treat anaerobic and protozoal infections; these organisms are not usually implicated in septic arthritis. Oral amoxicillin and oral erythromycin is a combination commonly used to treat community-acquired pneumonia. Amoxicillin targets the 'typical' organisms such as *Streptococcus pneumoniae* and *Haemophilus influenzae*, whereas erythromycin targets the 'atypical' organisms that can cause pneumonia, such as *Mycoplasma pneumoniae* and *Legionella pneumophila*.

The choice of antibiotics will be adjusted according to synovial fluid culture and blood culture results.

1.20

D – CT chest, abdomen and pelvis

This patient has not improved despite appropriate treatment for the initial clinical diagnosis of giant cell arteritis. Usually symptoms respond to high doses of oral prednisolone and the ESR falls. However, in this case an alternative diagnosis should be sought. There should be a high index of suspicion for a paraneoplastic musculoskeletal syndrome and so a CT scan of the chest, abdomen and pelvis should be performed in order to try and identify an underlying malignancy. Classically, a renal cell carcinoma is most associated with a paraneoplastic musculoskeletal syndrome. Paraneoplastic musculoskeletal syndromes can present with giant cell arteritis, myopathy, arthropathy or vasculitis. Steroids should be continued initially if a malignancy is found. Treatment of the malignancy should resolve the underlying secondary large-vessel vasculitis, which then allows for steroids to be withdrawn.

Aspirin can be given in temporal arteritis to reduce the increased risk of stroke secondary to increased blood viscosity. Azathioprine, methotrexate and cyclophosphamide may be used in patients who require high doses of corticosteroids to control symptoms in primary temporal arteritis. Temporal artery ultrasound can be performed to assess the degree of temporal artery inflammation; however, it has not yet replaced temporal artery biopsy as the gold standard for confirming a diagnosis of temporal arteritis.

1.21

B – Granulomatosis with polyangiitis (Wegener's granulomatosis)

This patient has granulomatosis with polyangiitis, a small- to medium-vessel, necrotizing, granulomatous vasculitis. The ear, nose and throat are affected in over 90% of patients, with nasal congestion and epistaxis being the most common symptoms. Perforation of the nasal septum and collapse of the nasal bridge causing a saddle-nose deformity also occur. The lung, kidney and skin are the other organs most commonly affected, although involvement of the eyes, joints and central nervous system also occurs. C-ANCAs are antibodies against the cytoplasmic antigen proteinase-3 and are most strongly associated with granulomatosis with polyangiitis.

Eosinophilic granulomatosis with polyangiitis is also a small- to medium-vessel vasculitis but it affects predominantly the lungs and the skin. Asthma and eosinophilia in the setting of vasculitis are associated with eosinophilic granulomatosis with polyangiitis. Patients often develop a mononeuritis multiplex. Eosinophilic granulomatosis with polyangiitis is most associated with p-ANCAs, which are antibodies against the perinuclear antigen myeloperoxidase. It is important to note that there is no ear, nose and throat involvement in eosinophilic granulomatosis with polyangiitis.

Histoplasmosis is caused by the fungus *Histoplasma capsulatum*, which is found in bird and bat droppings, and occurs in patients who spelunk (explore caves). Patients often are asymptomatic although fever, cough and in severe cases respiratory failure can occur. Chest X-ray reveals the presence of multiple calcified, nodular lesions. There is no renal involvement in histoplasmosis.

Sarcoidosis is a multisystem inflammatory condition of unknown cause that commonly presents with non-caseating, granulomatous pulmonary lesions. It would be unusual for sarcoidosis to present in the same way as this scenario.

Tuberculosis also produces cavitating lesions in the upper lobes of the lungs although it rarely causes renal involvement.

1.22

E – Anti-Ro

This patient has systemic lupus erythematosus. Anti-Ro antibodies can cross the placenta and cause congenital heart block in children born to mothers with this disease. Approximately 1 in 20 mothers with anti-Ro antibodies give birth to children with heart block. Anti-Ro and anti-La antibodies are found in 20% of patients with systemic lupus erythematosus, and are also strongly associated with Sjögren's syndrome.

Anti-dsDNA antibodies are almost exclusively found in patients with systemic lupus erythematosus, although only 60% of patients test positive. Anti-nuclear antibodies are found in more than 99% of patients with systemic lupus erythematosus; however, they are not specific as they are also found in many other autoimmune conditions. Anti-phospholipid antibodies are found in the anti-phospholipid syndrome; this occurs either as a stand-alone disease or secondary to systemic lupus erythematosus.

1.23

B – *Propionibacterium acnes*

Propionibacterium acnes is a Gram-positive bacillus that is associated with prosthetic joint infection. *Neisseria gonorrhoeae* is a Gram-negative intracellular diplococcus. *Pseudomonas aeruginosa* is a Gram-negative bacillus. *Staphylococcus aureus* is a Gram-positive coccus that appears in clusters when viewed under the microscope. *Streptococcus pneumoniae* is a Gram-positive coccus that appears in chains when viewed under the microscope.

1.24

B – CMV

This patient has developed CMV pneumonitis secondary to post-transplantation immunosuppression. As with all herpesviruses, CMV (HHV-5) can establish latency for long periods. CMV reactivation can occur if the host is placed under stress or becomes immunocompromised. Enlarged cells with 'owl's eye' viral inclusion bodies are pathognomonic of CMV infection. However, the diagnosis of CMV is now more commonly achieved by serology and polymerase chain reaction rather than histopathology.

VZV (HHV-3) can also cause pneumonitis. *Pneumocystis jiroveci* is a fungus that can cause a similar picture in the immunocompromised; however, in this case a biopsy would demonstrate characteristic cysts on silver staining. Invasive *Aspergillus fumigatus* is another fungal infection that can cause pneumonia in immunocompromised hosts, but lung biopsy would reveal fungal spores in this scenario. Epstein–Barr virus (HHV-4) can very rarely be complicated by a pneumonitis.

1.25

A – Cisplatin

Cisplatin is a chemotherapeutic agent that crosslinks DNA and is used to treat ovarian cancer and various other malignancies. It has many side effects including vestibulocochlear nerve palsy, neurotoxicity and nephrotoxicity. It is also highly emetogenic so should be given in combination with an antiemetic agent.

Doxorubicin is a second-line agent in the treatment of ovarian cancer and intercalates DNA; its most notable side effect is cardiotoxicity. Palclitaxel is a microtubule inhibitor also used in the treatment of ovarian cancer that can cause a peripheral neuropathy. It is not ototoxic. Tobramycin is an aminoglycoside antibiotic that is nephrotoxic and can cause deafness but is not used to treat malignancy. Topotecan is a topoisomerase I inhibitor also used for ovarian cancer whose side effect profile would not cause the presentation in this scenario.

1.26

A – Central retinal artery occlusion

This patient has developed a left central retinal artery occlusion. The retina has a characteristic appearance. The visibility of the vascular choroidal layer at the fovea is commonly referred to as a cherry red spot. Central retinal artery occlusion occurs most commonly as a result of cholesterol emboli from the carotid artery, termed Hollenhorst plaques, occluding blood flow. It should be thought of as a stroke affecting the retina.

Central retinal vein occlusion also causes a sudden painless loss of vision. The retina in these patients has a characteristic pattern of papilloedema, cotton wool spots, and flame, dot and blot haemorrhages. This is referred to as a 'stormy sunset' appearance. Central retinal vein occlusion occurs secondary to hypercoagulability, phlebitis or hypertension.

Giant cell arteritis gives rise to an arteritic anterior ischaemic optic neuropathy, and presents as a sudden, painful loss of vision. Retinal examination will reveal the presence of a pale, atrophic optic disc.

Optic neuritis presents with a gradual loss of vision, and the patient will often complain of pain on moving their eyeball. Retinal examination will reveal a normal or swollen optic disc. Causes include:

- Multiple sclerosis
- Lyme disease
- Systemic lupus erythematosus
- Diabetes mellitus
- Drugs, such as ethambutol and chloramphenicol.

Patients with vitreous haemorrhage will present with dark 'floaters' that suddenly appear and obscure their visual field. Retinal examination is difficult in these patients, as blood in the vitreous humour does not allow visualisation of the retina. Vitreous haemorrhage is a complication of proliferative diabetic retinopathy because the walls of the new vessels that form are of poorer calibre, are more friable and break more easily.

1.27

A – β-HCG

The most appropriate initial investigation for any female of child-bearing age that presents with nausea and abdominal pain is a pregnancy test. Exclusion of pregnancy is essential before necessary investigations that are harmful to a foetus can be performed, such as an abdominal CT or X-ray. Abdominal ultrasound may be helpful in this situation to investigate for ectopic pregnancy, renal or biliary stones, or appendicitis. Full blood count, urea and electrolytes, liver function tests and C-reactive protein may also form part of an appropriate management plan for this patient once a pregnancy test has been performed.

1.28

E – Spironolactone

Spironolactone competitively inhibits the intracellular aldosterone receptors of the cells lining the renal tubular collecting ducts. The result is a net loss of sodium and water and increased potassium reabsorption, blunting the effect of the renin-angiotensin-aldosterone system, which is overactive in patients with heart failure. Spironolactone has been shown to improve mortality and morbidity only in patients with heart failure who experience symptoms even on minimal activity (New York Heart Association stage III or IV). Gynaecomastia is a common side effect of spironolactone.

As with most causes of gynaecomastia, spironolactone reduces androgen levels in comparison to oestrogen levels. Androgen levels are reduced through inhibition of 17-alpha hydroxylase and 17,20-desmolase, enzymes involved in testosterone biosynthesis. Oestrogen levels are increased through peripheral conversion of testosterone to oestradiol and by displacement of oestrogen from sex hormone-binding globulin. Eplerenone is a newer alternative aldosterone antagonist with higher mineralocorticoid receptor selectivity and fewer anti-androgenic and oestrogenic effects.

Digoxin is a cardiac glycoside that can cause gynaecomastia due to its oestrogen-like structure. It has been shown to reduce morbidity and rate of hospitalisation in heart failure; however, it does not reduce mortality. It is more commonly used as an adjunct to maximise other therapies. It should be used with caution in heart failure as it is renally excreted and has a narrow therapeutic index.

Neither furosemide, bisoprolol, bumetanide nor enalapril cause gynaecomastia but are all recognised treatments for heart failure. Enalapril is an angiotensin-converting enzyme inhibitor and bisoprolol is a relatively cardioselective beta-adrenoreceptor antagonist; both of these medications have been shown to reduce mortality in heart failure. Furosemide and bumetanide are loop diuretics that are useful for symptomatic relief of fluid overload in patients with chronic heart failure, but do not improve mortality.

1.29

B – Dressler's syndrome

This patient is most likely to have Dressler's syndrome, a secondary pericarditis that occurs after injury to the myocardium or pericardium. It is most commonly associated with myocardial infarction and complicates around 7% of cases. It consists of a triad of fever, pleuritic chest pain and pericarditis with an effusion. The audible parasternal rub and shortness of breath in this patient are suggestive of a pericardial effusion. Dressler's syndrome typically occurs two to three weeks after a myocardial infarction and is due to an autoimmune reaction to myocardial antigens released as a consequence of the myocardial infarction.

Acute mitral regurgitation is another complication of a myocardial infarction, and is thought to be due to ischaemic damage and rupture of papillary muscles. However, this usually occurs within five days and is associated with a pansystolic murmur heard loudest at the apex. Pneumonia, pleural effusion and pulmonary embolism can all present with pleuritic chest pain; however, a normal chest X-ray and CT pulmonary angiogram make these unlikely diagnoses in this patient.

1.30

E – Turner syndrome

This patient's symptoms and the presence of an ejection systolic murmur heard loudest between the scapulae suggest aortic coarctation. In combination with primary amenorrhoea, Turner syndrome is the most likely diagnosis. This condition is due to a chromosomal abnormality in which females have one rather than two normal X chromosomes (45XO). Affected patients still display the female phenotype. Turner syndrome affects around 1 in 2000–5000 females and can manifest in many different ways, including short stature, broad chest, low hairline, low-set ears, short fourth and fifth metacarpals and neck webbing. However, patients also experience a range of other abnormalities including cardiovascular, renal, thyroid, reproductive and skeletal abnormalities. Reproductive abnormalities include primary amenorrhea (menstrual cycles never starting), premature ovarian failure, streak gonads (dysfunctioning ovaries comprised of fibrous tissue) and infertility. The most common cardiac abnormalities are bicuspid aortic valve (15%) and aortic coarctation (5–10%). The coarctation is usually just distal to the origin of the left subclavian artery. This presents with an ejection systolic murmur heard loudest between the scapulae, radiofemoral delay, upper limb hypertension and in severe cases signs of hypoperfusion of the lower limbs and intermittent claudication. If the coarctation is proximal to the left subclavian artery then blood flow to the left arm is compromised and patients will have an absent, weak or delayed left radial pulse in comparison to the right.

Primary hyperparathyroidism is most frequently due to a benign adenoma of the parathyroid glands that causes hypercalcaemia. This increases the risk of developing a calcified aortic valve and subsequent aortic stenosis. Down's syndrome is associated with numerous cardiac anomalies including atrioventricular canal defects, atrial and ventricular septal defects, tetralogy of Fallot and patent ductus arteriosus. Ebstein's anomaly is a congenital heart defect in which the opening of the tricuspid valve is displaced down towards the apex of the right ventricle. The major risk factor associated with Ebstein's anomaly is the use of lithium during the first trimester. Kallman's syndrome is a congenital condition in which the gonadotrophin-releasing hormone neurons fail to migrate from the olfactory bulb to the hypothalamus during embryogenesis. This results in primary amenorrhoea (due to a failure of the hypothalamic pituitary axis) and congenital anosmia (lack of smell).

1.31

A – Intravenous bumetanide

This patient's history, examination and investigation findings indicate a likely diagnosis of pulmonary oedema; a loop diuretic such as bumetanide or furosemide should be started immediately. Loop diuretics initially cause venous dilation (thereby reducing preload and relieving pulmonary venous congestion) and later produce a diuresis (further reducing preload by increasing renal fluid loss). This diuresis is due to sodium-potassium-chloride co-transporter inhibition in the ascending loop of Henle, and is delayed partly due to the impaired renal perfusion seen in such patients.

Spironolactone inhibits the intracellular mineralocorticoid receptors in the cells of the renal tubular collecting duct. As these effects target the distal nephron, urine volume can only be slightly modified. Therefore spironolactone is only a weak diuretic. It is therefore not used in the management of acute pulmonary oedema. However, its interruption of the renin-angiotensin-aldosterone system is useful in chronic heart failure when this system is known to be overactive.

Sildenafil is an inhibitor of phosphodiesterase type V. This enzyme is normally responsible for the degradation of cyclic-GMP in the smooth muscle cells lining the pulmonary arteries and the arteries supplying the corpus cavernosum of the penis. Sildenafil therefore increases concentrations of cyclic-GMP in these sites, causing a relative vasodilation, which has been clinically utilised in the management of pulmonary hypertension and erectile dysfunction, respectively. It is also used in the prevention and treatment of high-altitude pulmonary oedema. However, sildenafil has no role in the treatment of acute pulmonary oedema secondary to heart failure.

Pneumonia is an important differential in this patient; however, apyrexia and pulmonary vasculature engorgement make this diagnosis unlikely. In an unwell patient with severe community-acquired pneumonia intravenous co-amoxiclav can be used. Intravenous ceftriaxone (a third-generation cephalosporin) can also be used in combination with a macrolide.

1.32

C – Hepatitis B carrier of low infectivity

This patient's hepatitis B serology is highly suggestive of a carrier of low infectivity. Hepatitis B serology detects viral antigens and their respective antibodies that are subsequently produced by the host. The hepatitis B virus contains three key antigens that are important to understanding hepatitis B serology: the surface antigen (HBsAg), core antigen (HBcAg) and E antigen (HBeAg).

In acute infection the first detectable antigen is HBsAg, six weeks to three months after primary infection. The presence of HBsAg indicates current infection. If present for six months or more, this indicates chronic infection. The first detectable antibodies are anti-HBcAg IgM and these appear soon after HBsAg is detected. They are a marker of acute infection, throughout which their titres increase steadily until six months when they are replaced by anti-HBcAg IgG. If a patient is IgM negative but IgG positive it can be due to previous infection (when anti-HBsAg will be positive) or chronic infection (when HBsAg will be positive). Shortly after the appearance of the HBsAg, the HBeAg will appear. This is associated with high rates of viral replication; however, most patients quickly develop anti-HBeAg antibodies to reduce this. Those who do not are at an increased risk of becoming chronic carriers of high infectivity.

The only way to become anti-HBcAg or anti-HBeAg positive is through natural infection. Patients with anti-HBcAg and anti-HBsAg have suffered a previous infection. However, those with only anti-HBsAg have been successfully vaccinated (the vaccine contains large quantities of only HBsAg). Unfortunately, roughly 10% of patients that undergo the full course of hepatitis B vaccinations are non-responders. These patients will require hepatitis B immunoglobulin if they have a high-risk exposure to the virus.

The table below summarises hepatitis B serology:

	HBsAg	Anti-HBsAg	Anti-HBcAg IgG	Anti-HBcAg IgM	HBeAg	Anti-HBeAg
Never infected	–	–	–	–	–	–
Vaccinated	–	+	–	–	–	–
Immune (natural infection)	–	+	+	–	–	–
Acute infection						
Incubation phase	+	–	–	–	–	–
Later/ symptomatic	+	–	+	++	+	–
Chronic infection						
High infectivity	+	–	+	–	+	–
Low infectivity	+	–	+	–	–	+

1.33

A – Selective IgA deficiency

This patient has coeliac disease; however, the reason that she is negative for anti-tissue transglutaminase IgA antibodies is because she has selective IgA deficiency. Selective IgA deficiency occurs in approximately 1 in 500 Caucasians, but is found in approximately 1 in 50 patients with coeliac disease. It is therefore not uncommon for anti-tissue transglutaminase antibodies to be negative in patients with coeliac disease. Other causes of a negative anti-tissue transglutaminase antibody result in patients with coeliac disease are if their disease is well controlled and well treated (antibodies disappear when gluten is removed from the diet) or if it is long-standing (due to severe protein loss and subsequent inability to synthesise IgA). It is therefore important to check IgA levels and perform a small bowel biopsy, looking for subtotal villous atrophy, in patients in which there is a high index of suspicion of coeliac disease and anti-tissue transglutaminase antibodies are negative. Coeliac disease is characterised by gluten-induced inflammation of the upper small bowel that results in indigestion, bloating and diarrhoea or steatorrhoea. Mouth ulcers, infertility, polyneuropathy and neuropsychiatric symptoms can also occur. If the disease is left untreated, osteoporosis and gross malnutrition may result. Patients with coeliac disease may also develop dermatitis herpetiformis, an itchy, blistering rash most commonly found on the elbows. Dapsone, an antibacterial agent, improves the rash when applied topically.

Patients with scleroderma can develop malabsorption from bacterial overgrowth secondary to small bowel hypomotility and dilatation. The symptoms are mainly of diarrhoea and steatorrhoea. Bacterial overgrowth is confirmed by hydrogen breath test, with management centering on rotational courses of antibiotics to try and eradicate the bacteria.

Tropical sprue describes a condition in which patients who live in or have travelled to Asia, the Caribbean or South America develop chronic diarrhoea as a result of an as yet unknown infectious agent.

Whipple's disease is a rare cause of malabsorption due to infection with the bacteria *Tropheryma whipplei*. The majority of patients are Caucasian, middle-aged males who present with arthralgia, diarrhoea, weight loss and abdominal pain. Oculomasticatory myorhythmia describes pendular vergence oscillations of the eyes with concomitant contractions of the muscles of mastication, and is pathognomonic of Whipple's disease. However, diagnosis is usually made by small bowel biopsy, which reveals the presence of magenta-coloured periodic acid-Schiff-positive macrophages and the presence of trilaminar-walled *Tropheryma whipplei* bacteria within macrophages on electron microscopy.

Ulcerative colitis does not affect the small bowel and so would not present with features of malabsorption.

1.34

A – Initiate treatment with cabergoline

Prolactinomas are benign pituitary adenomas that contain prolactin-secreting lactotrophs. They usually lead to hyperprolactinaemia, which presents differently depending on gender. Males present with galactorrhoea, infertility and reduced libido. Females present with galactorrhoea, amenorrhoea and oligomenorrhoea. Although prolactinoma can be diagnosed when there is sustained hyperprolactinaemia, when other causes of hyperprolactinaemia have been excluded (e.g. pregnancy, use of dopamine antagonists) and when there is radiographic evidence of a pituitary mass (usually gadolinium-enhanced MRI), the definitive diagnosis is based either on a sustained reduction in prolactin levels in response to dopamine agonists or post-operative histological analysis. This is because any mass that compresses the pituitary stalk can impair the flow of dopamine to the lactotrophs, triggering prolactin release. In reality, prolactinomas are rarely surgically removed and are usually treated medically.

Prolactinomas are usually classified based on their size on imaging:

- Microprolactinoma = less than 10 mm
- Macroprolactinoma = 10–40 mm
- Giant pituitary adenoma = more than 40 mm.

The aim of treatment for patients with prolactinomas is to normalise prolactin levels, reduce symptoms and remove any mass effect of the tumour. All patients with giant and macropituitary adenomas need treatment whereas those with a microadenoma are only treated if there is a mass effect (e.g. optic chiasm compression) or symptomatic hyperprolactinaemia (e.g. gonadal dysfunction or galactorrhoea). First-line treatment is a dopamine agonist (e.g. cabergoline) because hypothalamic dopamine, via the portal vessels, normally inhibits the release of prolactin from the anterior pituitary lactotrophs. Medical treatment normalises prolactin levels in most patients; however, those with resistant prolactinomas may require further treatment (e.g. alternative dopamine agonist or surgery).

Transsphenoidal surgery is only successful in around 75% of patients with a microprolactinoma; much less for a macroprolactinoma. It is therefore only indicated in patients who do not respond to, or are intolerant of, dopamine agonists, have pituitary apoplexy (a neurosurgical emergency) or have a cystic macroprolactinoma. Radiotherapy is rarely used to treat prolactinomas since it is associated with major side effects including hypopituitarism, optic nerve damage, neurological damage and an increased risk of secondary brain tumours. It is therefore reserved for those who do not respond to dopamine agonists or surgical intervention, or in the rare case of malignant prolactinoma. Only once the patient's prolactin levels have normalized should they have their prolactin levels monitored annually to check for any recurrence. Clozapine is an atypical antipsychotic and is therefore a dopamine antagonist. It should therefore not be used in patients with a prolactinoma as it may reduce dopamine levels in the anterior pituitary and increase prolactin release.

1.35

D – Hoffman's syndrome

Proximal myopathy, sinus bradycardia and slow relaxing reflexes are characteristic of hypothyroidism. Hoffman's syndrome is a specific form of hypothyroid myopathy that causes painful proximal muscle weakness and muscular pseudohypertrophy; however, it can present in the absence of overt hypothyroid symptoms. Muscular symptoms are common in patients with hypothyroidism (myalgia, weakness, stiffness, cramps and fatigability); however, the hypertrophy and painful proximal myopathy of Hoffman's syndrome is uncommon.

Graves' disease is an autoimmune hyperthyroid condition caused by autoantibodies that overactivate the thyroid-stimulating hormone receptor, triggering thyroid hormone synthesis and secretion. It can cause a proximal myopathy but unlike Hoffman's syndrome it is typically painless and is accompanied by hyperthyroidism.

Two types of amiodarone-induced thyroid disease exist. Type I results in hyperthyroidism and usually occurs in patients with pre-existing thyroid disorders or in those who are iodine deficient. Type II results in the patient becoming hypothyroid and occurs in patients with a previously normal thyroid. This patient is hypothyroid and therefore amiodarone-induced hyperthyroidism is unlikely.

De Quervain's thyroiditis is the most common cause of painful thyroid. It is a transient inflammation of the thyroid thought to be post-viral in origin (e.g. coxsackievirus, Epstein–Barr virus). It presents with hyperthyroidism, followed by hypothyroidism, followed by complete recovery within weeks/months.

1.36

E – Systemic lupus erythematosus

This patient has a haemolytic anaemia, as evidenced by their anaemia, raised reticulocyte count and raised serum unconjugated bilirubin. Haemolytic anaemias can be classified according to whether the haemolysis is mediated by antibodies directed against a patient's own erythrocytes (autoimmune) or not. The Coombs test is useful for distinguishing between these two, whereby a positive test occurs in the setting of autoimmune haemolytic anaemia. There are two types of Coombs test: direct and indirect. In the direct Coombs test, the patient's erythrocytes are mixed with antibodies against human antibodies. If this causes erythrocyte agglutination then there are antibodies that are bound to the surface of the erythrocytes. In the indirect test, the patient's serum is mixed with other human erythrocytes. If agglutination occurs in this scenario it suggests that the patient's serum contains antibodies that bind to erythrocytes.

There are two broad categories of autoimmune haemolytic anaemia: warm and cold. This depends upon the temperature at which the erythrocytes agglutinate during the Coombs test. The following table highlights the differences between warm and cold autoimmune haemolytic anaemias:

	Warm autoimmune haemolytic anaemia	Cold autoimmune haemolytic anaemia
Site of haemolysis	Extravascular	Intravascular
Type of antibody	IgG	IgM
Temperature at which agglutination of erythrocytes occurs	37 °C	4 °C
Causes	• Idiopathic • Chronic lymphocytic leukaemia • Lymphoma • Systemic lupus erythematosus • Rheumatoid arthritis • Drugs, e.g. methyldopa	• Idiopathic • Lymphoma • EBV • *Mycoplasma pneumoniae* • HIV • Occasionally systemic lupus erythematosus

Sickle cell disease and glucose-6-phosphate disease are both causes of a haemolytic anaemia but they are not antibody mediated. Therefore, they are non-autoimmune haemolytic anaemias and will have a negative Coombs test.

1.37

A – Acute myeloid leukaemia

This female has polycythaemia rubra vera, a type of myeloproliferative disorder in which there is primarily an increase in erythrocyte production; thrombocytosis can also occur. The myeloid proliferative disorders are a spectrum of disorders in the myeloid lineage of the bone marrow (the precursors to all mature non-lymphocytic blood cells). They can be divided into those which are Philadelphia chromosome positive or Philadelphia chromosome negative, whereby chronic myeloid leukaemia comprises the former group and polycythaemia rubra vera, essential thrombocytosis and myelofibrosis comprise the latter. The Philadelphia chromosome is a reciprocal translocation in which the long arms of chromosome 9 and 22 are exchanged, which forms the *BCR-ABL* fusion gene on chromosome 22. The Philadelphia chromosome negative myeloproliferative disorders are associated with the JAK2 kinase mutation, particularly polycythaemia rubra vera, of which 80% are JAK2 kinase positive. Given their neoplastic and myeloid nature, a rare but important complication of all the myeloproliferative disorders is acute myeloid leukaemia. Referred to as a 'blast crisis' in the case of chronic myeloid leukaemia, this is where the pre-existing clonal expansion of mature myeloid cells is complicated by additonal mutations that trigger malignant accumulation of immature blood cells ('blast cells'). This is associated with a very poor prognosis.

The patient in this scenario has developed aquagenic pruritus. This describes an intense pruritus after exposure to warm water. It is likely that this is due to the release of excess histamine or prostaglandins. Patients with multiple sclerosis may have Uhthoff's phenomenon which is characterised by increasing weakness with increasing body temperature. Multiple sclerosis is unlikely in this patient as there are no other neurological features in the history.

Chronic lymphocytic leukaemia is the most common form of leukaemia, and as opposed to the myeloproliferative disorders it is a disorder of the lymphoid lineage. It typically affects people older than 50 and has a slow progression. As for the myeloproliferative conditions, it too has the ability to transform into more aggressive haematological dysplasias, such as Richter's syndrome (a fast-growing diffuse large B-cell lymphoma), prolymphocytic leukaemia, Hodgkin's lymphoma or acute lymphoblastic leukaemia.

1.38

C – *Salmonella typhi*

The history suggests femoral head osteomyelitis. Patients with sickle cell disease who are older than around five years are prone to hyposplenia due to infarction of the splenic vasculature. This puts them at risk of infection from encapsulated organisms, such as *Salmonella typhi*. It is therefore a common cause of osteomyelitis in patients with sickle cell disease.

Klebsiella pneumoniae is also an encapsulated organism and is also known to be a cause of osteomyelitis in patients with sickle cell disease, but is implicated much less frequently than *Salmonella typhi*. The other common encapsulated bacteria are:

- *Haemophilus influenzae*
- *Streptococcus pneumoniae*
- *Neisseria meningitidis*.

In the general population, *Staphylococcus aureus* is the most common organism implicated in osteomyelitis; it is thought to be due to the presence of a collagen receptor on some strains. After *Staphylococcus aureus* the most common causative organism of osteomyelitis is *Pseudomonas aeruginosa*, a part of the normal skin flora. It is for this reason that *Pseudomonas aeruginosa* osteomyelitis is particularly prevalent in intravenous drug users.

The viridans group of streptococci are a much less common cause of osteomyelitis. They are usually implicated when a patient has had a recent dental extraction because they are a part of the normal oral flora. Gastrointestinal or genitourinary infections may lead to osteomyelitis involving Gram-negative organisms, such as *Escherichia coli*.

Finally, although a rare cause of osteomyelitis, *Staphylococcus epidermidis* is a part of the normal skin flora and is well known for its ability to form biofilms over prosthetic materials. It is for this reason that it is particularly associated with infections in prosthetic joints, prosthetic heart valves and indwelling lines.

1.39

A – Diabetic nephropathy

The presence of persistent microalbuminuria and stage II chronic kidney disease (glomerular filtration rate of 60–90 mL/min/1.73 m^2) in a patient with postural hypotension is suggestive of poorly controlled diabetes mellitus. The postural hypotension is likely to be secondary to diabetic neuropathy of the autonomic nervous system and the presence of microalbuminuria and reduced glomerular filtration rate are suggestive of diabetic nephropathy. These are features of poor diabetic control. The diagnosis of diabetic nephropathy is further supported by the presence of nodular glomerulosclerosis. Patients with diabetic nephropathy typically have a nodular glomerulosclerosis on renal biopsy, more commonly referred to as the presence of Kimmelstiel–Wilson nodules. In this patient, nodular glomerulosclerosis is most likely to be caused by poorly controlled diabetes mellitus; however, it can also be idiopathic in nature.

In addition to idiopathic nephropathy, hypertensive nephropathy is also unlikely as there is no suggestion of persistent hypertension, or the complications thereof (e.g. hypertensive retinopathy, myocardial hypertrophy). Hypertensive nephropathy produces a secondary focal segmental glomerulosclerosis on renal biopsy.

HIV causes a collapsing focal segmental glomerulosclerosis on renal biopsy; however, there is no suggestion of poorly controlled HIV in this patient.

Multiple myeloma is a less common cause of chronic kidney disease and postural hypotension than diabetes mellitus. There are many causes of renal damage in multiple myeloma, mainly a result of hypercalcaemia and excretion of large quantities of light chain immunoglobulins (also known as Bence Jones proteins or paraproteins). Postural hypotension is a rare complication of multiple myeloma too, which occurs secondary to deposition of light chain immunoglobulins in the peripheral nerves (as a cause of AL amyloidosis).

1.40

E – T2-weighted MRI brain

Episodic vomiting and progressive headaches which are worse after lying for prolonged periods (e.g. in the morning) is suggestive of a slow-onset rise in intracranial pressure. It is therefore very important to perform an MRI brain to rule out the possibility of a space-occupying lesion. In this scenario, an MRI scan is preferred to head CT because MRI is more sensitive and specific for abnormalities within the brain, and depicts the anatomy in greater detail. MRI also allows delineation of the margins of any lesions found more accurately than a CT scan. If a patient has a contraindication for an MRI scan, such as a metal prosthesis or claustrophobia, then a CT head would be the first choice investigation. In patients with symptoms suggestive of raised intracranial pressure, a lumbar puncture is contraindicated as the removal of cerebrospinal fluid from the lumbar spine may cause herniation of the medulla through the foramen magnum. Vomiting in association with a progressive headache is more likely to be of neurological origin rather than abdominal. As a result, abdominal imaging (CT or ultrasound) is unlikely to be of benefit in this patient initially.

1.41

B – Frontotemporal lobe dementia

This patient's symptoms are characteristic of frontotemporal lobe dementia, which is a clinical syndrome caused by degeneration of the frontal and temporal lobes of the brain. Symptoms of frontotemporal dementia are classified into three groups which comprise three functions of the frontal and temporal lobes. First, behavioural symptoms, which include lethargy, mood swings and disinhibition. Disinhibited patients make inappropriate comments or perform inappropriate acts. Second, speech symptoms which include the development of a progressive non-fluent aphasia. This is characterised by the breakdown in speech fluency due to articulation difficulty, but with preservation of word comprehension. This is probably due to the involvement of Broca's area, which is located in the posterior inferior frontal gyrus of the brain. Finally, cognitive symptoms. Patients increasingly lose semantic memory (the memory of meanings, understandings and other concept-based knowledge unrelated to specific experiences) and executive function (the ability to perform skills that require complex planning or sequencing). Some cases of frontotemporal lobe dementia are associated with motor neuron disease, particularly amyotrophic lateral sclerosis.

Lewy body dementia is associated with visual hallucinations and significant variations in cognition and attention. It is also associated with Parkinsonian symptoms; if the onset of dementia is either before or within one year of the onset of Parkinsonian symptoms then Lewy body dementia is diagnosed. If dementia occurs later than one year from the onset of Parkinsonism then Parkinson's disease with dementia is diagnosed.

Alzheimer's disease is the most common form of irreversible dementia and the early symptoms are often mistakenly put down to ageing. The early symptoms of Alzheimer's is the inability to remember recent events due to involvement of the hippocampus, which is responsible for this form of memory. As the disease progresses symptoms can include confusion, irritability, mood swings, progressive aphasia and long-term memory loss.

Vascular dementia is a common form of progressive dementia and can mimic Alzheimer's disease. Patients typically have a step-wise decline due to small ischaemic events, whereas patients with Alzheimer's disease decline at a steady rate. Patients with vascular dementia may have a history of previous cerebral infarctions and risk factors for arterial disease (e.g. hypertension, hypercholesteraemia, smoking, diabetes mellitus).

In all patients with symptoms suggestive of cognitive impairment it is essential to first exclude reversible causes of dementia. Particularly in older patients, hypothyroidism can cause a form of dementia that is usually reversible on initation of thyroxine treatment. These patients would be likely to have other features typical of hypothyroidism (e.g. hair loss, cold intolerance, weight gain). Other causes of a reversible dementia in older patients include vitamin deficiencies (niacin (B_3), B_{12}, folate), electrolyte imbalances and normal pressure hydrocephalus.

1.42

D – Anti-GQ1B

This patient has Miller Fisher syndrome, a variant of Guillain–Barré syndrome. Unlike the more common form of Guillain–Barré syndrome, Miller Fisher syndrome presents in a descending fashion. It is characterised by a triad of ophthalmoplegia, ataxia (predominantly truncal and gait) and areflexia. Guillain–Barré syndrome is thought to be the result of molecular mimicry, whereby an immune response to foreign antigens (e.g. infectious agents) generates antibodies that cross-react with peripheral nervous tissue, particularly molecules called gangliosides which are present in high quantities in these tissues. The most common preceding infection is *Campylobacter jejuni*, which is characterised by a history of bloody diarrhoea. The anti-ganglioside antibody anti-GQ1B is present in over 90% of patients with Miller Fisher syndrome.

The classical and most common form of Guillain–Barré syndrome is an acute inflammatory demyelinating polyneuropathy, presenting with ascending weakness. The closely related condition of chronic inflammatory demyelinating polyneuropathy is thought to be the chronic counterpart to Guillain–Barré syndrome. Classical Guillain–Barré syndrome is not associated with a specific anti-ganglioside antibody; however, if a case has been preceded by infection with *Campylobacter jejuni* then anti-GM1 antibodies may be positive (GM1 is an antigen present on this microorganism).

Another variant of Guillain–Barré syndrome is an acute motor axonal neuropathy. Unlike classical Guillain–Barré syndrome, this variant is due to an autoimmune response against the axoplasm of peripheral nerves. This variant of Guillain–Barré syndrome is associated with anti-GD3 and anti-GD1a antibodies, which seem to target the axon rather than the myelin sheath.

Anti-MuSK antibodies are associated with patients who have myasthenia gravis who are anti-AchR seronegative.

1.43

B – MRI cervical, thoracic and lumbar spine

This patient has spinal cord compression secondary to metastatic breast cancer. All patients with suspected metastatic spinal cord compression should undergo an urgent MRI of the whole spine. The presence of neurological symptoms such as difficulty in walking or bladder/bowel dysfunction is suggestive of spinal cord compression. This is an oncological emergency and an MRI should be performed within 24 hours. Patients with spinal cord compression should be immediately referred for a neurosurgical assessment.

Spinal X-rays can be performed in conjunction with MRI. However, spinal X-rays alone are often unreliable in diagnosing a patient with spinal cord compression.

Initiating high-dose dexamethasone treatment (16 mg per day) is a priority and should be given before imaging. Administration of corticosteroids helps to reduce any oedema around the lesion and provides extra time to form a definitive management plan. Patients started on high-dose corticosteroid treatment must be given a prophylactic proton pump inhibitor to reduce the risk of peptic ulceration. Intravenous bisphosphonates should also be given to reduce the osteoclast hyperactivity, which causes the painful bone lesions found in patients with bone metastases.

1.44

C – Erythromycin

Prescription of a macrolide antibiotic for a chest infection has resulted in inhibition of the CYP450 system, which is responsible for the metabolism of warfarin. As a result, accumulation of warfarin has inhibited the patient's vitamin K–dependent clotting factors, and she has become over-anticoagulated.

Rifampicin, a commonly prescribed antibiotic for tuberculosis, is an inducer of the CYP450 system and can therefore reduce the effectiveness of warfarin.

Amoxicillin, ampicillin and penicillin V (all penicillins) do not affect warfarin metabolism.

1.45

C – The murmur is loudest at the apex

The causes of a pansystolic murmur include tricuspid regurgitation, mitral regurgitation and ventricular septal defect. Of these, this patient has mitral regurgitation, which is best heard at the apex. Patients with mitral regurgitation may present with shortness of breath, fatigue, asymptomatically with a pansystolic murmur or during the assessment of a patient with atrial fibrillation (which occurs commonly in patients with mitral regurgitation secondary to left atrial dilatation).

All other options refer primarily to diagnoses that cause ejection systolic murmurs. Severe anaemia can result in pale conjunctiva, shortness of breath and an early systolic murmur. This is a flow murmur which represents a cardiovascular compensation to the reduced oxygen-carrying capacity of the blood. Pregnancy can result in a similar murmur as the cardiac output increases to cope with the demands of the developing foetus. Aortic stenosis causes an early systolic murmur which radiates to the carotids. Finally, squatting is useful to differentiate between the ejection systolic murmur of aortic stenosis and hypertrophic obstructive cardiomyopathy. Squatting increases venous return as blood drains away from the legs. This increases flow though a stenosed aortic valve resulting in the murmur of aortic stenosis getting louder. In contrast, squatting decreases the murmur volume in hypertrophic obstructive cardiomyopathy because the enlarged obstructive interventricular septum has less effect on left ventricular outflow. The murmur in mitral regurgitation gets louder on squatting because the increase in venous return increases both anterograde and retrograde flow through the incompetent mitral valve.

1.46

B – Cystic fibrosis

Cystic fibrosis is an autosomal recessive disorder that predominantly affects the lungs, pancreas and intestines. This patient is suffering recurrent chest infections due to underlying bronchiectasis, and pancreatic insufficiency that is causing fat malabsorption resulting in steatorrhoea.

Although many mutations have been described in cystic fibrosis, the most common form is caused by the deletion of the codon for the amino acid phenylalanine from the cystic fibrosis transmembrane regulator gene. In exocrine glands the cystic fibrosis transmembrane regulator protein is responsible for the transport of chloride from inside to the outside of the cell in order to form secretions. The mutation causes an increased concentration of intracellular chloride, and subsequently other positively charged ions and water enter the cells. As a consequence, pulmonary, pancreatic and intestinal secretions are thickened, leaving the patient prone to chest infections. Obstruction of the pancreatic ducts leads to accumulation of pancreatic digestive enzymes, which can destroy the gland and cause pancreatic diabetes mellitus. There is reduced secretion of pancreatic lipase (resulting in steatorrhoea and malabsorption, particularly of the fat-soluble vitamins A, D, E and K), proteases and amylase (leading to defective digestion of protein and starch, respectively). Patients are given pancreatic enzyme supplements to reduce this nutritional deficiency. Obstruction of the small airways results in recurrent pneumonias from an early age, progressing to bronchiectasis as a result of chronic pulmonary inflammation. The long-term bronchial changes can result in chronic hypoxia, pulmonary hypertension and ultimately right-sided heart failure. Impaired exocrine secretions in the intestines can cause meconium ileus in the neonate, and obstruction due to constipation in later life. Finally, impaired hepatic secretions can impair liver function, which may obstruct the bile ducts and lead to liver fibrosis. Males are infertile.

The second main function of the cystic fibrosis transmembrane regulator protein is in the skin, where it is responsible for transporting chloride from the sweat to the sweat glands (the reverse process to exocrine glands). Therefore, chloride and various positive ions (e.g. sodium) accumulate in the sweat, increasing water loss through osmosis and making affected infants taste salty to their parents (a common initial presentation). This is the basis of the sweat test, a diagnostic test used in cystic fibrosis which is positive if the sweat contains a high concentration of chloride (>60 mmol/L). A positive test is followed by genetic testing to confirm the diagnosis.

Sarcoidosis, gastroesophageal reflux, asthma and Kartagener's syndrome may present with a cough; however, they are not associated with steatorrhoea.

1.47

C – 10 ml 1:10000 intravenous adrenaline

The dosage required in situations of cardiac arrest is 10 ml 1:10000 intravenous adrenaline.

Securing the airway is the main priority in this scenario. Intramuscular adrenaline (0.5 ml of 1:1000) and securing IV access (large-bore cannulae) for the administration of antihistamines (e.g. 10 mg intravenous chlorpheniramine), corticosteroids (e.g. 200 mg intravenous hydrocortisone) and 0.9% sodium chloride solution (titrated against blood pressure) are also part of the initial emergency management. Adrenaline acts on alpha-adrenoreceptors to initiate peripheral vasoconstriction (to raise blood pressure) and also on beta-adrenoreceptors to initiate bronchodilation, and should be repeated every 5 minutes as guided by the patient's observations (blood pressure, pulse and respiratory function).

Salbutamol may be required to treat the patient's wheeze or instead of adrenaline if patients are taking a beta-blocker.

1.48
A – Abdominal CT scan

Painless jaundice with a palpable mass in the right upper quadrant is the classical presentation of carcinoma of the head of the pancreas. Diagnosis can be made by ultrasound; however, views of the tail or small lesions are poor and therefore abdominal CT is the gold standard investigation.

Endoscopic retrograde cholangiopancreatography is the investigation of choice for suspected cholelithiasis; however, this patient's symptoms and lack of risk factors do not support this diagnosis. A full blood count and peripheral blood film would be useful if haemolysis is the suspected cause of jaundice; however, this patient's abdominal examination suggests an obstructive cause of jaundice. Alpha fetoprotein is useful in the diagnosis of suspected hepatocellular carcinoma. Almost all cases of hepatocellular carcinoma develop on a background of liver cirrhosis, and again the lack of relevant risk factors from the patient's history makes hepatocellular carcinoma less likely.

1.49
D – Hypochloraemic hypokalaemic metabolic alkalosis

The clinical picture is that of congenital pyloric stenosis. This typically affects boys and they present with early projectile vomiting some six weeks after birth; hydrochloric acid and potassium are lost in the vomitus. The patient is dehydrated and at presentation paradoxically passes an acidic urine as the body conserves sodium by increasing distal renal tubular absorption of sodium. For each molecule of sodium reabsorbed (under the influence of aldosterone) either a molecule of hydrogen or potassium has to be excreted; potassium levels are low in prolonged vomiting so hydrogen is exchanged and excreted. With intravenous rehydration the kidneys will correct the acid base disturbance and the pH of the urine will increase. Pyloric stenosis has a polygenic inheritance pattern but environmental factors such as maternal ingestion of erythromycin during pregnancy may play a role. In adults, acquired pyloric stenosis is seen as a complication of pyloric peptic ulcer disease with structuring. It is also seen with pyloric tuberculosis, malignancy and as a complication of ferrous sulphate toxicity. The same metabolic picture is seen in other causes of intractable vomiting, such as hyperemesis gravidarum, severe gastroenteritis and certain severe drug reactions.

1.50

A – Serum amylase

Due to leakage of pancreatic enzymes, serum amylase levels do increase in pancreatitis. However, amylase is of diagnostic value only, and is of no use prognostically. Lipase is more sensitive and specific than amylase because amylase is more readily excreted than lipase, and, unlike lipase, amylase is increased in other conditions such as abdominal perforation (e.g. perforated peptic ulcer), anorexia, burns, salivary adenitis, intestinal ischaemia, ruptured or torted ovarian cyst and renal disease.

Serum glucose, white blood cell count, lactate dehydrogenase and calcium are important factors in assessing prognosis in acute pancreatitis. Pancreatitis and leakage of pancreatic enzymes causes inflammation and damage to the pancreas and surrounding tissues, resulting in an elevated serum lactate dehydrogenase and a raised white blood cell count. Hypocalcaemia can occur as a result of the complexing of serum calcium with necrotic fatty acids generated by pancreatic lipase. Hyperglycaemia occurs as a result of systemic shock and damage to the islet cells.

1.51

B – Intramuscular glucagon

Severe hypoglycaemia can cause convulsions, which can progress to permanent damage, coma and death as the cerebral neurons progressively become completely electrically dysfunctional. It is therefore vital to initiate emergency measures to increase this patient's blood glucose immediately. In the convulsing or uncooperative patient, medications cannot be administered orally, and if there is no intravenous access, the most appropriate immediate management is intramuscular glucagon. Glucagon is an endogenous peptide hormone secreted by the pancreatic endocrine alpha islet cells, which acts initially by promoting hepatic glycogenolysis, and renal and hepatic gluconeogenesis thereafter. This treatment is therefore ineffective in hypoglycaemia caused by one of the glycogen storage disorders. Intramuscular glucagon can be issued to parents/carers of children with type I diabetes mellitus who administer subcutaneous insulin, for use in severe hypoglycaemic episodes.

1.52

D – Serum insulin-like growth factor 1 levels

This is the classical presentation of a patient with acromegaly (excess growth hormone). As an outpatient, insulin-like growth factor levels should be measured. A high level will support the diagnosis and should be followed by an oral glucose tolerance test and measurements of growth hormone level. Failure of growth hormone levels to fall during an oral glucose tolerance test is the gold standard test for diagnosis. The oral glucose tolerance test is preceded by consumption of a normal diet for three days, followed by an overnight water-only fast for 10 hours. Then, after measuring the initial blood glucose level, the patient consumes a 75 g glucose drink in under 5 minutes. The blood glucose is then measured 30 minutes, 1 hour, 2 hours and 3 hours after consumption of the drink. The 2-hour result is the most important. During the test the patient should be relatively inactive, and should be prohibited from smoking.

Ninety-nine percent of cases of acromegaly are caused by a growth hormone–secreting pituitary adenoma, and therefore if acromegaly is suspected an MRI scan of the pituitary fossa should be the first-line imaging investigation of choice. Although the hypertrophic anterior pituitary is very slow growing, it can become large enough to cause bitemporal hemianopia by placing pressure on the optic chiasm. Therefore a visual field and acuity assessment should be performed.

1.53

E – Raised total iron-binding capacity, pencil cells and anisocytosis

This woman is most likely to be suffering from iron deficiency anaemia secondary to menorrhagia. Longstanding iron deficiency in women is usually due to menorrhagia and results in an anaemia where the red blood cells are small (microcytic) and hypochromic (reflecting a reduced mean corpuscular haemoglobin concentration). In addition, inspection of the blood film may find other abnormalities such as target cells (cells appear target-like when there is excessive membrane relative to haemoglobin), pencil cells (thin, elongated red blood cells) and nucleated red blood cells (during a regenerative anaemia, red blood cells are produced rapidly and may be released prematurely, prior to anucleation). This increased variation in the shape of red blood cells is called poikilocytosis. A dimorphic picture is where there are two discrete populations of cells, and is seen after treatment of a deficiency anaemia, in a mixed deficiency, after blood transfusion or in primary sideroblastic anaemia. On the other hand, increased variation in the size of red blood cells is called anisocytosis and is quantified by calculating the red cell distribution width. The red cell distribution width can be increased in iron deficiency anaemia because red blood cells have a lifespan of around 120 days, and therefore there may be a mixture of normocytic cells (produced prior to iron deficiency) and microcytic cells (produced during iron deficiency). The platelet count is often elevated too. This is thought to be due to high erythropoietin levels, which can activate thrombopoietin receptors in megakaryocytes to increase platelet production. Although this mechanism has not been confirmed, raised platelets are no danger and provide a useful diagnostic indicator.

Iron studies typically demonstrate a decreased serum ferritin (due to depleted iron stores), decreased serum iron, increased total iron-binding capacity and decreased transferrin saturation. A bone marrow aspirate biopsy, stained with Perls' Prussian blue stain for iron, would show decreased iron concentrations, but this is rarely necessary.

Spherocytes are typically seen in hereditary spherocytosis, the commonest hereditary cause of a haemolytic anaemia in the United Kingdom, but they may also be seen in other causes of haemolysis.

The underlying cause of iron deficiency anaemia must always be sought. The most common cause of iron deficiency anaemia world-wide is hookworm infestation. However, in the West, chronic blood loss secondary to gastrointestinal haemorrhage (as a result of a bleeding peptic ulcer or a carcinoma of the stomach/intestine) and menorrhagia are the commonest causes.

1.54

E – Minimal change glomerulonephritis

The presence of generalised oedema and heavy proteinuria suggests a diagnosis of the nephrotic syndrome. Nephrotic syndrome is a triad of:

- Proteinuria greater than 3.5 g per 24 hours
- Oedema
- Hypoalbuminaemia.

The oedema occurs as a result of hypoalbuminaemia, which reduces oncotic pressure and enables fluid to extravasate from blood vessels.

In young children, minimal change disease is by far the most common cause of nephrotic syndrome, and classically presents after a viral upper respiratory tract infection. Childhood nephrotic syndrome is assumed to be due to minimal change glomerulonephritis and treatment with oral prednisolone is started empirically. Renal biopsy is reserved for those cases that either do not respond or relapse.

1.55

C – Renal cell carcinoma

This man has developed a left-sided varicocoele secondary to renal cell carcinoma. A varicocoele is a collection of engorged veins (the pampiniform venous plexus, which drains into the testicular vein) around the testis that, like varicose veins in the legs, occurs due to impaired venous drainage. They therefore enlarge when abdominal pressure increases (e.g. straining, standing up) and disappear when the patient is lying down. Varicocoeles do not transilluminate (unlike a testicular hydrocoele, light shone through will not be visible on the other side), are largely asymptomatic and, on palpation, feel like a soft, twisted mass (classically a 'bag of worms'). Ninety-eight percent occur on the left side due to the anatomical arrangement of the testicular (gonadal) veins; the left testicular vein drains into the left renal vein at a right angle, whereas the right testicular vein drains into the much larger inferior vena cava at a shallower angle. Therefore, a right varicocoele should raise suspicion of a mass compressing the right testicular vein, such as a pelvic or intra-abdominal malignancy. Initially the General Practitioner rightly suspected that this patient was suffering an idiopathic varicocoele, which is only treated if it starts to cause problems. However, in addition to left-sided varicocoele this patient then developed frank, painless haematuria throughout his urinary stream which should alert suspicion towards the possibility of more sinister causes of haematuria such as malignancy in the kidneys, bladder or ureters (painless frank haematuria only at the start of micturition suggests urethral or prostatic lesions). This feature points away from a urinary tract infection, which would typically cause painful, usually microscopic haematuria. Therefore a renal cell carcinoma (a rare but important cause of a left-sided varicocoele) which is compressing the left testicular vein, as well as generating frank, painless haematuria, is the most likely cause of this male's symptoms.

1.56

E – Transrectal ultrasound

This patient has suspected prostatic adenocarcinoma and therefore he should be urgently referred for further investigation with a transrectal ultrasound and biopsy. The patient's symptoms include both obstructive and irritative symptoms of bladder outflow obstruction, of which the two main causes are benign prostatic hyperplasia and prostate cancer (because the prostate surrounds the proximal urethra). Prostatitis can also cause such symptoms but symptoms such as fever, malaise and pain (e.g. in the abdomen, pelvis, perineum, lower back, prostate and/or urethra) would also be expected. Obstructive symptoms include poor stream, interrupted flow, terminal dribbling, incomplete emptying and hesitancy (because higher urinary pressures are needed to overcome the obstruction). Irritative symptoms (of which the aetiologies are unclear) include frequency, urgency, urge incontinence and nocturia, symptoms which are also features of bladder pathology (cystitis, malignancy and calculi).

The prostate gland is comprised of a peripheral zone (the posterior aspect of the gland which lies adjacent to the anterior rectal wall), a central zone and a transition zone (the anterior portion of the prostate that surrounds the proximal urethra). The digital rectal examination is therefore a useful test in patients with suspected prostatism. However, prior to performing a digital rectal examination a sample of prostate-specific antigen, a protein produced by the acinar cells of the prostate, should be taken because the prostate-specific antigen rises after a digital rectal examination. In addition, more prostate-specific antigen is produced as the prostate enlarges, as occurs in benign prostatic hyperplasia and prostate cancer. Benign prostatic hyperplasia is a nodular enlargement of the transition (periurethral) zone of the prostate that, on digital rectal examination, is entirely normal (smooth surface and palpable midline sulcus) except that it is enlarged. In contrast, the majority of prostate cancers affect the peripheral zone, whereby the digital rectal examination is more likely to reveal an enlarged, hard, nodular, irregular, 'craggy' prostate surface. In this scenario, an urgent referral for transrectal ultrasound and biopsy should be made (only once malignancy is confirmed should a CT scan be organised).

If benign prostatic hypertrophy is supected (based on the digital rectal examination and prostate-specific antigen result) then mild symptoms may be managed by watchful waiting. However, if symptoms are severe or there is evidence of complications (recurrent urinary tract infections, urinary retention, hydronephrosis), then either medical or surgical treatment is required. Medical treatments include alpha-1-adrenoreceptor antagonists such as tamsulosin (which can also be used to manage co-morbid hypertension) or 5-alpha-reductase inhibitors such as finasteride. The mainstay of surgical treatment is transurethral resection of the prostate, which removes the prostate piece by piece.

1.57

B – Malaria

Malaria is the most important differential diagnosis in anyone returning from a malaria-endemic country with a fever. The life cycle of the parasite takes at least eight days from inoculation by the mosquito so any fever arising within the first week of exposure is not due to malaria. Malaria chemoprophylaxis is at best 70–90% effective. The diagnosis is made either with antigen stick testing or by looking at the blood films. A single negative blood film does not exclude malaria but malaria is unlikely after three negative films.

Malaria is an infectious, mosquito-borne parasitic disease caused by protozoa of the *Plasmodium* species. Haemoglobinopathies do provide a degree of protection against the severe systemic manifestations. Malaria can be divided into two broad groups: benign (*Plasmodium vivax, Plasmodium ovale, Plasmodium malariae*) and malignant types (*Plasmodium falciparum*). Falciparum malaria (classically in sub-Saharan Africa) is responsible for the majority of malaria mortality. Death is commonly due to cerebral involvement, disseminated intravascular coagulation and multi-organ failure.

Following the bite of an infected female *Anopheles* mosquito, the inoculated sporozoites migrate to the liver within 1 to 2 hours. Individuals are asymptomatic for 12 to 35 days (depending on parasite species), until the erythrocytic stage of the parasite life cycle. Release of merozoites from infected red cells when they rupture causes fever and the other manifestations of malaria. Red cell rupture obstructs the microcirculation in critical organs. The release of toxins leads to rigors. The relapsing species *Plasmodium vivax* and *Plasmodium ovale* can present as a new infection weeks or months after the initial illness due to activation of residual parasites in the liver.

Importantly, the initial symptoms of malaria are often non-specific. Tachypnoea, chills, malaise, fatigue, diaphoresis, headache, cough, anorexia, nausea, vomiting, abdominal pain, diarrhoea, arthralgia and myalgia are all symptoms of malaria. Classically, the fever in *Plasmodium vivax* and *Plasmodium ovale* occurs every third day, and the fever in *Plasmodium malariae* occurs every fourth day. The fever in *Plasmodium falciparum* is less predictable and can be continuous due to asynchrony of parasite development.

Treating benign malaria: Chloroquine followed by primaquine (to destroy residual liver parasites in *P. vivax* and *P. ovale*) is the recommended treatment. If there is chloroquine resistance, malarone (atovaquone plus proguanil) or mefloquine is recommended. Do not use primaquine in patients with glucose-6-phosphate dehydrogenase deficiency.

Treating mild malignant malaria: Oral quinine (three to seven days) followed by seven days of doxycline or clindamycin is recommended. Side effects of oral quinine include cinchonism (ringing in the ears), deafness, nausea and vomiting.

Treating severe malaria: High-level care is required. It is necessary to measure glucose, lactate and arterial blood gases, send off for coagulation studies, cross-match blood from the outset and meticulously assess fluid balance. Classically, intravenous quinine is the recommended treatment. Side effects include hypoglycaemia and arrhythmias. Artesunate has a better safety profile but does not have a product licence in Europe (but may be used on a named-patient basis). This treatment is followed with either doxycycline or clindamycin. Finally, exchange transfusion can be considered if parasitaemia exceeds 30% or in those who are pregnant or elderly.

1.58

D – Flucloxacillin and clindamycin

This male has developed toxic shock syndrome, a potentially fatal illness caused by toxin-producing *Staphylococcus aureus* or Group A streptococcus (*Streptococcus pyogenes*). The site of infection here was the abrasion on his shin. An important source of infection in females of childbearing age is tampon use, and it is therefore important in such patients to check for and remove this source of infection, if present. The toxin is a superantigen which directly activates T-cells, causing a cytokine storm and multisystem disease characterised by high fever, a characteristic sunburn-like rash (which progresses to desquamation of the palms, soles, fingers and toes one to two weeks later), hypotension and subsequent end-organ dysfunction. After acute resuscitation it is important to treat the infective cause by using a combination of antibiotics both to clear the infection and to turn off toxin protein production. Inhibition of bacterial protein production can be achieved by the administration of clindamycin, which binds to and inhibits the 50S ribosome subunit of the bacteria. Intravenous immunoglobulin can also be given to neutralise the circulating toxin.

1.59

D – *MSH2*

This patient has hereditary non-polyposis colorectal cancer, an autosomal dominant genetic condition associated with a markedly increased risk of colorectal cancer, along with malignancies of the uterus, ovary, stomach, kidney, small intestine or pancreas. In over 60% of patients with hereditary non-polyposis colorectal cancer, there is a mutation in *MSH2*, a gene that encodes for a DNA mismatch repair protein. Lifetime risk for colorectal cancer in this group of patients is 60%; females who carry the mutation have a 40% lifetime risk of endometrial cancer. It is advised that family members of affected individuals should undergo surveillance colonoscopy or genetic testing.

Some of the other cancer syndromes associated with specific genetic mutations are listed in the table below:

Cancer syndromes	Genetic mutation
Hereditary breast ovarian cancer syndrome	*BRCA1, BRCA2*
Familial adenomatous polyposis	*APC*
Multiple endocrine neoplasia type I	*MEN1*
Mulitiple endocrine neoplasia type II	*RET*
Retinoblastoma	*Rb*
Li–Fraumeni syndrome	*TP53*

Patients with familial adenomatous polyposis have multiple polyps throughout the colon from adolescence.

1.60

E – MRI venography and lumbar puncture

This patient has been treated with long-term tetracycline for acne and has developed idiopathic intracranial hypertension as a result. The best initial set of investigations are MRI venography to exclude space-occupying lesions and cerebral venous thrombosis as a cause for the examination findings, followed by a lumbar puncture, which will show a markedly raised cerebrospinal fluid pressure.

Idiopathic intracranial hypertension is most commonly seen in obese young females; risk factors include:

- Pregnancy
- Drugs (tetracycline, combined oral contraceptive pill)
- Cerebral venous thrombosis
- Head injury.

Treatments for idiopathic intracranial hypertension include:

- Repeated therapeutic lumbar punctures
- Pharmacological agents:
  - o Diuretics (e.g. acetazolamide)
  - o Steroids
- Surgical methods:
  - o Optic nerve sheath fenestration
  - o Ventriculoperitoneal shunting.

It is essential to assess visual fields for any enlargement of the blind spot or central scotoma, as this may signify optic nerve compression.

Paper 2

Chapter 2

Paper 2: Questions

2.1 You are called by the nursing staff to review a 66-year-old female. Her blood pressure has been found to be 223/112 mmHg.

Which one of the following is the most appropriate initial step in this patient's management?

A   24-hour urine collection for vanillylmandelic acid test
B   Bendroflumethiazide
C   Blood test for urea and electrolytes
D   Fundoscopy and urine dipstick
E   Labetalol

2.2 A 54-year-old female who was commenced on ramipril for hypertension one week ago has now developed severe facial oedema and dyspnoea. The skin is non-erythematous and there is no pruritus.

Which one of the following is the most likely explanation for this?

A   Anaphylactic reaction
B   Anaphylactoid reaction
C   C1 esterase inhibitor deficiency
D   Nephrotic syndrome
E   Renal artery stenosis

2.3 A 33-year-old pregnant female develops sudden-onset shortness of breath and pleuritic chest pain. She has a swollen, tender right calf.

Which one of the following ECG findings is most likely?

A   Deep S waves in I, Q waves in III, inverted T waves in III
B   P pulmonale

C   Right-axis deviation
D   Saddle-shaped ST elevation
E   Sinus tachycardia

2.4 A 29-year-old female is diagnosed with pulmonary tuberculosis and is about to be commenced on rifampicin, isoniazid, pyrazinamide and ethambutol.

Which one of the following is used to decrease the incidence of isoniazid-induced peripheral neuropathy?

A   Vitamin A
B   Vitamin B_1
C   Vitamin B_6
D   Vitamin B_{12}
E   Vitamin D

2.5 A 67-year-old male presents with a six-week history of generalised joint pain which is worse in the lower limbs. The patient also describes malaise, fever and weight loss. The patient has a 50-pack year smoking history. On examination, the patient has clubbing of the fingers and toes, with painful swollen knee and ankle joints bilaterally. The distal tibiae are tender to palpation bilaterally. A chest X-ray is performed and is normal. X-rays of the ankles show a bilateral periosteal reaction of the distal tibiae.

Which one of the following is the most likely unifying diagnosis?

A   Bone metastases from a primary malignancy
B   Hypertrophic osteoarthropathy
C   Parathyroid hormone-related peptide-secreting squamous cell lung carcinoma
D   Pott's disease
E   Systemic lupus erythematosus

2.6 A 23-year-old male presents with a three-month history of chest tightness, shortness of breath, wheeze and cough that is worse at night. On examination, a widespread expiratory wheeze is heard throughout.

Which one of the following pathological features is most likely to be found in this patient?

A Curschmann's spirals
B Grey hepatisation
C Kulchitsky cells
D Lines of Zahn
E Red hepatisation

2.7 A 74-year-old female with COPD presents with dyspnoea, confusion, flushing and central cyanosis. On examination there is a coarse tremor of the hands and papilloedema is seen on fundoscopy. Her observations are as follows:

Heart rate	115 beats per minute
Respiratory rate	28 breaths per minute
Temperature	36.8 °C

Which one of the following arterial blood gas profiles is most likely to be found in this patient?

A pH 7.25, PaO_2 7.3 kPa, $PaCO_2$ 5.3 kPa
B pH 7.25, PaO_2 6.2 kPa, $PaCO_2$ 9.0 kPa
C pH 7.35, PaO_2 7.3 kPa, $PaCO_2$ 4.8 kPa
D pH 7.45, PaO_2 7.3 kPa, $PaCO_2$ 5.3 kPa
E pH 7.45, PaO_2 15 kPa, $PaCO_2$ 1.8 kPa

2.8 A 63-year-old female who has attended the Emergency Department with an acutely swollen, tender right calf is found collapsed on the floor in the waiting room. During an initial assessment the airway is clear but the patient is making no respiratory effort and no carotid pulse can be palpated. Cardiopulmonary resuscitation is started and a defibrillator is attached. The ECG monitor shows ventricular tachycardia; one shockis administered using a defibrillator and chest compressions are resumed. A cannula is *in situ*.

Which one of the following is the most appropriate initial medication to administer?

A 0.5 ml intramuscular 1:1000 adrenaline
B 1 mg intravenous atropine

C 10 ml intravenous 1:10000 adrenaline
D 300 mg intravenous amiodarone
E 50 mg intravenous alteplase

2.9 A 35-year-old male with dyspepsia is commenced on triple therapy (omeprazole, metronidazole and clarithromycin) for *Helicobacter pylori* infection. He does not improve and further microbiological investigation demonstrates clarithromycin resistance. Consequently clarithromycin is stopped.

Which two drugs is it most appropriate to add to this patient's regimen?

A Amoxicillin and levofloxacin
B Bismuth and amoxicillin
C Bismuth and tetracycline
D Ranitidine and amoxicillin
E Ranitidine and bismuth

2.10 A 54-year-old female presents with weight loss, drenching night sweats and general malaise. Clinical examination reveals massive splenomegaly. Investigations are as follows:

Haemoglobin	7.1 g/dL
Platelets	63×10^9/L
White cell count	106×10^9/L (raised numbers of polymorphonuclear leukocytes)
Cytogenetic analysis	Translocation in chromosomes 9 and 22

Which one of the following medications is the most appropriate first-line management in this patient?

A All-trans-retinoic acid
B Cyclophosphamide
C Imatinib
D Interferon alpha
E Rituximab

2.11 A 57-year-old female is commenced on warfarin treatment as an inpatient following a diagnosis of pulmonary embolus. She is maintained on heparin in conjunction with warfarin for five days until her international normalised ratio is stable and within the normal range.

Which one of the following anticoagulant clotting factors is inhibited by warfarin?

A Antithrombin III
B Factor V Leiden
C Factor IX
D Factor X
E Protein C

2.12 A 23-year-old female presents with a painless, firm, rubbery cervical lymph node. She also complains of weight loss, night sweats and fever. Lymph node biopsy reveals the presence of Reed–Sternberg cells. CT scan shows involvement of cervical and inguinal lymph nodes. Bone marrow biopsy shows no abnormality.

Which one of the following stages of disease does this patient have?

A Stage IIA
B Stage IIB
C Stage IIIA
D Stage IIIB
E Stage IV

2.13 A 52-year-old female with sarcoidosis presents with suprapubic tenderness, dysuria and frequency. Midstream urine culture shows bacteruria. Abdominal X-ray imaging identifies the presence of multiple well-demarcated bilateral radio-opaque phenomena just lateral to the transverse processes of the lumbar spinal vertebrae.

Which one of the following is the most likely organism implicated?

A *Escherichia coli*
B *Klebsiella* species

C *Proteus mirabilis*
D *Pseudomonas aeruginosa*
E *Staphylococcus saprophyticus*

2.14 A 43-year-old male presents with fever, arthralgia and 5 kg weight loss. His blood pressure is 188/102 mmHg. His skin has a mottled, lace-like appearance and there is loss of sensation and motor function in the distribution of the radial and sural nerves. Subsequent angiography reveals the presence of renal artery aneurysms and a diagnosis of polyarteritis nodosa is made.

Which one of the following is most associated with polyarteritis nodosa?

A Asthma and eosinophilia
B C-ANCAs
C Granulomatous inflammation
D Hepatitis B infection
E X-ANCAs

2.15 A 35-year-old female presents with fever, a palpable purpuric rash and confusion. Her blood tests are as follows:

Haemoglobin	8.9 g/dL
Platelet count	19×10^9/L
Serum creatinine	350 μmol/L
ADAMTS13 level	3% of normal

The blood film report identifies the presence of schistocytes.

Which one of the following is the most likely diagnosis?

A Acute intermittent porphyria
B Haemolytic uraemic syndrome
C Henoch–Schönlein purpura
D Meningococcal septicaemia
E Thrombotic thrombocytopaenic purpura

2.16 A 68-year-old male presents to the Emergency Department with sudden onset of dizziness, vomiting, ataxia and dysphagia.

On examination there is a right-sided Horner's syndrome, a right-sided loss of pain and temperature sensation on the face and a left-sided loss of pain and temperature sensation on the body.

Which one of the following arteries is most likely to be affected?

A Anterior inferior cerebellar artery
B Lacunar artery
C Middle cerebral artery
D Posterior cerebral artery
E Posterior inferior cerebellar artery

2.17 A 50-year-old female undergoes a dual-energy X-ray absorptiometry bone scan that reveals a T-score of −2.6. She has been treated for breast cancer and has a 30-pack year smoking history.

Which one of the following treatment options is most appropriate for this patient?

A Alendronic acid
B Calcitonin
C Raloxifene
D Strontium ranelate
E Zoledronic acid by intravenous infusion

2.18 A 38-year-old female with known rheumatoid arthritis presents with a history of shortness of breath, easy bruising and recurrent chest infections. On clinical examination there is splenomegaly.

Which one of the following is the most likely explanation for this presentation?

A AL amyloid
B Azathioprine
C Felty's syndrome
D Idiopathic thrombocytopaenic purpura
E Methotrexate

2.19 A 49-year-old male suddenly experiences severe pain in his left ankle while walking. His past medical history is unremarkable, except for a recent course of antibiotics for severe gastroenteritis. Clinical examination reveals an inability to plantar flex the left foot.

Which one of the following antibiotics was the patient most likely to have been taking?

A Amoxicillin
B Cephalexin
C Ciprofloxacin
D Erythromycin
E Metronidazole

2.20 A 48-year-old male with a history of scleroderma develops worsening shortness of breath. On general inspection, the patient has sclerodactyly, microstomia, skin calcification, numerous telengiectasia and also a history of Raynaud's phenomenon. On further examination there is a raised jugular venous pressure, a left parasternal heave, pedal oedema and hepatomegaly.

Which one of the following is contraindicated?

A Captopril
B Cyclophosphamide
C Prednisolone
D Propranolol
E Prostacyclin

2.21 An 88-year-old man with longstanding Paget's disease presents with a two-month history of bone pain in his left femur that is worse on movement. On examination a tender mass is palpable over the left distal femur. X-ray of the femur reveals the presence of a destructive lytic lesion with surrounding new bone formation and periosteal reaction. A visible soft tissue mass is also present.

Which one of the following is the most likely diagnosis?

A Background Pagetic bone change
B Ewing's sarcoma
C Osteoblastoma

D Osteochondroma
E Osteosarcoma

2.22 A 32-year-old woman who is HIV positive has a routine blood test, which reveals a CD4 cell count of 180 cells/ml.

Which one of the following medications is the gold standard prophylactic treatment for this patient?

A Aciclovir
B Amphotericin B
C Co-trimoxazole
D Nystatin
E Primaquine

2.23 A 19-year-old male student presents to his General Practitioner with sore throat, cervical lymphadenopathy and malaise. The patient has no drug allergies and is prescribed amoxicillin. He returns two days later complaining of a widespread maculopapular rash.

Regarding the likely diagnosis, which one of the following statements is most correct?

A Complications include thrombocytopaenia and Guillain–Barré syndrome
B Diagnosis can be confirmed by the Mantoux test
C Most patients experience further complications
D Reed–Sternberg cells are found on bone marrow biopsy
E The patient should never be given amoxicillin again

2.24 A 47-year-old male on chemotherapy for high-grade non-Hodgkin's lymphoma presents with dysuria and haematuria.

Which one of the following medications is most likely to be the cause of his symptoms?

A Cyclophosphamide
B Doxorubicin
C Prednisolone

D Rituximab
E Vincristine

2.25 A 35-year-old male with central chest pain is admitted to the Emergency Department. On further questioning it is also noted that he has a severe headache that was sudden in onset. An initial ECG reveals widespread ST elevation throughout chest and limb leads.

Which one of the following is the most appropriate investigation to perform in this patient?

A 12-hour troponin
B Cardiac angiogram
C CT head
D Echocardiogram
E Serum urea and electrolytes

2.26 A 54-year-old female presents to her General Practitioner complaining of a lump in her neck which has been enlarging over the previous three months. The remainder of the history, including the family history, is unremarkable aside from tiredness, 7kg unintentional weight loss, diarrhoea, a change in voice and numerous episodes of facial flushing and sweating, all of which she felt to be climacteric in origin. On examination there is a discrete 2cm nodule at the base of the neck which elevates on swallowing. Blood test results are as follows:

Creatinine	87 micromol/L
Corrected calcium	2.14 mmol/L
Free T_4	13 nmol/L
Thyroid-stimulating hormone	0.5 mU/L

Fine-needle aspiration is arranged, after which the following histological report is provided:

'Uniform nests of cells with peripheral nuclei separated by bands of stroma that stain positively with Congo red stain and demonstrate yellow/green birefringence. Absence of thyroid follicular cells.'

Which one of the following is the most likely diagnosis?

A Medullary thyroid carcinoma
B Papillary thyroid carcinoma
C Parathyroid hyperplasia
D Phaeochromocytoma
E Toxic thyroid adenoma

2.27 A 45-year-old male is admitted to hospital with a fever that has lasted several weeks and has been accompanied by increasing shortness of breath on exertion. He has also had a change in bowel habit over the last four months. On auscultation of the precordium there is a pansystolic murmur heard loudest at the apex.

Which one of the following is the most likely causative agent in this patient?

A *Bartonella quintana*
B *Staphylococcus aureus*
C *Staphylococcus epidermidis*
D *Streptococcus bovis*
E *Streptococcus viridans*

2.28 A 50-year-old male with a penicillin allergy is being treated for osteomyelitis. Seven days later he complains of increasingly loose stools along with colicky abdominal pain and is noted to have a fever of 37.9 °C.

Which one of the following is the most appropriate first-line treatment in this patient?

A Intravenous metronidazole
B Intravenous vancomycin
C Oral loperamide
D Oral metronidazole
E Oral vancomycin

2.29 A 36-year-old male with a 20-year history of type I diabetes mellitus, background diabetic retinopathy, diabetic nephropathy and peripheral sensory neuropathy presents with a three-month history of nausea and vomiting. The vomit is mainly undigested food and bile and he has lost 6 kg during this time. Further questioning reveals that the patient is also being treated for a prolactinoma. On examination, there is mild abdominal distension but no epigastric tenderness. Lying and standing blood pressures reveal a drop of 30 mmHg in both the diastolic and systolic readings.

Which one of the following medications is most likely to provide this patient with symptomatic relief?

A Domperidone
B Erythromycin
C Metoclopramide
D Morphine
E Oxybutynin

2.30 A 70-year-old male with COPD presents with persistent breathlessness despite smoking cessation and inhaled ipratropium bromide. He has a good inhaler technique and lung function testing reveals that his FEV_1 is 45% of predicted.

Which one of the following is the best combination of inhalers to offer in addition to his current prescription?

A Fluticasone, salmeterol and tiotropium bromide
B Fluticasone and salmeterol
C Salmeterol
D Salmeterol and tiotropium bromide
E Tiotropium bromide

2.31 A 54-year-old male who has recently moved to the UK from Sudan develops atrial fibrillation. He is started on amiodarone. On examination, there is a goitre and an initial blood test reveals low serum iodine levels.

Which one of following is this patient most likely to develop?

A Epididymitis
B Hepatitis

C Hyperthyroidism
D Hypothyroidism
E Peripheral neuropathy

2.32 A 26-year-old female has a routine set of blood tests. The results are given below:

Haemoglobin   11.6 g/dL
Mean corpuscular volume   68 fL
Serum ferritin   39 µg/L

Which one of the following is the most likely cause of this finding?

A β-thalassaemia trait
B Bleeding from peptic ulcer
C Chronic kidney disease
D Iron deficiency anaemia
E Menorrhagia

2.33 A 36-year-old female has recently started a new medication after she developed a painful and swollen left calf. Routine blood tests reveal a platelet count of 46×10^9/L.

Which one of the following medications is most likely to be responsible?

A Alteplase
B Fondaparinux
C Low-molecular-weight heparin
D Unfractionated heparin
E Warfarin

2.34 A 55-year-old female with autosomal dominant polycystic kidney disease on haemodialysis complains of 'tingling' in her right thumb and index finger during a routine outpatient appointment. On examination of the right hand there is wasting of the thenar eminence, dry skin over the lateral three fingers and a positive Durkan's test.

Which one of the following is the most likely explanation for these findings?

A Acromegaly
B Amyloidosis
C Diabetes mellitus
D Hypothyroidism
E Pregnancy

2.35 A 22-year-old male presents to the Emergency Department complaining of progressively worsening leg weakness and numbness which started two days previously. Three weeks earlier he suffered an episode of febrile exudative tonsillitis with severe fatigue and tender cervical lymphadenopathy.

Which of the following is the most important initial investigation?

A Anti-streptolysin O titre
B Creatine kinase levels
C Paul–Bunnell test
D Spirometry
E Urine dipstick

2.36 A 20-year-old male student with a previous history of juvenile cataracts presents with progressive bilateral hearing loss. He has also noticed a small lump in his right popliteal fossa which has been getting progressively larger over the past two years.

Which one of the following is the most likely diagnosis?

A Acoustic neuroma
B Astrocytoma
C Meningioma
D Neurofibromatosis type I
E Neurofibromatosis type II

2.37 A 65-year-old male presents to his General Practitioner with increasing difficulty in walking. He feels that both of his legs have become gradually weaker. He also states that he has a headache that is worse lying down and is gradually getting worse. On examination there is bilateral hypertonia of the lower limbs, muscle weakness, a positive Babinski sign and hyperreflexia of both the ankle and knee reflexes bilaterally. Sensory examination is normal.

Which one of the following is the most appropriate investigation to perform in this patient?

A Contrast CT head
B Lower limb nerve conduction studies
C Lumbar puncture
D Spinal angiography
E Whole spine MRI

2.38 A 43-year-old female veterinary surgeon with no past medical history arrives in the Emergency Department. For the last 12 hours she has been suffering from bilateral facial droop, hyperacusis, difficulty speaking and altered taste sensation. For three weeks she has been experiencing painful, swollen joints; initially her left knee and now her left wrist. The day before her presentation she had a mild headache and vomited three times. On examination her upper and lower limb neurology is normal. An initial chest X-ray is unremarkable.

Which one of the following is the most likely diagnosis?

A EBV infection
B Guillain–Barré syndrome
C Lyme disease
D Moebius syndrome
E Sarcoidosis

2.39 A 35-year-old female with recently diagnosed Raynaud's syndrome presents to her General Practitioner with headaches. They are unilateral and throbbing in nature, and are preceded by hyperacusis and flashing zig-zag patterns in her vision. The headaches last roughly 72 hours and occur four times per month. Her neurological examination is normal.

Which one of the following medications should this patient be given for prophylaxis?

A Amitriptyline
B Pizotifen
C Propranolol
D Sodium valproate
E Topiramate

2.40 A 43-year-old female has a history of arthritis, thrombocyto-paenia and a malar rash. Her General Practitioner is considering the diagnosis of systemic lupus erythematosus.

Which one of the following antibodies is the most specific test for non-drug-induced systemic lupus erythematosus?

A Anti-dsDNA antibody
B Anti-histone antibody
C Anti-nuclear antibody
D Anti-Ro antibody
E Anti-Sm antibody

2.41 A 50-year-old previously well female presents with a two-month history of diarrhoea, fatigue and arthralgia with intermittent episodes of facial flushing. On examination there is a polyphonic expiratory wheeze, a mid-diastolic murmur well localised to the lower left sternal edge and a desquamating, erythematous, scaly rash with keratosis on the sun-exposed areas of her body.

Which one of the following is the most likely underlying diagnosis in this patient?

A Dermatomyositis
B Malignant carcinoid
C Pellagra
D Porphyria cutanea tarda
E Urticaria pigmentosa

2.42 A depressed 24-year-old female has taken an overdose of aspirin.

Which one of the following is the most likely initial metabolic change to occur?

A Hyperkalaemia
B Hypoglycaemia
C Metabolic acidosis
D Metabolic alkalosis
E Respiratory alkalosis

2.43 A General Practitioner performs fundoscopy on a 72-year-old female with longstanding type II diabetes mellitus and observes new dot and blot haemorrhages on the temporal retina. Her private ophthalmologist confirms these findings.

Which one of the following is the next most appropriate course of action?

A Improve glycaemic control
B LASER photocoagulation
C Reassure and continue regular checkups
D Start a beta-blocker
E Start a statin

2.44 A 74-year-old female is in hospital after undergoing a right-sided total hip replacement. After not opening her bowels for four days she now complains of incontinence of watery diarrhoea with abdominal discomfort and bloating. On examination there is generalised abdominal distension and tenderness with a hard, compressible mass in the left lower quadrant. Digital rectal examination reveals the presence of a large, hard stool in the rectum with no masses, blood or mucous. She is encouraged to increase her oral intake of bran fibre and fluid. The physiotherapists are asked to increase her mobilisation and, where appropriate, all constipating medications are stopped or reduced.

Which one of the following is the most appropriate next step in management?

A Ispaghula husk after meals
B Lactulose as required
C Magnesium sulphate
D Polyethylene glycol
E Senna every morning

2.45 A 62-year-old female with hypercalcaemia is found to have a right upper parathyroid adenoma.

Which one of the following is most likely to be seen in this setting?

A Hypertonia
B Perioral paraesthesiae
C Positive Chvostek's sign
D Positive Trousseau's sign
E Shortened QT interval

2.46 A 27-year-old male has come to his General Practitioner saying that he constantly feels hungry, thirsty and is passing urine more often. The patient says that he feels 'very tired and unwell', but mentions that his friends say he looks 'tanned and healthy'. After some basic investigations, the General Practitioner finds that the man has deranged liver function tests and a random blood glucose of 14.2 mmol/L.

Which one of the following is the most likely underlying diagnosis?

A Glucagonoma
B Hereditary haemochromatosis
C Mature-onset diabetes of the young
D Type II diabetes mellitus
E Wilson's disease

2.47 A 43-year-old female is brought into the Emergency Department after being found unconscious on the street. The paramedics found an empty blister pack of paracetamol along with several empty cans of high-strength lager beer. She appears cachectic and underweight.

The doctor on call suspects paracetamol overdose and measures her blood paracetamol levels, which is found to be 120 mg/L.

Which one of the following is the most appropriate first-step in management?

A Administer vitamin K
B Gastric lavage
C Give 50 g oral activated charcoal
D Refer to psychiatry
E Start *N*-acetylcysteine infusion

2.48 A 72-year-old male has been suffering from recurrent pneumonias over the past 18 months, as well as worsening lower back pain. Blood tests reveal impaired renal function. He is referred to the haematologist, and, following investigation of his immunoglobulin profile and bone marrow aspiration, a diagnosis of multiple myeloma is made.

Which one of the following is the most likely cause of kidney disease in such a patient?

A Bence Jones protein
B Cholelithasis
C Hypocalcaemia
D Hypouricacmia
E Rhabdomyolysis

2.49 A 75-year-old male who has been attending his General Practitioner complaining of lower back pain has recently developed bilateral pain down the backs of the legs which is worse during prolonged standing and walking on the flat, such that he has to stop walking after only 200 metres. However, he finds that his pain is improved when walking up the stairs and when cycling.

Which one of the following is the most likely diagnosis?

A Abdominal aortic aneurysm
B Atheromatous peripheral vascular disease
C Lumbar canal stenosis

D Osteoarthritis of the hips and knees
E Thromboangiitis obliterans

2.50 A 54-year-old female who has been admitted for elective cholecystectomy has been complaining of worsening right upper quadrant pain. She is later examined and appears drowsy and confused,
with signs of jaundice. Her observations are as follows:

Temperature	38.1 °C
Respiratory rate	18 breaths per minute
Blood pressure	95/65 mmHg
Oxygen saturations on room air	99%
Heart rate	110 beats per minute

Which one of the following is the most likely diagnosis?

A Ascending cholangitis
B Choledocolithiasis
C Cholelithiasis
D Liver abscess
E Right lower lobe pneumonia

2.51 A 67-year-old male with poorly controlled type II diabetes mellitus presents to the Emergency Department with increasing episodes
of feeling dizzy over the last 12 months and multiple near falls. His
symptoms have not improved since he was asked to increase his oral
fluid intake, reduce his alcohol intake, switch to eating smaller meals
more frequently and stop his anti-hypertensives. His symptoms tend
to occur when standing up, and cause visual blurring and lighthead-
edness. He experiences no seizures, loss of consciousness, vertigo,
nausea or hearing disturbance, and he improves after sitting or lying
down for a few minutes. His past medical history includes peripheral
neuropathy, chronic kidney disease and rheumatic heart disease. His
regular medications include metformin, gliclazide and simvastatin.
On examination his heart and respiratory sounds are normal and he
appears well hydrated. His observations are as follows:

Temperature	36.8 °C
Heart rate	79 beats per minute
Respiratory rate	14 breaths per minute
Blood pressure (lying)	154/82 mmHg
Blood pressure (standing)	121/59 mmHg
Oxygen saturations on room air	98%

The following blood tests are performed:

Haemoglobin	14.1 g/dL
White cell count	5.7×10^9/L
Serum sodium	137 mmol/L
Serum potassium	4.2 mmol/L
Serum urea	7.7 mmol/L
Serum creatinine	116 μmol/L
Serum cortisol (0 minutes)	242 nmol/L
Serum cortisol (30 minutes after synacthen)	614 nmol/L

Which one of the following is the most appropriate next step in management?

A Bumetanide
B Ferrous sulphate
C Fludrocortisone
D Midodrine
E Propranolol

2.52 A 69-year-old male has been brought into the Emergency Department with a suspected myocardial infarction. The ECG shows ST elevation in leads II, III and aVF and, although the P waves are regular, there is a lengthening PR interval, which culminates in a dropped beat every four beats.

Which one of the following complications of myocardial infarction has this patient developed?

A First-degree atrioventricular block
B Mobitz type II second-degree atrioventricular block
C Third-degree atrioventricular block
D Three-to-one atrioventricular block
E Wenckebach's phenomenon

2.53 A 33-year-old male with abdominal pain and recurrent afebrile bloody diarrhoea is referred for colonoscopy ± biopsy for suspected ulcerative colitis.

Which one of the following laboratory reports is most congruent with a diagnosis of ulcerative colitis?

A Cobblestone appearance with full-thickness inflammation and non-caseating granulomatous formation on biopsy
B Erythematous, friable, inflamed mucosa with mucosal crypt inflammation and crypt distortion
C Islands of residual mucosa separating inflamed areas containing transmural inflammatory infiltration
D Patchy inflammation containing serpiginous, deep fissuring 'rose thorn' ulcers of the colonic mucosa with non-necrotising epithelioid granuloma formation on biopsy
E Skip lesions of marked inflammation of the lamina propria and muscularis propria with crypt abscesses

2.54 A 61-year-old female with stage V chronic kidney disease is about to start on dialysis.

Which one of the following causes of end-stage renal failure is most associated with a normal haemoglobin concentration?

A Autosomal dominant polycystic kidney disease
B Diabetic nephropathy
C Glomerulonephritis
D Hypertensive nephropathy
E Multiple myeloma

2.55 A 65-year-old male presents with a two-hour history of central chest pain which is tearing in nature and radiates to his back.

Which one of the following is the most important predisposing factor for this presentation?

A Diabetes mellitus
B Essential hypertension

C Granulomatosis with polyangiitis
D Hypercholesterolaemia
E Secondary syphilis

2.56 A 35-year-old male attends an endocrinology outpatients clinic three months after having new treatment for his Graves' disease. He states that over the last two months his eyes appear to have started to protrude more than they had previously.

Which one of the following treatment options is most likely to have worsened this patient's exophthalmus?

A Carbimazole
B Propranolol
C Propylthiouracil
D Radioactive iodine
E Total thyroidectomy

2.57 A 14-year-old male presents to his General Practitioner with increasing fatiguability and shortness of breath on exertion. This has been getting worse over the last three years. On inspection there is severe clubbing of the hands and feet, central cyanosis and a raised jugular venous pressure. Palpation reveals a right ventricular heave and auscultation reveals a loud second heart sound but no added sounds. Basic investigations are as follows:

Temperature	36.5 °C
Haemoglobin	19.2 g/dL

Which one of the following is the most likely diagnosis?

A Atrial myxoma
B Eisenmenger's syndrome
C Subacute bacterial endocarditis
D Tetralogy of Fallot
E Uncomplicated patent ductus arteriosus

2.58 A 32-year-old female presents to her General Practitioner complaining of a rash on her elbows and knees. On inspection, the lesions are raised, well circumscribed, salmon-pink in colour and covered in a silvery-white scale. The General Practitioner notices bilateral nail pitting and lines going across the nails of both hands. The patient explains that the lesions have evolved over the past few weeks, and aside from a slight improvement whilst she was on a summer holiday abroad, the history reveals no other relieving or exacerbating factors, such as a change in her lifestyle, occupation, drug regimen, diet or hygiene routine.

Which of the following is the most likely diagnosis?

A Contact dermatitis
B Hypertrophic lichen planus
C Inverse psoriasis
D Plaque psoriasis
E Psoriaform drug reaction

2.59 A 25-year-old male presents to the Emergency Department with an episode of extreme muscle weakness. He has had multiple such episodes over the past two years, each of which resolved spontaneously. He reports that he often has these episodes post-prandially. An ECG is performed and reveals generalised peaked T waves.

Which one of the following is the most likely finding in this patient?

A Hypercalcaemia
B Hyperkalaemia
C Hypocalcaemia
D Hypokalaemia
E Hypomagnesaemia

2.60 A 68-year-old male with hypertension and type II diabetes mellitus presents with a one-week history of palpitations and dizziness. His ECG shows that his heart rate is 89 beats per minute, his heart rhythm is irregularly irregular and there are no P waves.

Which one of the following is the most appropriate treatment for this patient?

A Atenolol and aspirin
B Digoxin and warfarin
C Flecainide and warfarin
D Sotalol and aspirin
E Verapamil and warfarin

Paper 2: Answers

2.1

D – Fundoscopy and urine dipstick

This patient has significantly raised blood pressure and the most appropriate initial investigation is to perform fundoscopy and urine dipstick to look for signs of hypertensive damage to the eyes and kidneys. Routine blood tests should be reviewed and this will guide future management. Bendroflumethiazide may be used in order to lower the patient's blood pressure in this scenario. Labetalol may be given intravenously if the patient develops symptoms suggestive of hypertensive encephalopathy, such as headache, focal neurology or seizures. Testing of urinary vanillylmandelic acid is used to screen for phaeochromocytoma. Phaeochromocytoma is rare (it accounts for less than 0.1% of all cases of hypertension) and usually presents with episodic bouts of hypertension with associated anxiety and flushing.

2.2

C – C1 esterase inhibitor deficiency

This patient is most likely to have C1 esterase inhibitor deficiency, also known as hereditary angioedema. C1 esterase inhibitor is a member of the serpin (*serum protease inhibitor*) family of protease inhibitors and acts to inhibit activation of the classical pathway of the complement cascade. In the absence of C1 esterase inhibitor, activation of the complement cascade leads to increased levels of vasoactive peptides that increase capillary permeability, most notably bradykinin. Bradykinin is usually inactivated by ACE; however, in patients taking ACE inhibitors, such as ramipril, this level can rise such that it causes facial and laryngeal oedema with subsequent airway obstruction. These patients do not experience pruritus or erythema because there is no release of histamine in this process. This explains why anaphylactic and anaphylactoid reactions are incorrect responses, as these processes involve the release of histamine as a result of mast cell degranulation. IgE binding to mast cells mediates anaphylactic reactions; a drug that binds directly to mast cells mediates anaphylactoid reactions. It should be noted that ACE inhibitors may directly cause angioedema.

Patients with renal artery stenosis who are commenced on ACE inhibitors can develop dyspnoea but this is due to pulmonary oedema as a result of acute kidney injury rather than laryngeal oedema. Acute kidney injury occurs because angiotensin II normally constricts the efferent arteriole to maintain glomerular filtration pressure. Loss of this effect, in the setting of already impaired renal perfusion (renal artery stenosis), causes a reduction in glomerular filtration rate.

Nephrotic syndrome is a triad of:

- Proteinuria greater than 3.5 g per 24 hours
- Oedema
- Hypoalbuminaemia.

The oedema occurs as a result of hypoalbuminaemia, which reduces oncotic pressure and enables fluid to extravasate from blood vessels.

Only oedema is found in this patient, the other features are absent. In addition, ACE inhibitors are usually given to help reduce proteinuria as they lower blood pressure and decrease leakage of protein out of the glomerular capillaries.

2.3

E – Sinus tachycardia

The primary purpose of the ECG in suspected pulmonary embolism is to exclude other diagnoses, such as acute myocardial infarction. Sinus tachycardia is the ECG finding most commonly associated with pulmonary embolus. The classical $S_I Q_{III} T_{III}$ pattern and right-axis deviation can occur but are much less common. These ECG changes represent acute pressure and volume overload of the right ventricle, and can also therefore be seen in other acute lung conditions such as bronchospasm and pneumothorax.

P pulmonale are peaked P waves often found in the context of right atrial hypertrophy. This change is characteristic of chronic right heart strain, for example in patients with pulmonary hypertension. Global saddle-shaped ST elevation is associated with pericarditis.

2.4

C – Vitamin B$_6$

Pyridoxine (vitamin B$_6$) should be given while the patient is taking isoniazid in order to decrease the chances of developing a peripheral neuropathy.

Ethambutol can cause optic neuritis. Vision should be tested with Ishihara plates as colour vision is the first to deteriorate in such patients.

Patients starting on anti-tuberculosis medication should also be told to have routine full blood count, urea and electrolytes, and liver function tests performed regularly. They should also be told:

- To look at the whites of their eyes every morning (if yellow, seek medical attention)
- That their secretions will turn red and contact lenses will be stained permanently
- To pay attention to colours (if red is less bright, seek medical attention)
- To look out for tingling in the toes (continue with the tablets; tell doctor at next visit)
- That the oral contraceptive pill may fail (use barrier contraception)
- That compliance is vital to help them and to prevent the spread of resistance.

2.5

B – Hypertrophic osteoarthropathy

This patient has hypertrophic osteoarthropathy, a paraneoplastic syndrome of unknown aetiology most commonly associated with adenocarcinoma of the lung. It is characterised by a triad of arthritis, which is often painful and symmetrical, clubbing of the fingers and toes, and periostitis of the distal ends of long bones. Hypertrophic osteoarthropathy may pre-date the discovery of an underlying malignancy by several months.

Bone metastases from a primary malignancy occur most commonly in breast, kidney, lung, prostate and thyroid cancer. They are seen as predominantly osteolytic lesions on X-ray (dark, osteoclastic lesions), except in the case of prostate cancer, where the majority of the lesions are osteosclerotic (white, osteoblastic lesions). Pott's disease is infection of the spine with *Mycobacterium tuberculosis*. Squamous cell carcinoma of the lung is associated with the production of parathyroid hormone-related peptide. Increased levels lead to a rise in serum calcium levels through increased renal reabsorption of calcium and increased bone turnover. The presenting complaint of patients with hypercalcaemia is usually one or more of 'stones (renal or biliary colic), bones (bone pain), groans (abdominal pain, nausea and vomiting) and moans (fatigue, confusion and depression)'. Systemic lupus erythematosus is a disease characterised by autoimmune-mediated, systemic inflammation that can affect multiple organs.

2.6

A – Curschmann's spirals

Curschmann's spirals are whirls of shed respiratory epithelium that form within mucous plugs and can be seen in the sputum of patients with asthma. They are sometimes seen in association with Charcot–Leyden crystals that are produced by eosinophils.

Red and grey hepatisation are seen in pneumonia. Red hepatisation refers to the stage where there is extravasation of erythrocytes and neutrophils into the alveoli. The subsequent filling of the airspaces with inflammatory exudate gives the lung parenchyma the appearance of the liver (hence the term 'hepatisation' is used). Grey hepatisation occurs once the erythrocytes have died, and only the neutrophils and inflammatory exudate are left behind.

Kulchitsky cells are non-pathological; they are neuroendocrine cells that occur in the respiratory and gastrointestinal tract and are responsible for the release of 5HT in these organs.

Lines of Zahn are found within thrombi and delineate the boundaries between platelets mixed with fibrin and erythrocytes.

2.7

B – pH 7.25, PaO_2 6.2 kPa, $PaCO_2$ 9.0 kPa

This patient is displaying clinical features of hypoxia and hypercapnia, and her arterial blood gas measurement is likely to reflect these features. Hypoxia and hypercapnia combined constitute type II respiratory failure. Causes of type II respiratory failure can be divided into failure of drive or respiratory pump failure. Failure of drive is caused by brainstem abnormalities or suppression by sedative drugs. Respiratory pump failure is either due to neurological abnormalities (myopathies, neuropathies or neuromuscular junction abnormalities), chest wall deformities (secondary to obesity or scoliosis) or airway obstruction (asthma or COPD). It is most likely that this patient has an acute exacerbation of COPD, which also explains the acidotic state.

2.8

E – 50 mg intravenous alteplase

The clinical picture is compatible with a massive pulmonary embolism and subsequent cardiac arrest secondary to intravenous embolisation of a thrombosis from the deep veins of the legs. The most appropriate initial medication is a recombinant tissue plasminogen activator such as alteplase, which should be followed by an intravenous heparin bolus/infusion. Plasminogen is a proenzyme produced in the liver that can be activated to produce plasmin, a serine protease enzyme. Plasmin rapidly breaks down the fibrin mesh and degrades thrombi. Where the benefits outweigh the risks, activation of plasminogen by fibrinolytic agents (e.g. alteplase, streptokinase) can be utilised in managing many thromboembolic disorders (e.g. myocardial infarction, acute ischaemic stroke and pulmonary embolism). However, the benefits of fibrinolytic therapy in massive pulmonary embolism associated with cardiac arrest (possible restoration of haemodynamic function) must be balanced against the risks (bleeding from intracranial haemorrhage and rib fractures). Furthermore, it must be considered that the initiation of fibrinolytic medication during cardiac arrest will necessitate a further 60–90 minutes of resuscitation to allow time for the medication to work. Initiating a fibrinolytic bolus is therefore a complex decision, especially given the uncertainty of the diagnosis (the diagnosis of pulmonary embolism would usually be based on clinical suspicion, possibly after excluding other reversible causes of cardiac arrest).

The reversible causes of cardiac arrest are classically divided into the 'Hs and Ts':

- Hypovolaemia
- Hypoxia
- Hypothermia
- Hyperkalaemia/hypokalaemia
- Hyperglycaemia/hypoglycaemia
- Toxins
- Tamponade
- Tension pneumothorax
- Thrombus (e.g. myocardial infarction, pulmonary embolism)
- Trauma (either commotio cordisor structural damage).

Adrenaline has been used in cardiac arrests as a vasopressive sympathomimetic agent for over 40 years. The beneficial effects of adrenaline occur through its effects on alpha-adrenergic (systemic vasoconstriction, increasing cerebral and coronary perfusion pressures) and beta-adrenergic adrenoreceptors (inotropy and chronotropy may further enhance these perfusion pressures). However, these advantages may be partly offset by the risks, which include increased myocardial oxygen demands, ectopic ventricular arrhythmias and transient arteriovenous shunting, impaired systemic microcirculation and worsened post-arrest myocardial dysfunction. All in all, although the evidence for long-term benefits from adrenaline administration are lacking, improved short-term survival continues to warrant its use in cardiac arrest situations.

In the case of ventricular fibrillation or pulseless ventricular tachycardia the administration of adrenaline is delayed until after three defibrillation attempts because these rhythms are more amenable to defibrillation, and also because of the risks of administering adrenaline. The volume and type of adrenaline solution given depends on the situation. During cardiac arrests adrenaline is given intravenously in a more dilute solution (1:10000, 0.01%, 0.1 mg/mL) and flushed through with 20 mL of 0.9% saline. For anaphylaxis adrenaline is given intramuscularly in a more concentrated solution (1:1000, 0.1%, 1 mg/mL). Because the amount of adrenaline solution given in cardiac arrest (10 ml) is greater than the volume given in anaphylaxis (0.5 ml) the actual dose of adrenaline given in cardiac arrest (1 mg) is only double that used in anaphlylaxis (0.5 mg).

Amiodarone is a membrane-stabiliser and anti-arrhythmogenic that lengthens both the action potential and the refractory period of the myocardial cells. It is used in managing ventricular fibrillation and pulseless ventricular tachycardia that is refractory to defibrillation. A dose of 300 mg is given intravenously alongside adrenaline after three attempts at defibrillation. Lignocaine can be given instead when amiodarone is unavailable. In situations of cardiac arrest with pulseless electrical activity or asystole, adrenaline is given from the outset as these rhythms are not amenable to defibrillation. In addition, although atropine has previously been utilised in the management of these 'non-shockable' rhythms to block the negative chronotropic and inotropic effects of the parasympathetic vagus nerve on the atrioventricular and sinoatrial nodes, it is no longer routinely recommended because vagal drive is not thought to contribute enough to these rhythms to justify its use. Instead, primary myocardial pathology is the usual cause of asystole. Finally, it is important to note that the evidence for the use of medications in cardiac arrest situations is limited. The only two treatments that have been shown to improve mortality and morbidity are good quality chest compressions and the appropriate use of cardiac defibrillation.

2.9

C – Bismuth and tetracycline

If it is demonstrated that a patient has a clarithromycin-resistant *Helicobacter pylori* infection, the clarithromycin should be stopped and bismuth and tetracycline should be added to the patient's regimen. Bismuth is a chemical element, and the bismuth compounds bismuth subsalicylate and bismuth subcitrate can be used to treat peptic ulcers. They act by accelerating peptic ulcer healing and have also been shown to inhibit *Helicobacter pylori* virulence factors. Tetracycline inhibits protein synthesis by binding to the 30S ribosome subunit.

Amoxicillin and levofloxacin are antibiotics that, in conjunction with a proton pump inhibitor, constitute third-line treatment for *Helicobacter pylori* infection. This is used in situations where repeated attempts at *Helicobacter pylori* eradication using triple and quadruple therapy have failed. Ranitidine is a histamine-2-receptor antagonist that reduces gastric acid production but is only used if proton pump inhibitors (e.g. omeprazole) are not tolerated.

2.10

C– Imatinib

This patient has chronic myeloid leukaemia. The massive splenomegaly, the raised numbers of polymorphonuclear cells in the blood count, and the presence of the Philadelphia chromosome (a reciprocal translocation involving the long arms of chromosome 9 and 22, which forms the *BCR-ABL* fusion gene on chromosome 22) are all indicative of chronic myeloid leukaemia. Treatment is with imatinib, which specifically inhibits the BCR-ABL tyrosine kinase protein and induces apoptosis.

Treatment with imatinib has revolutionised the management of chronic myeloid leukaemia and it has been shown to be much more effective at preventing disease progression than the previous first-line therapy, interferon-alpha. Rituximab is an anti-CD20 monoclonal antibody that acts to reduce B-cell proliferation and plays an important role in the treatment of lymphomas and autoimmune diseases. All trans-retinoic acid is a vitamin A derivative used in the treatment of acute promyelocytic leukaemia (acute myeloid leukaemia subtype M3). Cyclophosphamide is an alkylating agent used in the management of patients with lymphoma and certain other malignancies and autoimmune diseases.

2.11

E – Protein C

Protein C (along with protein S) is a vitamin K–dependent anticoagulant factor and is therefore inhibited by warfarin. Warfarin inhibits vitamin K epoxide reductase, an enzyme that recycles oxidised vitamin K to its reduced form after it has participated in the carboxylation of vitamin K–dependent anticoagulant (and coagulant) factors. It is important to note that warfarin takes three to five days to attain its maximum effect and that protein C and protein S can be depleted before the coagulant factors II, VII, IX and X. Therefore, patients commenced on warfarin can become thrombophilic before its anticoagulant effect takes place, if they have low levels of protein C or protein S. As a result, patients are adminstered the anticoagulant heparin alongside warfarin until their international normalised ratio is stable and within the therapeutic range.

Antithrombin III is an anticoagulant that acts to inhibit factors IIa and Xa. Its action is markedly enhanced by heparins and inhibited by protamine. Acquired antithrombin III deficiency occurs in nephrotic syndrome, which means that these patients are thrombophilic and may require anticoagulation. Factor V Leiden is an abnormal form of factor V, and is the most common inherited thrombophilia. Factor V is usually deactivated by protein C. However, factor V Leiden is less easily degraded and so these patients have an increased tendency to thrombotic events.

2.12

D – Stage IIIB.

This patient has stage IIIB Hodgkin's lymphoma, as she has involvement of lymph nodes above and below the diaphragm and the presence of 'B' symptoms: weight loss, night sweats and fever. Hodgkin's lymphoma is characterised by the presence of Reed–Sternberg cells and is most commonly found in young adults. Most patients present with a painless, non-tender, asymmetrical, firm, discrete, rubbery enlargement of superficial lymph nodes, with the cervical lymph nodes being involved most commonly. Staging for Hodgkin's lymphoma is based on the Ann Arbour staging method:

Stage	Site of disease
I	Lymph node involvement in one area
II	Lymph node involvement in two or more areas on the same side of the diaphragm
III	Lymph node involvement above and below the diaphragm
IV	Extranodal involvement such as the bone marrow, liver or other extranodal sites

The suffixes 'A' and 'B' are used to indicate the absence and presence of 'B' symptoms, respectively. The spleen is counted as a lymph node for staging purposes. If there is splenic involvement, the suffix 'S' is used.

2.13

C –*Proteus mirabilis*

In sarcoidosis, granulomatous lesions convert 1-alpha hydroxylate 25-hydroxycholecalciferol (calcidiol) to its active form, 1,25-dihydroxycholecalciferol (calcitriol). An increased level of calcitriol leads to a rise in serum calcium levels through increased gut and renal reabsorption of calcium and increased bone turnover. Increased serum calcium levels puts patients at risk of renal calculi. These can be found in the renal parenchyma, renal pelvis, ureters, bladder or urethra. The ureters run parallel to the lumbar transverse processes.

Patients with renal calculi can develop a co-existing urinary tract infection, with *Proteus mirabilis* being the main organism implicated in this group. In uncomplicated urinary tract infections, *Escherichia coli* is the most common organism implicated, with *Klebsiella* species and *Staphylococcus saprophyticus* being amongst the less common protagonists. *Pseudomonas aeruginosa* is most commonly found in urinary tract infections associated with indwelling catheters.

2.14

D – Hepatitis B infection

Thirty percent of patients with polyarteritis nodosa are HBsAg positive. Polyarteritis nodosa is a medium-vessel vasculitis associated with renal artery aneurysms and skin, nerve and gut involvement. Patients are often hypertensive and can present with livedo reticularis and a mononeuritis multiplex. Polyarteritis nodosa is not associated with the ANCA-positive small-vessel vasculitides and should be considered distinct from these diseases. Granulomatous inflammation is not a feature of polyarteritis nodosa.

C-ANCAs are antibodies against the cytoplasmic antigen proteinase-3 and are most strongly associated with granulomatosis with polyangiitis (Wegener's granulomatosis). X-ANCAs are antibodies against lactoferrin and are most strongly associated with ulcerative colitis. Asthma and eosinophilia in the setting of vasculitis are associated with eosinophilic granulomatosis with polyangiitis (Churg–Strauss syndrome), a small- to medium-vessel vasculitis that affects predominantly the lungs and the skin. Eosinophilic granulomatosis with polyangiitis is most associated with p-ANCAs, which are antibodies against the perinuclear antigen myeloperoxidase.

2.15

E – Thrombotic thrombocytopaenic purpura

Thrombotic thrombocytopaenic purpura is one of the thrombotic microangiopathies and is classically characterised by a pentad of fever, microangiopathic haemolytic anaemia (which is characterised by a low haemoglobin and the presence of fragmented red cells, or schistocytes), consumptive thrombocytopaenic purpura, renal failure and neurological abnormalities. Microvascular platelet thrombus formation causes tissue ischaemia and is responsible for the renal and neurological manifestations, along with the microangiopathic haemolytic anaemia and consumptive thrombocytopaenia. Levels of the proteinase ADAMTS13 are found to be low in thrombotic thrombocytopaenic purpura; this is either due to an inherited mutation, or secondary to the formation of autoantibodies against ADAMTS13. ADAMTS13 is a zinc metalloproteinase that cleaves von Willebrand factor from its larger form into its smaller proteins. In the absence of ADAMTS13, the larger form of von Willebrand factor enters the circulation and binds and activates platelets. This leads to platelet aggregation and platelet thrombi formation. The platelet thrombi are then capable of embolising to microvessels downstream causing a microangiopathy that leads to end-organ ischaemia. Treatment is with plasma exchange to remove the larger form of von Willebrand factor and any autoantibodies that may be present, and to replace ADAMTS13 using fresh frozen plasma or cryosupernatant.

Haemolytic uraemic syndrome is also a thrombotic microangiopathy and is closely related to thrombotic thrombocytopaenic purpura. However, in haemolytic uraemic syndrome ADAMTS13 levels are normal and organ damage is limited to the kidneys. Haemolytic uraemic syndrome is either congenital, due to deficiency in the complement regulatory protein factor H, or, more commonly, acquired as a result of *Escherichia coli* O157 infection. *Escherichia coli* O157 is an enterohaemorrhagic bacterium that produces the Shiga-like toxin, which causes release of the larger forms of von Willebrand factor and other prothrombotic factors from affected endothelial cells.

In the thrombotic microangiopathies the prothrombin time, the activated partial thromboplastin time and fibrinogen levels are all normal.

Meningococcal septicaemia can often present with fever, purpura and generalised confusion. Patients develop disseminated intravascular coagulation in meningococcal septicaemia as a result of endothelial damage and subsequent release and consumption of coagulation factors. Release of intravascular thrombin causes widespread platelet aggregation; this consumption of platelets leads to thrombocytopaenia. A microangiopathic haemolytic anaemia can also occur as red cells pass through strands of fibrin found in small vessels. However, as with haemolytic uraemic syndrome, there is no change in ADAMTS13 levels in meningococcal septicaemia.

Acute intermittent porphyria is a rare autosomal dominant metabolic disorder associated with a deficiency in the enzyme porphobilinogen deaminase, one of the enzymes involved in haem synthesis. Patients present with abdominal pain, neurological abnormalities, and urine that darkens on standing. Hyponatraemia may also be found.

Henoch–Schönlein purpua is a systemic vasculitis that mainly affects children and presents with a combination of abdominal pain, arthralgia, a palpable purpuric rash most commonly found on the arms and buttocks, and renal involvement.

2.16

E – Posterior inferior cerebellar artery

This patient has had an infarct affecting the right posterior inferior cerebellar artery. Stroke presents with a sudden, focal neurological deficit that causes loss of, rather than gain of, function. Patients often have vascular risk factors such as increasing age, hypertension, diabetes, hypercholesterolaemia and atrial fibrillation. A posterior inferior cerebellar artery stroke (lateral medullary syndrome or Wallenberg syndrome) affects the nuclei of cranial nerves V, VIII, IX and X, the descending sympathetic fibres, cerebellum and the spinothalamic tract (the fibres of which have already decussated). Clinical features include dysarthria, dysphagia, dysphonia, unilateral Horner's syndrome, unilateral cerebellar signs, loss of pain and temperature on the same side of the face and the opposite side of the body (with respect to the side of the lesion).

An anterior inferior cerebellar artery infarct presents with ipsilateral ataxia due to cerebellar involvement, contralateral hemiparesis due to damage to the corticospinal tract and contralateral loss of pain and temperature sensation on the body due to spinothalamic tract damage.

The middle cerebral artery is the most common site for cerebral infarction. A middle cerebral artery infarct will have varying presentations depending on the extent of the infarction and the side of the lesion. Common features of a middle cerebral infarct include varying degrees of drowsiness (an intact cerebral cortex is required for consciousness), contralateral hemiparesis, contralateral hemisensory loss (worse in the upper limb and face than the lower limb), contralateral homonymous hemianopia and contralateral neglect and inattention. If the infarct occurs in the dominant hemisphere there may also be aphasia. This can be a Broca's aphasia, Wernicke's aphasia or global aphasia depending upon the extent of the infarct.

The posterior cerebral artery supplies the occipital lobe, the inferomedial temporal lobe, a large portion of the thalamus and the midbrain. Symptoms will vary depending upon the location of the infarct. A proximal infarct will affect all of the areas supplied by the artery whereas more distal infarcts will result in more limited deficits. Common features of a proximal posterior cerebral infarct include a contralateral homonymous hemianopia with macular sparing, cortical blindness, memory difficulties, post-stroke (thalamic) pain, contralateral hemiplegia and oculomotor nerve palsy. The contralateral hemiplegia and oculomotor nerve palsy occur due to occlusion of the paramedian branches, which supply the midbrain. Infarction of the paramedian vessels is known as Weber's syndrome (medial medullary syndrome).

A lacunar stroke is a collective term given when there is occlusion of one of the penetrating arteries that provides blood to the subcortical structures. There are many different types of lacunar infarct depending upon the penetrating arteries affected. The most common lacunar strokes are a pure motor stroke and a pure sensory stroke. A pure motor stroke causes a contralateral hemiparesis and is due to infarction of the striate arteries that supply the posterior limb of the internal capsule through which the corticospinal tract passes. A pure sensory stroke presents with unpleasant sensations on one side of the body and is due to infarction of the arteries that supply the ventral posterolateral nucleus of the thalamus.

2.17

C – Alendronic acid

This woman has osteoporosis, as her dual-energy X-ray absorptiometry bone scan has revealed a bone density of greater than 2.5 standard deviations below the average value for a healthy 30-year-old (T-score of less than −2.5; the Z-score is relative to the value age-matched value). She should be commenced on alendronic acid, a bisphosphonate, which inhibits bone reabsorption. Zoledronic acid is given intravenously and is used if patients can't tolerate bisphosphonates. It is important to ensure that vitamin D levels are normal and dietary calcium is adequate, and to supplement these if necessary.

2.18

C – Felty's syndrome

Felty's syndrome is the triad of rheumatoid arthritis, splenomegaly and leukopaenia. In these patients hypersplenism leads to sequestration of red blood cells (anaemia) and platelets (thrombocytopaenia), which has caused this patient to develop shortness of breath and easy bruising, respectively. The low white cell count in Felty's syndrome leaves the patient susceptible to infections. Patients who are taking disease-modifying agents (e.g. azathioprine, methotrexate) may also develop symptoms consistent with low platelets, red blood cells and white cells (i.e. aplastic aneamia) due to the myelosuppressive effect of these medications. However, these medications do not cause splenomegaly.

AL (primary) amyloid is not a recognised complication of rheumatoid arthritis but AA (secondary) amyloid is.

Idiopathic thrombocytopaenic purpura is associated with other autoimmune diseases but does not cause anaemia or leukopaenia. Platelets coated in IgG are removed by the spleen but the spleen is seldom enlarged.

2.19

C – Ciprofloxacin

It is most likely that this patient had been prescribed ciprofloxacin, a member of the quinolone family of antibiotics. Quinolones act by inhibiting bacterial DNA gyrase and can be used to treat severe gastrointestinal infections. Quinolone antibiotics are associated with tendon rupture; in this scenario the patient has ruptured his Achilles tendon. Before a patient is commenced on a quinolone, the clinician should always enquire about previous tendonopathy and to avoid quinolone prescription where possible if there is a positive history. The risk of tendon rupture is increased in patients taking corticosteroids. Other adverse effects associated with quinolones include irreversible peripheral neuropathy, Stevens–Johnson syndrome, lowering of the seizure threshold in epilepsy and increased susceptibility to *Clostridium difficile* infection. Ciprofloxacin, along with erythromycin (a macrolide antibiotic) and metronidazole (an antibiotic used to treat anaerobic infections), also inhibits the CYP450 enzymes and thus potentiates the activity of drugs such as warfarin.

2.20

D – Propranolol

This patient has developed pulmonary hypertension in association with limited cutaneous systemic sclerosis. Pulmonary hypertension may complicate pulmonary fibrosis but more commonly occurs in isolation. Pulmonary hypertension causes pressure overload in the right side of the heart, resulting in right ventricular hypertrophy (left parasternal heave) and vena caval congestion (pedal oedema and hepatomegaly). Treatment with parenteral prostacyclin, a prostaglandin analogue, decreases pressure in the pulmonary vasculature and improves symptoms. Pulmonary disease is the leading cause of death in patients with scleroderma, therefore such patients should have annual echocardiography and lung function tests to detect for subclinical pulmonary hypertension. High-resolution chest CT scanning is also strongly advocated to detect pulmonary fibrosis.

ACE inhibitors, such as captopril, play an important role in the management of scleroderma renal crisis. Cyclophosphamide, often given with corticosteroids such as prednisolone, plays an important role in trying to reduce lung fibrosis in scleroderma.

Non-selective beta-blockers, such as propranolol, must be avoided in scleroderma as they can precipitate vasoconstriction and worsen Raynaud's phenomenon.

2.21

E – Osteosarcoma

Osteosarcoma is 30 times more common in patients with Paget's disease and is more common in patients with longstanding disease. This population is responsible for the second peak in incidence of this tumour, after the first peak in young children.

Background Pagetic bone change is identified radiologically by sclerosis (osteoblast activity), bone expansion, and coarse, disorganised trabecular bone. Ewing's sarcoma is most commonly found in teen-agers and adolescents whose bones are still growing. Osteoblastoma is a rare benign tumour of the bone. Osteochondroma is also benign and is the most common skeletal tumour. It involves growth of both cartilage and bone.

2.22

C – Co-trimoxazole

Patients with a CD4 cell count of less than 200 per ml are at an increased risk of developing *Pneumocystis jirovecii* pneumonia. *Pneumocystis jirovecii* is a yeast-like fungus and *Pneumocystis jirovecii* pneumonia is one of the AIDS-defining illnesses. To reduce this risk, such patients should be given prophylactic co-trimoxazole, an antibiotic consisting of one part trimethoprim to five parts sul-phamethoxazole. Co-trimoxazole is contraindicated in patients with glucose-6-phosphate dehydrogenase deficiency as it can pre-cipitate a haemolytic anaemia. Other side effects include Stevens–Johnson syndrome and myelosuppression.

Aciclovir is an anti-viral agent used for, amongst other things, her-pes simplex virus infections. Amphotericin B is used to treat severe systemic fungal infections but is not usually used in the setting of *Pneumocystis jirovecii* pneumonia. Nystatin is an anti-fungal drug most commonly used to treat oral *Candida* infection. Primaquine is a second-line agent used to treat *Pneumocystis jirovecii* pneumonia, and is used in patients with glucose-6-phosphate dehydrogenase deficiency.

2.23

A – Complications include thrombocytopaenia and Guillain–Barré syndrome

This patient has experienced a drug reaction by taking amoxicillin whilst having EBV infection. EBV is a member of the HHV family (group IV) that infects B-lymphocytes and causes a proliferation of atypical T-lymphocytes. Atypical T-lymphocytes are CD8-positive cells that have reacted against virally infected B-cells. Complications of EBV infection include thrombocytopaenia and Guillain–Barré syndrome, along with meningitis, encephalitis and facial nerve palsy. Nevertheless, the vast majority of patients recover uneventfully.

Diagnosis is confirmed by the Paul–Bunnell (Monospot) test identifying the presence of heterophile antibodies, which are produced in response to the infection. These antibodies are present in 90% of patients by week three of the infection, and disappear after approximately three months. The Mantoux test is a test for tuberculosis infection, whereby an extract of the tubercle bacillus ('tuberculin') is injected into the skin. A good immune response 48–72 hours later indicates prior infection. Although this patient's rash is diffuse, erythematous and pruritic, it does not denote a true allergy and will not occur if amoxicillin is taken in the absence of EBV. Therefore this patient can be given amoxicillin again in the future and it should not be documented as an allergy.

2.24

A – Cyclophosphamide

Haemorrhagic cystitis is a well-known complication of cyclophosphamide therapy. Cyclophosphamide is an alkylating agent used in the management of patients with lymphoma, other malignancies and autoimmune diseases. Cyclophosphamide is broken down to acrolein, a urotoxic metabolite, which causes this adverse effect on the urinary tract. Cyclophosphamide is usually co-prescribed with mesna, which binds acrolein and reduces the incidence of haemorrhagic cystitis.

Rituximab, cyclophosphamide, doxorubicin (hydroxydaunorubicin), vincristine (oncovin) and prednisolone compose the R-CHOP treatment regimen for non-Hodgkin's lymphoma. Rituximab is an anti-CD20 monoclonal antibody that acts to reduce B-cell proliferation. Doxorubicin intercalates DNA; its most notable side effect is cardiotoxicity (dilated cardiomyopathy). Vincristine is a microtubule inhibitor, which is associated with peripheral neuropathy. Predniso-lone is a corticosteroid and is associated with a wide range of side effects including acne, diabetes mellitus and central obesity.

2.25

C – CT head

This patient needs an urgent CT head as the history of severe sudden-onset headache is highly suggestive of subarachnoid haemorrhage. The classical presentation of a subarachnoid haemorrhage is a thun-derclap headache, which is the worst headache the patient has ever experienced and is maximal within seconds. However, subarach-noid haemorrhages can have an atypical presentation in which central chest pain and ST elevation are the predominant features; this can easily be mistaken for a myocardial infarction. However, the presence of the severe headache in this patient should raise the suspicion of subarachnoid haemorrhage, which would be potenti-ated if treated as a myocardial infarction with thrombolysis and anti-platelet agents. It is essential in this patient to arrange for a CT head to exclude a subarachnoid haemorrhage.

Subarachnoid haemorrhage is one of many conditions that may mimic an STEMI and are important to consider before proceeding with treatment. Non-vascular cardiac conditions such as pericardi-tis and myocarditis can present with ST elevation and chest pain. If suspected, an echocardiogram should be performed to exclude these conditions. Non-cardiac conditions such as acute cholecysti-tis, pancreatitis or hyperkalemia may also mimic an STEMI.

In patients with a likely diagnosis of STEMI, treatment involves reperfusion of the myocardium preferably by percutaneous coro-nary angioplasty, which is performed during a cardiac angiogram. The angiogram can initially confirm the diagnosis of myocardial infarction and then angioplasty can be undertaken to reperfuse the blocked vessel. Cardiac angiograms are also used to help in the diagnosis of NSTEMI, unstable angina and stable angina. If angio-plasty is not an option then thrombolysis is the next best option.

2.26

A – Medullary thyroid carcinoma

The development of a solitary thyroid nodule in a patient with flushing, sweating, weight loss and altered voice is highly suspicious of medullary thyroid carcinoma. Medullary thyroid carcinoma is a malignancy of the parafollicular C-cells of the thyroid, which are cells of neuroendocrine origin that produce the hormone calcitonin. They can therefore be associated with hypocalcaemia. Medullary thyroid carcinomas are well-differentiated, functional tumours that are highly secretory. In addition to calcitonin (which is of diagnostic and symptomatic importance) they can produce large amounts of carcioembryonic antigen, adrenocorticotropin-releasing hormone and 5HT (e.g. producing paraneoplastic Cushingoid and carcinoid syndromes, respectively).

As for breast lumps, thyroid lumps should undergo thorough investigation based on the triple assessment:

- Clinical (thorough history and examination)
- Radiological (ultrasound investigation)
- Cytological (biopsy and histological examination).

The majority of medullary thyroid carcinomas present with a neck mass, usually in the posterior thyroid, that can invade local structures such as the recurrent laryngeal nerve (causing vocal cord paralysis and hoarse voice), oesophagus (causing dysphagia) and airway (causing respiratory difficulty). A third of patients also have lymphadenopathy. High levels of circulating calcitonin cause flushing, weight loss, nausea, vomiting and a secretory diarrhoea (calcitonin lowers serum calcium levels partly by reducing gastrointestinal calcium absorption, causing diarrhoea). The menopause ('climacteric') can produce the following effects:

- Vasomotor (hot flushes, palpitations, night sweats)
- Psychological (depression, anxiety, reduced libido)

- Gastrointestinal (diarrhoea, constipation, bloating)
- Genitourinary (atrophic vaginitis, oligomenorrhoea, urinary symptoms).

This patient's tumour histology demonstrates the characteristic pathological findings of medullary thyroid carcinoma; absence of thyroid follicles and stromal amyloid. Procalcitonin is deposited in the tumour stroma as amyloid fibrils (beta-pleated sheets) which characteristically demonstrate apple-green birefringence when stained with the Congo red stain and viewed under polarised light.

Thyroid cancers can be categorised based on their tissue type. Histologically the thyroid gland is made up of spherical thyroid follicles that contain thyroglobulin colloid and are lined by follicular epithelial cells. Tumours of the follicular cells include papillary (70% of primary thyroid cancers), follicular (20%) and anaplastic (1%) thyroid carcinoma varieties. Interspersed between the follicular cells are the parafollicular 'C' cells that are responsible for medullary carcinomas (5% of primary thyroid cancers). Other types of thyroid tumours include lymphoma (rare; associated with Hashimoto's thyroiditis) and secondary metastases (most commonly haematogenous spread from malignant melanoma, lung, gastrointestinal, breast and renal cell carcinomas). Most patients with thyroid cancers are euthyroid; however, patients with toxic thyroid adenoma, by definition, display clinical evidence of hyperthyroidism. Seventy-five percent of medullary thyroid carcinomas are sporadic (these tend to occur in older patients); however, 25% are associated with the familial cancer syndrome type II multiple endocrine neoplasia. There are two types:

- Multiple endocrine neoplasia type IIa: medullary thyroid carcinoma, phaechromocytoma and parathyroid hyperplasia (which would cause hypercalcaemia)
- Multiple endocrine neoplasia type IIb: medullary thyroid carcinoma, phaeochromocytoma, mucosal neuroma and marfanoid body habitus.

2.27

D –*Streptococcus bovis*

The history of fever, shortness of breath on exertion and a new-onset murmur is highly suggestive of subacute bacterial infective endocarditis. Change of bowel habit also raises the possibility a colonic malignancy. In patients with infective endocarditis and symptoms suggestive of colonic malignancy, the most likely causative organism is *Streptococcus bovis*. This is a group D beta-haemolytic streptococci and, although a rare cause of infective endocarditis, it is associated with bowel cancer. Due to the risk of colonic malignancy, all patients with *Streptococcus bovis* endocarditis should undergo a colonoscopy even if there are no gastrointestinal symptoms.

Streptococcus viridans is the name for a large group of alpha-haemolytic streptococci that are a normal part of the mouth flora. They produce a green ('viridans') colouration on blood agar. *Streptococcus viridans* are the most frequently implicated organisms in native valve endocarditis and are often associated with infective endocarditis after a tooth extraction.

In patients with prosthetic valves infective endocarditis the organism implicated differs depending upon the amount of time since surgery. Within six months, the most likely causative agents are *Staphylococcus aureus* and coagulase-negative staphylococcus (*Staphylococcus epidermidis*). Outside six months, the organisms are the same as for a native valve infective endocarditis.

Bartonella quintana is an aerobic Gram-negative bacillus and a cause of infective endocarditis in homeless patients with substandard hygiene. It must be considered to be the causative organism in such patients.

2.28

D – Oral metronidazole

This patient has been given intravenous clindamycin (a lincosamide antibiotic) which is an antibiotic used in the treatment of osteomyelitis. A well-recognised complication of clindamycin is the development of *Clostridium difficile* infection, which can lead to a pseudomembranous colitis. This patient's symptoms are typical of a mild to moderate *Clostridium difficile* infection, for which the first-line treatment is oral metronidazole.

The glycopeptide antibiotics (e.g. vancomycin, teicoplanin) are used as second-line therapy in patients with a mild or moderate infection when oral metronidazole has failed or is contraindicated (e.g. in pregnancy). Because the glycopeptides are relatively large and hydrophilic molecules, they cross membranes poorly. Therefore oral preparations remain exclusively in the gastrointestinal tract and intravenous preparations remain in the blood. This feature is well utilised in the treatment of a penicillin-resistant Gram-positive sepsis (e.g. as methicillin-resistant *Staphylococcus aureus*). Metronidazole is also poorly absorbed from the gastrointestinal tract and therefore, as with the glycopeptide antibiotics, by using oral preparations high concentrations of the antibiotic can be achieved at the site of the infection in the colon. Monitoring of glycopeptide levels is clearly not necessary in such patients.

Intravenous metronidazole and vancomycin are usually reserved for more severe infections or when the oral preparations have failed to treat the infections.

Loperamide is an opioid receptor agonist that does not cross the blood brain barrier and can be used to reduce bowel motility and episodes of diarrhoea but it has no use in the treatment of *Clostridium difficile* infection.

2.29

B – Erythromycin

This patient has poorly controlled type I diabetes mellitus, and has now developed symptoms highly suggestive of gastroparesis. This occurs as a result of autonomic neuropathy due to poor glycaemic control. If the vagus nerve is affected delayed gastric emptying can occur. Common symptoms of gastroparesis include vomiting undigested food, nausea, weight loss and early satiety. Treatment for gastroparesis includes dietary changes such as a low-fibre diet and restriction of fats or solids. Prokinetic agents are also used in the treatment of gastroparesis as they promote antral contractility and improve antroduodenal coordination. They can also accelerate small bowel and colon transit leading to better gut transit time. Examples of prokinetic agents include dopamine antagonists (e.g. domperidone and metoclopramide) and macrolide antibiotics (e.g. erythromycin). Erythromycin is the preferred treatment in this patient as domperidone and metoclopramide should be avoided in patients with a prolactinoma.

Dopamine is synthesised in the hypothalamus and travels to the anterior pituitary via the portal vessels to inhibit the release of prolactin. Consequently, dopamine antagonists will increase the release of prolactin and may lead to worsening of symptoms in patients with a prolactinoma. Oxybutynin is an anticholinergic that reduces the action of the parasympathetic nervous system. It should therefore be avoided in patients with gastroparesis as it reduces the rate of gastric emptying. Opioid receptor agonists such as morphine should also be avoided in patients with gastroparesis as they delay gastric empyting.

2.30

B – Fluticasone and salmeterol

In addition to the short-acting muscarinic antagonist ipratropium bromide, this patient should be started on a combination inhaler containing corticosteroid and long-acting beta-2-adrenoreceptor agonist (e.g. Fostair, Seretide and Symbicort).

All patients with newly diagnosed COPD should start first-line therapy with either an inhaled short-acting beta-2-adrenoreceptor agonist (e.g. salbutamol) or an inhaled short-acting muscarinic receptor antagonist (e.g. ipratropium bromide). These cause smooth muscle relaxation and bronchiolar dilation. If patients remain symptomatic then add-on therapy should be commenced. The choice depends on the FEV_1:FVC ratio. Patients with an FEV_1:FVC ratio less than 50% (as in this patient) should be started on a long-acting beta-2-adrenoreceptor agonist and inhaled corticosteroid in a combination inhaler (e.g. Seretide). Combination inhalers are used frequently as they improve patient compliance. Inhaled corticosteroids are used in the treatment of COPD because they reduce bronchiolar inflammation. Due to systemic side effects, oral corticosteroids are usually not indicated in the long-term management of COPD. Patients with an FEV_1:FVC ratio of less than 50% could be started on a long-acting muscarinic receptor antagonist (e.g. tiotropium bromide) instead of the above combination; however, in this scenario it is important to stop the inhaled short-acting muscarinic receptor antagonist. This patient is continuing their ipratropium bromide and therefore tiotropium bromide is not an appropriate option. If patients continue to have severe breathlessness despite second-line therapy, further treatment is required. Triple therapy with an inhaled long-acting beta-2-adrenoreceptor agonist, inhaled long-acting muscarinic antagonist and inhaled corticosteroid should be initiated.

2.31

C – Hyperthyroidism

This patient is most likely to develop amiodarone-induced hyperthyroidism. Amiodarone, a class III anti-arrhythmic agent, is structurally similar to thyroxine and has a very high iodine content. As a result, abnormalities of the thyroid gland are common in patients on amiodarone.

Two types of amiodarone-induced thyroid disorders exist. Type I results in hyperthyroidism and usually occurs in patients with either pre-existing thyroid disorders or iodine deficiency. Normally, if a patient is given a large dose of iodine (e.g. amiodarone) then there is an autoregulatory reduction in thyroid hormone synthesis.

Patients with an underlying thyroid disorder or who are iodine deficient cannot autoregulate effectively and there is an increase in production and hyperthyroidism. This is known as the Jod-Basedow phenomenon. Amiodarone may also cause thyrotoxicosis by releasing preformed thyroxine from the thyroid gland. Type II results in the patient becoming hypothyroid and occurs in patients with a previously normal thyroid gland. This is due to the above autoregulatory reduction in thyroid hormone synthesis, and is known as the Wolff–Chaikoff effect.

Non-thyroid side effects are also common in patients on amiodarone. Abnormal liver function tests are common and can progress to hepatitis and even cirrhosis in a minority of patients. Peripheral neuropathies also occur, most commonly manifesting as a distal symmetrical sensorimotor polyneuropathy. This usually presents over a long period but can present acutely, where it may mimic Guillain–Barré syndrome. Finally, amiodarone can cause epididymitis, a dose-dependent accumulation of amiodarone in the head of the epididymis due to high serum concentrations of the drug.

2.32

A –β-thalassaemia trait

This patient has severe microcytosis that is out of proportion to the borderline anaemic haemoglobin concentration. Undiagnosed β-thalassaemia trait is the most likely explanation. In patients with β-thalassaemia trait there is approximately a 50% decrease in beta-globin protein synthesis, which accounts for the severe microcytosis. The obvious assumption is that the haemoglobin concentration should also be reduced; however, over time there is a gradual compensation due to increased production of erythropoietin. This normalises haemoglobin levels.

Iron deficiency anaemia, of which two common causes are gastrointestinal haemorrhage and menorrhagia, is the most common cause of microcytic anaemia. However, this is unlikely given the normal ferritin result. Chronic kidney disease in a young, previously well person is unlikely and, due to reduced erythropoietin, causes a normocytic normochromic anaemia.

2.33

D – Unfractionated heparin

Heparin-induced thrombocytopaenia is a well-known side effect of heparin, particularly unfractionated heparin. It is thought to occur as a result of antibody formation against the complex of heparin and platelet factor IV. The immune complex of antibody, heparin and platelet factor IV causes platelet activation, resulting in a prothrombotic state and consumption of platelets. Therefore the most common presenting symptom is thrombosis, rather than haemorrhage. Unlike most causes of thrombocytopaenia the physical number of platelets in heparin-induced thrombocytopaenia is not low. Instead, the platelets are active and clumped together, and are therefore not detected by laboratory tests. Heparin-induced thrombocytopaenia is much less common with low-molecular-weight heparin.

Fondaparinux is a synthetic factor Xa inhibitor that is chemically related to low-molecular-weight heparin but does not trigger autoimmune thrombocytopaenia. Warfarin is an inhibitor of vitamin K epoxide reductase. This enzyme recycles oxidised vitamin K to its reduced form after its participation in the carboxylation of the vitamin K-dependent clotting factors. It therefore inhibits the production of the clotting factors II, VII, IX and X. The major side effect is over-anticoagulation and haemorrhage, which can be precipitated by the administration of drugs that displace warfarin from serum albumin or decrease its metabolism by the hepatic CYP450 system. Warfarin is highly teratogenic and is contraindicated in pregnancy, and like heparin can also increase the risk of developing osteoporosis. However, unlike heparin, warfarin does not lead to autoimmune thrombocytopaenia.

Alteplase is a tissue plasminogen activator. Tissue plasminogen is a protein involved in the breakdown of blood clots. Alteplase is therefore used as a thrombolytic agent in cases of acute thrombotic ischaemia (e.g. acute cerebral infarction). The major risk of alteplase are the complications from secondary haemorrhage, and therefore bleeding must be excluded prior to its administration. Alteplase is not known to cause an immune-mediated thrombocytopaenia.

2.34

B – Amyloidosis

This female has developed a median nerve entrapment, also known as carpal tunnel syndrome. The most likely cause is amyloidosis. In the hand the median nerve has motor, sensory and autonomic functions.

Motor functions (these can be remembered by the mnemonic 'LOAF'):

- Lateral two lumbricals
- Opponens pollicis brevis
- Abductor pollicis brevis
- Flexor pollicis brevis.

The lumbricals flex the metacarpophalangeal joints but extend the fingers. The latter three muscles ('OAF') comprise the thenar eminence, which become wasted in patients with carpal tunnel syndrome.

The median nerve supplies sensation to the skin overlying the palmar aspect of the thumb, index finger, middle finger, half the ring finger and the nail bed of these fingers. Patients with carpal tunnel syndrome experience altered sensation in this distribution, with the exception of the lateral part of the palm. This area is spared because the palmar cutaneous branch of the median nerve, which arises proximal to the carpal tunnel, supplies it. Finally, disruption of the autonomic sympathetic fibres results in reduced sweating and dry skin.

Various tests for carpel tunnel syndrome exist. The most common are Phalen's test (both wrists and hands held in flexion for one minute) and Tinel's test (tapping over the median nerve at the wrist), both of which are positive if they temporarily exacerbate the sensory symptoms of carpal tunnel syndrome. However, Durkan's test, in which direct pressure is applied over the carpal tunnel for 30 seconds, has been shown to be more sensitive and specific than Phalen's and Tinel's test.

All of the answers in this question are recognised causes of carpal tunnel syndrome and should be excluded by appropriate investigation. However, the most likely cause here is amyloidosis because haemodialysis does not filter out β2-microglobulin from the bloodstream. This protein is amyloidogenic (aggregates in tissue) and is deposited in the peripheral nerves of patients with chronic kidney disease who are on long-term haemodialysis.

2.35

D –Spirometry

This patient's history is suggestive of Guillain–Barré syndrome secondary to EBV infection. Guillain–Barré syndrome is an acute polyneuropathy that causes a symmetrical ascending paralysis starting at the feet and moving upwards towards the arms and respiratory muscles. The most important initial investigation in a patient with Guillain–Barré syndrome is spirometry. A falling FVC indicates respiratory muscle involvement, which may prompt the need for intubation in the Intensive Care Unit.

The patient's previous history of fever, tonsillitis and cervical lymphadenopathy are classical features of EBV infection, which can be diagnosed using the Paul–Bunnell test.

Anti-streptolysin O titres are useful in streptococcal infections, which may present with severe exudative tonsillitis. However, streptococcal infections are not usually associated with the development of Guillain–Barré syndrome. EBV and *Campylobacter jejuni* are the most common pathogens associated with the development of Guillain–Barré syndrome. *Campylobacter jejuni* produces a lipolysaccharide that exhibits molecular similarity to gangliosides. These are molecules involved in cell signalling that are present in high concentrations in nervous tissue. This molecular mimicry is thought to be responsible for the production of pathogenic anti-ganglioside antibodies that mediate Guillain–Barré syndrome.

Urine dipstick would be useful if you suspected that this patient was suffering a post-streptococcal phenomenon, such as a post-streptococcal glomerulonephritis. However, there is no mention of any renal impairment in this patient's history.

Creatine kinase levels are a useful screening blood test for muscle damage (which is a cause of weakness in the legs). However, in this instance, the history is classical for Guillain–Barré syndrome, which involves the peripheral nerves and not the muscles, as would be the case for a myositic process.

2.36

E – Neurofibromatosis type II

It would be uncommon for a 20-year-old to develop noise-induced hearing loss and as a result, an alternative diagnosis should be considered. In this patient the most likely diagnosis is neurofibromatosis type II, which is caused by a defect in a gene on chromosome 22 that codes for the protein schwannomin. Such patients develop multiple schwannomas, benign tumours of the nerve sheath of Schwann cells (the myelinating cells that are normally responsible for insulating peripheral nerves). In neurofibromatosis type II they most commonly form on the vestibulocochlear nerve (cranial nerve VIII); however, any peripheral nerve can be affected (e.g. in this patient's popliteal fossa). On the vestibulocochlear nerve, tumours are frequently bilateral and form at the junction of the cerebello-pontine angle. These tumours are vestibular schwannomas; however, they are often called acoustic neuromas. This is a misnomer as they are neither acoustic (they rarely form on the cochlear portion of the nerve), nor are they neuromas (they are tumours of Schwann cells, not nerve tumours). Vestibular schwannomas can also develop in patients without neurofibromatosis type II; however, they are more commonly unilateral and affect older patients. They tend to present with hearing loss and tinnitus. In addition to cranial nerve VIII, cranial nerves V (trigeminal) and VII (facial) also arise in the region of the cerebellopontine angle (the anatomical space between the cerebellum and the pons) and can be compressed by vestibular schwannomas. Another common presentation in young patients with neurofibromatosis type II is cataracts.

Neurofibromatosis type I is caused by a mutation in the gene which encodes for the protein neurofibromin. These patients typically develop cutaneous signs, including café au lait spots (more than six), axillary/inguinal freckling and Lisch nodules in the iris (pigmented hamartomas of dendritic melanocytes). These patients are at increased risk of developing neurofibromas (benign tumours of non-myelinating Schwann cells) but only very rarely develop bilateral vestibular schwannomas (these are instead the hallmark of neurofibromatosis type II).

Meningiomas are benign tumours of the meninges. They occur near venous sinuses, most commonly over the superior sagittal sinus in the region of the frontal and parietal lobes ('parasagittal meningiomas'). They present with either a focal neurological deficit (e.g. bilateral lower limb hemiparesis if both frontal lobe primary motor cortices are affected) or signs of raised intracranial pressure (if large enough to cause mass effect).

Astrocytomas are brain tumours arising from astrocytes (a form of glial cell) and are therefore a type of glioma. Glial cells are found within the white and grey matter of the central nervous system and occur within the brain and the spinal cord. Originating in one region, astrocytomas present with either a focal neurological deficit, seizure activity associated with that region or signs of raised intracranial pressure (due to mass effect of a non-communicating hydrocephalus). Astrocytomas may occur at the cerebellopontine angle causing deafness and tinnitus due to compression of the vestibulocochlear nerve. However, it would be incredibly rare for astrocytomas to occur within the cerebellopontine angle bilaterally.

2.37

A – Contrast CT head

This patient has upper motor neuron signs in his legs and a high pressure headache. This is highly suggestive of a parasagittal meningioma and therefore this patient requires a contrast CT head scan. A parasagittal meningioma is in the midline superiorly between the two hemispheres. If it compresses the primary motor cortex, the legs will be affected first as the lower body is represented superio-medially. The upper body is represented inferio-laterally.

A lesion in the spinal cord would not produce a high pressure headache. Whole spine MRI would be required if spinal cord injury or compression was suspected, and spinal angiography would be required if spinal cord infarction was suspected. Cord damage/ compression below the level of upper limb innervation would produce a bilateral lower limb upper motor neuron pattern as seen here. However, involvement of the major long sensory tracts (dorsal columns and spinothalamic tracts) and a 'sensory level' would be expected. This patient has a normal sensory examination. Spinal cord infarction can cause upper motor neuron signs. The artery of Adamkiewicz arises from a left posterior intercostal artery (a branch from the aorta) and supplies the lower two thirds of the ventral spinal cord via the anterior spinal artery. It therefore supplies the corticospinal and spinothalamic tracts (not the dorsal columns). Infarction of this artery will cause a bilateral lower limb upper motor neuron lesion as well as loss of pain and temperature sensation. Again, this is excluded by this patient's normal sensory examination. Nerve conduction studies are useful in the investigation of patients with lower motor neuron signs, and are therefore not appropriate in this instance. Finally, in the absence of meningitic signs a lumbar puncture is unlikely to aid diagnosis. This procedure may in fact be harmful in a patient with raised intracranial pressure, due to the risk of herniation of the brainstem through the foramen magnum ('coning').

2.38

C – Lyme disease

This patient's history of bilateral facial droop, hyperacusis, difficulty speaking and altered taste sensation is highly suggestive of bilateral facial nerve palsy. The facial nerve contains the motor supply to the muscles of facial expression and the middle ear stapedius muscle (which is important in minimising the effect of loud sounds), as well as afferent sensory fibres from the anterior twothirds of the tongue (via the chorda tympani branch). Loss of these functions account for this patient's symptoms.

Bilateral facial nerve palsy is unusual and represents less than 2% of all cases of facial nerve palsy. However, because almost all cases are associated with serious underlying medical conditions, it is an important diagnosis to consider. Given her occupation, the most likely cause in this patient is Lyme disease, the most common infectious cause of bilateral facial nerve palsy. Lyme disease is a tick-borne infection caused by the spirochaete *Borrelia burgdorferi*. The classic early sign is an outwardly expanding circular rash with a central clearing (erythema chronicum migrans) which occurs 3 to 30 days after at the site of a tick bite. However, the rash can go unnoticed (it is classically painless and doesn't occur in all patients) so many patients may first present weeks to months after initial infection with disseminated disease (via haematogenous spread). The most common systems to be affected are neurological (facial nerve palsies, meningitis and radiculoneuritis) and musculoskeletal (intermittent migratory polyarthritis followed by a large joint monoarthritis). Without treatment patients develop severe, chronic symptoms in many parts of the body (e.g. brain, nerves, eyes, joints and heart). A course of doxycycline cures Lyme disease if given at an early stage. However, treatment during the latent phase has variable outcomes.

EBV is a known cause of facial nerve palsy, and 10% of cases are bilateral. However, this patient demonstrates none of the typical features (e.g. exudative tonsillitis, lymphadenopathy, hepatitis, splenomegaly). One of the neurological effects of sarcoidosis is bilateral facial nerve palsy; however, this patient's normal chest X-ray makes this diagnosis less likely. Guillain–Barré syndrome is a post-infectious acute inflammatory demyelinating polyneuropathy that usually presents with ascending weakness and lower motor neuron signs. This patient's normal upper and lower limb neurology makes this diagnosis unlikely. Finally, Moebius syndrome is a rare congenital syndrome characterised by underdevelopment of the facial and abducens nerves bilaterally. The cause is unknown.

2.39

A – Amitriptyline

This patient's history is highly suggestive of migraine. Management is divided into acute management and prophylaxis. Prophylaxis is indicated if patients have frequent (more than two per month) disabling attacks lasting for three days or more. Amitriptyline (a tricyclic antidepressant) and propranolol (a beta-adrenoreceptor antagonist) are both first-line medications for migraine prophylaxis; however, propranolol (through inhibition of vasodilatory beta-2-adrenoreceptors) worsens Raynaud's syndrome and is therefore contraindicated in this scenario. Amitriptyline is therefore the correct answer. Topiramate and sodium valproate are anti-epileptics that are considered second-line treatments for migraine prophylaxis. Pizotifen, a 5HT-receptor antagonist, is a third-line medication.

2.40

E – Anti-Sm antibody

The anti-Sm (anti-Smith) antibody is the most specific antibody for non-drug-induced systemic lupus erythematosus. It must not be confused with the anti-SM (anti-smooth muscle) antibody, which is characteristic of type I autoimmune hepatitis. Anti-nuclear anti-bodies are a group of antibodies that target various autoantigens within the cell nucleus. As a whole they are positive in over 98% of patients with systemic lupus erythematosus (highly sensitive); however, they are also positive in many other connective tissue diseases (e.g. Sjögren's syndrome, systemic sclerosis, polymyositis), as well as 5% of the normal population. Anti-nuclear antibody is therefore not a very specific test for systemic lupus erythematosus. However, analysis of the various subtypes of anti-nuclear antibod-ies is more useful. One subgroup of anti-nuclear antibodies is the extractable nuclear antigens, so named because they can all be extracted from the nucleus with saline. The anti-Smith antibody has a specificity of around 99% for systemic lupus erythematosus (i.e. it is virtually diagnostic). However, it is only positive in 30% of patients and therefore has a low sensitivity. Anti-Ro antibodies can be positive in systemic lupus erythematosus but they are not sensi-tive or specific as they are often positive in Sjögren's syndrome and primary biliary cirrhosis. In pregnancy, anti-Ro antibodies can cross the placenta and bind to proteins required in the development of the cardiac conduction system. Offspring of anti-Ro-positive moth-ers have a 1 in 20 chance of developing heart block. Another sub-type of anti-nuclear antibodies is anti-dsDNA. Anti-dsDNA is also highly specific (95%) for systemic lupus erythematosus but is not as specific as anti-Smith antibody. However, testing for anti-dsDNA is performed more frequently than anti-Smith because it is positive in 70% of patients (it is more sensitive than anti-Smith antibody). Titres of anti-dsDNA are also useful as they correlate well with disease flare-ups. Anti-histone antibody is another autoantigen tar-get within the cell nucleus. It is highly sensitive and specific for drug-induced systemic lupus erythematosus.

2.41

B – Malignant carcinoid

This patient's symptoms and signs are highly suggestive of malig-nant carcinoid. Carcinoid tumours are neuroendocrine tumours, of which twothirds occur in the gastrointestinal tract (mainly the small intestine). They secrete various compounds, including bradykinin and 5HT, which will only cause carcinoid syndrome if they reach the systemic circulation. In order for this to occur gastrointestinal tract carcinoid tumours have to metastasise so that they can bypass hepatic first-pass metabolism.

The classic features of carcinoid syndrome therefore tend to involve the right side of the heart and the pulmonary circulation, as the compounds released act locally. Bronchospasm, diarrhoea, skin flushing and right-sided valvular heart defects (due to endocardial fibrosis) are most common. If the tumour originates in the lungs, or there are lung metastases present, then left-sided valvular lesions may occur.

Tryptophan is an essential amino acid and a precursor to both 5HT and niacin. Normally only 1% of dietary tryptophan is converted to 5HT; however, this increases dramatically in carcinoid syndrome such that patients may develop niacin deficiency ('pellagra'). The clinical manifestation of pellagra is classically described as the 'four Ds': dementia, dermatitis, diarrhoea and death. The rash is photosensitive.

Porphyria cutanea tarda is the most common form of porphyria and unlike other forms it is nearly always acquired, rather than inherited. Causes include alcohol abuse, oestrogens, iron overload and hepatitis C infection. It results from low levels of the enzyme uroporphyrinogen III decarboxylase, which is responsible for the fifth step in haem production. Uroporphyrinogen accumulates and is toxic to the skin. Patients present with a photosensitive rash and bullae.

Dermatomyositis is a connective-tissue disorder characterised by inflammation of the muscles and skin. Patients classically have symmetrical proximal muscle weakness, Gottron's papules (scaly eruptions over the metacarpophalangeal and interphalangeal joints), a heliotrope rash (a pruritic violet rash on the upper eyelids) and a photosensitive shawl-like rash over the back and shoulders.

Urticaria pigmentosa is a rare condition. It is a form of cutaneous mastocytosis (an accumulation of mast cells in the skin and histamine release). The symptoms can be mild (flushing and urticaria requiring no treatment), moderate (diarrhoea, tachycardia, nausea, vomiting, headache and fainting), or life threatening (vascular collapse).

2.42

E – Respiratory alkalosis

Aspirin overdose is not uncommon. The combination of a respiratory alkalosis and high anion gap metabolic acidosis (due to the addition of organic anions) is the hallmark of salicylate toxicity. However, the initial metabolic disturbance is respiratory alkalosis. This occurs because of uncoupling of mitochondrial oxidative phosphorylation in the central and peripheral nervous system, which results in reduced cellular respiration. In the medullary respiratory centres this is interpreted as hypoxaemia, which triggers an increase in respiratory rate, carbon dioxide exhalation and a respiratory alkalosis.

With time, a high anion gap metabolic acidosis develops. This occurs because ketone bodies are produced (due to salicylic inhibition of fatty acid metabolism) and also due to uncoupling of oxidative phosphorylation and inhibition of the Krebs cycle in the kidneys, which impairs renal function and results in the accumulation of more organic acids (phosphate and sulphate).

Hyperthermia also occurs because without effective aerobic respiration, less efficient anaerobic pathways are utilised, resulting in the loss of energy as heat. Hyperthermia increases insensible fluid losses, which, as well as the direct tachypnoeic and emetogenic effects of salicylic acid, worsens the state of dehydration and further impairs renal function. Hypoglycaemia occurs because more glucose is utilised in the less efficient anaerobic pathways. The glucose is replaced through lipolysis, which generates more ketones and worsens the state of metabolic acidosis.

2.43

A – Improve glycaemic control

'Dots' are retinal venous microaneurysms. If these microaneurysms rupture in the deeper layers of the retina then 'blots' of haemorrhage form. 'Dots' and 'blots' are therefore signs of background diabetic retinopathy. They occur due to a weakening of the retinal vessel walls caused by hyperglycaemia-induced high retinal perfusion. As long as the macula is not involved, management involves strict glycaemic and blood pressure control with regular surveillance fundoscopy. If any signs of retinal ischaemia develop, or the macula is involved, the ophthalmologist may decide to use LASER photocoagulation to reduce the risk of visual loss.

2.44

D – Polyethylene glycol

This patient is suffering from faecal impaction with overflow incontinence. Faecal impaction is where there is a solid, immobile mass of hard, dry faeces in the rectum due to constipation. The rectum should normally be almost empty. The most appropriate initial management of faecal impaction is to administer a regular oral osmotic laxative (e.g. lactulose, polyethylene glycol) with or without a per rectum counterpart (e.g. sodium phosphate enema, glycerine suppository). These act to increase water content in the large bowel, softening the stool and encouraging its natural expulsion. Polyethylene glycol is an inert polymer of ethylene glycol that retains fluid in the bowel through osmotic pressure. Branded preparations include Movicol® and Laxido®. Lactulose is another osmotic laxative. It is a non-absorbable disaccharide of fructose and galactose that works through its fermentation to lactic acid by colonic bacterial beta-galactosidase. This acidifies stool to increase its water content through osmotic pressure. However, lactulose also produces large quantities of gas. Although this can improve peristalsis and increase the need to defecate, it commonly causes uncomfortable bloating and flatulence for patients. This is the same effect as that of sorbitol due to excessive consumption of chewing gum. Lactulose should only be administered regularly as it is far less effective when given 'as required'. Magnesium sulphate is another osmotic laxative that can be used orally for rapid bowel evacuation; however, it is more widely used either topically ('Epsom salts') or intravenously for the treatment of hypomagnesaemia, pre-eclampsia, torsades de pointes and severe asthma.

Ispaghula husk, the active ingredient in Fybogel®, is, alongside methylcellulose and sterculia, a bulk-forming laxative. These should only be used in patients who cannot tolerate oral forms of bran, which is the preferred alternative. Indeed, a balanced diet, adequate mobilisation and adequate fluid intake are the mainstay of constipation prevention. Bulk-forming laxatives should be taken with meals and relieve constipation over a number of days by increasing faecal mass, thereby stimulating peristalsis. They are therefore most useful for managing small, hard stools and not fae-cal impaction. Senna, as well as dantron and aloe vera, is a member of the anthraquinone group of stimulant laxatives. Other stimulant laxatives include bisacodyl (Dulcolax®), sodium docusate, sodium picosulphate (Dulcolax® Pico) and glycerine suppositories (which are both osmotic and mildly irritant). When used for constipation stimulant laxatives are preferably administered at night because they can take over 12 hours to induce a bowel motion. Stimulant laxatives work by irritating the intestinal mucosa to stimulate motility. They can therefore cause abdominal cramps and should be avoided in intestinal obstruction. Excessive use can cause diarrhoea and hypokalaemia. Prolonged use can cause dependence, whereby patients lose the ability to pass stool without the laxative.

If faecal impaction fails to respond to oral or rectal laxatives, man-ual disimpaction may be required with or without sedation or general anaesthesia.

2.45

E – Shortened QT interval

Eighty percent of cases of primary hyperparathyroidism are due to a single parathyroid adenoma. Parathyroid hormone acts to increase plasma calcium and decrease plasma phosphate by stimulating osteoclastic bone resorption, decreasing renal calcium excretion and increasing renal phosphate excretion. Therefore, raised parathyroid hormone levels result in hypercalcaemia and hypophosphataemia. Although hypophosphataemia can contribute to a patient's lethargy and general malaise, the symptoms of hyperparathyroidism are mainly due to hypercalcaemia. Raised extracellular calcium concentrations hyperpolarise cell membranes, resulting in slower depolarisation of the neuromuscular membranes (muscle weakness, constipation and hypotonia) as well as faster repolarisation of neuromuscular membranes (shortened QT interval). Classically, the symptoms of hypercalcaemia are remembered as 'bones (bone pain and increased fracture risk due to resorption), stones (formation of kidney stones), abdominal groans (abdominal pains associated with constipation, pancreatitis, nausea and vomiting) and psychiatric moans (central nervous system effects; depression, delirium and coma)'.

Hypopolarisation (partial depolarisation) of cell membranes is caused by low extracellular calcium levels, and results in membrane hyperexciteability. This results in tetany, paraesthesiae (classically around the mouth), a positive Chvostek's sign and a positive Trousseau's sign. Other causes of membrane hyperexciteability include hyperkalaemia, hypoxia, respiratory alkalosis and hypomagnesaemia.

2.46

B – Hereditary haemochromatosis

This patient has hereditary haemochromatosis, an autosomal recessive condition associated with mutations in the *HFE* gene on chromosome 6. This gene encodes for the HFE protein, which contributes to regulation of intestinal iron absorption. Homozygous individuals absorb increased quantities of iron. Although small amounts of iron are excreted each day through physiological sloughing of both keratinised (skin) and non-keratinised (gastrointestinal tract, genital tract, cornea) stratified squamous epithelial surfaces, the only significant physiological route for iron excretion is menstruation. Ergo males present much earlier in life than females and venesection is the mainstay of treatment. Patients with hereditary haemochromatosis deposit excessive amounts of iron in various tissues in the form of haemosiderin. Such tissues include the skin (where it stimulates melanin production and leads to 'tanning'), the liver (signs of chronic liver disease and cirrhosis develop; there is also a 200 times increased risk of hepatocellular carcinoma), the pancreas (islet cell failure leads to 'bronze diabetes', referring to diabetes mellitus with skin hyperpigmentation), heart (restrictive or dilated cardiomyopathy), pituitary (hypopituitarism), joints (arthralgia, arthritis) and the gonads (testicular/ovarian failure).

2.47

E – Start *N*-acetylcysteine infusion

This patient has taken a paracetamol overdose. Although the time of paracetamol ingestion is unknown, any value greater than 100 mg/L is over the treatment line. *N*-acetylcysteine should be started immediately. Normally, 90% of ingested paracetamol is conjugated by sulphation or glucuronidation and then excreted in bile; this is a harmless process. However, metabolism of the remaining 10% is dependent on the CYP450 system, which produces the toxic metabolite NAPQI. Inactivation of NAPQI is glutathione-dependent. During paracetamol overdose, the conjugation pathway of paracetamol metabolism becomes saturated, and shunting of paracetamol through the CYP450 system occurs, depleting the glutathione stores and causing NAPQI to accumulate. In order to replenish glutathione stores, *N*-acetylcysteine, a polar molecule that is de-acetylated to cysteine once inside the hepatocytes, is given. Cysteine is then utilised to increase glutathione levels and therefore increase the rate of NAPQI inactivation.

In certain patients, NAPQI concentrations increase more readily. They include patients with chronic alcoholism, or those taking CYP450-inducing medications. In such patients, higher percentages of their serum paracetamol is metabolised by the CYP450 system and they therefore produce more toxic NAPQI. In addition, if glutathione stores are depleted then a patient is less able to break down NAPQI. This is the case in patients with HIV, cystic fibrosis and malnourishment. All these patients were previously classified as high risk and, in comparison to low-risk individuals, were given N-acetylcysteine at half the serum paracetamol levels of low-risk individuals. However, all patients are now classified high risk.

Referral to psychiatry is indicated once the patient has been stabilised. Vitamin K is only given if there is evidence of active bleeding. Gastric lavage and oral-activated charcoal are both forms of gastric decontamination, and are only useful if initiated within an hour of the overdose.

2.48

A – Bence Jones protein

Multiple myeloma is characterised by an uncontrolled proliferation of a single clone of B-cells in the bone marrow, which impairs bone marrow function and can cause bone pain and fractures. The monoclonal B-cells produce a monoclonal protein (IgG is commonest followed by IgA and then IgM), with or without suppression of the other immunoglobulins. Renal impairment in multiple myeloma is common and multifactorial in origin.

A Bence Jones protein is a free immunoglobulin light chain, which is found in the urine and can deposit in the renal tubules. This impairs kidney function. Immunoparesis increases the susceptibility to infections (pyelonephritis and chronic kidney infections contribute to impaired renal function). Hypercalcaemia is often encountered in patients with multiple myeloma, which leads to dehydration and contributes to renal impairment. Calcium levels are increased due to hyperstimulation of osteoclasts, which break down bone and predispose patients to pathological fractures. Hypercalcaemia also puts patients at increased risk of developing calcium oxalate renal stones (nephrolithiasis). Hyperuricaemia is commonly encountered in patients with multiple myeloma. Uric acid levels are raised due to increased purine and pyrimidine metabolism, as a result of rapid monoclonal B-cell proliferation. Uricosuria is highly nephrotoxic, and therefore may also contribute to renal impairment. In addition, multiple myeloma is a recognised cause of a proximal (type II) renal tubular acidosis, which impairs absorption of potassium, glucose, amino acids, phosphate and bicarbonate resulting in dehydration, hyperphosphataemic osteo-malacia, and a normal anion gap hyperchloraemic hypokalaemic metabolic acidosis. In rhabdomyolysis, rapid and massive release of intracellular myoglobin from muscle cells quickly saturates its serum binding protein, haptoglobin. Unbounded myoglobin sub-sequently results in renal damage through its deposition in the renal tubules. However, this is not a feature of multiple myeloma.

2.49

C – Lumbar canal stenosis

This patient is suffering from neurogenic claudication, which occurs when there is compression of the lumbar spinal cord and/or lum-bosacral nerve roots. Compression typically occurs with ageing; however, specific causes include osteoarthritis, rheumatoid arthri-tis, hypertrophy of the surrounding ligaments (e.g. ligamentum flavum), spondylolisthesis (where one vertebrae slips over another), tumours, trauma and other hereditary structural deformities. Compression causes lower back pain that progresses to leg pain and weakness, which is typically relieved when the spinal canal is opened up as a result of bending forward, walking up a hill/stairs, pushing and cycling. Although vascular claudication (which occurs secondary to atheromatous peripheral vascular disease) can mimic spinal stenosis (as it also causes pain on exercise), vascular claudica-tion is due to muscle ischaemia and is therefore relieved by rest, regardless of whether the spinal canal is open or not.

2.50

A – Ascending cholangitis

Ascending cholangitis is an infection in an obstructed biliary system. The most common cause is gallstones in the biliary tree (choledocolithiasis). Other causes include tumours, sclerosing cholangitis and indwelling biliary stents. This lady, who is awaiting cholecystectomy, has an obstructed biliary system due to a gallstone with a secondary Gram-negative infection of the bile (e.g. *Escherichia coli*, *Klebsiella* species). Classical symptoms are fever, right upper quadrant pain and jaundice ('Charcot's triad') and in more severe cases, shock and deranged mentation (known collectively as 'Reynolds' pentad'), which can lead to death. Ascending cholangitis is a medical emergency and must be treated rapidly with intravenous broad-spectrum antibiotics (e.g. ciprofloxacin, or cefuroxine and metronidazole) followed by a procedure to drain the infected bile (often with endoscopic retrograde cholangiopancreatography).

2.51

C – Fludrocortisone

This patient is experiencing episodes of orthostatic hypotension and conservative measures have failed. The most appropriate initial medication is fludrocortisone. Postural hypotension is defined as a drop of 20 mmHg (systolic) or 10 mmHg (diastolic) when rising from the lying (supine) to the standing (orthostatic) position (or sitting if standing is intolerable). However, it is important to exclude other causes of dizziness and perform a falls assessment. Dizziness can mean ataxia (sensory or cerebellar), vertigo or presyncope (e.g. postural hypotension).

Falls in the elderly are usually either mechanical (non-medical; due to the environment) or multifactorial. Factors contributing to falls are:

- Cardiovascular: postural hypotension, arrhythmias, structural heart disease

- Neurological: stroke, delirium, dementia, Parkinsonism, neuropathy
- Visual: retinopathy, glaucoma, cataracts
- Musculoskeletal: osteoporosis, osteoarthritis, joint replacements
- Iatrogenic: polypharmacy, sedatives, anti-hypertensives.

Initial conservative management of postural hypotension involves excluding/treating reversible causes, increasing salt and fluid intake, reducing alcohol intake and taking contributory medications at night (e.g. anti-hypertensives). Common reversible causes of orthostatic hypotension include anaemia (ferrous sulphate if iron deficient), hypovolaemia (e.g. dehydration, bleeding), alcoholism, prolonged bed rest (due to reduced muscle tone), drugs (e.g. anti-hypertensives, antidepressants, levo-dopa) and Addisonian disease.

In this scenario, conservative measures have failed and all reversible causes have been excluded, therefore the most likely cause is diabetic neuropathy of the autonomic nervous system, which can affect the genitourinary (bladder incontinence, urinary retention, impotence), gastrointestinal tract (gastroparesis, dysphagia, nausea, vomiting, altered bowel habit) and/or cardiovascular (tachy/ bradycardia, orthostatic hypotension, masking of hypoglycaemic symptoms, sweating) systems.

First-line management is to increase sodium and water retention with fludrocortisone (a mineralocorticoid receptor agonist), for which the main side effect is peripheral oedema and hypokalaemia. Midodrine is an alpha-adrenoreceptor agonist, which can be used where fludrocortisone is inappropriate (e.g. hypokalaemia). It is also used in intensive care to wean patients off intravenous vasopressors. Propranolol (a beta-adrenoreceptor antagonist) and bumetanide (a loop diuretic) are both hypotensive medications that should be avoided in cases of orthostatic hypotension.

2.52

E – Wenckebach's phenomenon

A regular P wave with progressive prolonging of the PR interval resulting in dropped beats is Mobitz type I second-degree atrioventricular block, otherwise known as the Wenckebach phenomenon. It is important to be aware that myocardial infarction can cause arrhythmias due to damage to the conduction system (e.g. atrioventricular node, bundle of His, Purkinje fibres). In first-degree heart block atrioventricular conduction is delayed (>0.2s); however, the PR interval is constant and each P wave is associated with a QRS complex. Second-degree heart block occurs when some atrial depolarisations fail to conduct to the ventricles. There are two types. Type I (described above) and type II. Type I is a primarily a disease of the atrioventricular node whereas type II is a disease of the His-Purkinje system. In type II some P waves are not associated with QRS complexes, but the PR interval is constant. Mobitz type I is usually a benign condition only requiring treatment if symptomatic. Mobitz type II can rapidly progress to complete heart block and risk of asystole. It therefore requires pacemaker insertion.

2.53

B – Erythematous, friable, inflamed mucosa with mucosal crypt inflammation and crypt distortion

Definitive distinction of ulcerative colitis and Crohn's disease ultimately requires colonoscopy and biopsy, and all options except the correct answer represent changes seen in Crohn's disease. Crohn's disease causes inflammation of all layers of the intestinal wall, including the mucosa (neutrophils enter the crypts of Lieberkuhn to cause inflammation), the muscular mucosa (causing hyperplasia and stricturing/obstruction) and the serosa (causing adhesions, fat-wrapping and fistula formation to other organs), with deep, snake-like (serpiginous) fissuring ulcers and non-caseating granuloma formation (specific to Crohn's). In Crohn's disease this inflammation occurs mainly in the small intestine and colon (though technically it can occur anywhere from mouth to anus) and there are characteristic islands of normal mucosa ('skip lesions') that are surrounded by ulcers (giving a cobblestone appearance). In contrast, ulcerative colitis is a non-granulomatous condition that extends continuously and proximally from the rectum with no skip lesions (although extensive ulceration can lead to islands of normal mucosa called pseudopolyps). The inflammation in ulcerative colitis is limited to the mucosa and therefore there is no fat-wrapping, fistula formation, fissuring and bowel wall hyperplasia as seen in Crohn's disease. The cryptitis in ulcerative colitis is superficial.

2.54

A – Autosomal dominant polycystic kidney disease

Anaemia of chronic kidney disease predominantly occurs as a result of insufficient production of erythropoietin in the kidneys (although other factors include reduced red blood cell survival, folate and iron deficiencies and uraemic accumulation of toxic inhibitors of erythropoiesis). However, if the cause of severe chronic kidney disease is autosomal dominant polycystic kidney disease then, unlike other causes (above), the degree of anaemia is moderated, such that the haemoglobin concentration can be maintained at normal levels. This is thought to be due to the production of erythropoietin in the cells lining the renal cysts. Anaemia in chronic kidney disease (of which the highest prevalence is found in patients with diabetic nephropathy) can be corrected with administration of recombinant human erythropoietin.

2.55

B – Essential hypertension

This patient has presented with a classic history of aortic dissection, which is a tear in the innermost of the three layers of the arterial wall (the tunica intima). This tear allows blood into the middle layer (tunica media), which forces the layers apart, allowing the tear to expand. Rupture of the outermost layers (tunica adventitia) can sometimes occur, resulting in massive and rapid exsanguination. Therefore aortic dissection is a medical emergency (the mortality rate is 80%). Patients typically present with severe, sharp, sudden-onset tearing/stabbing pain that is maximal at onset and moves as the tear expands. The site of pain radiation can depend on the area affected by the tear; anterior chest pain occurs in ascending aortic dissection, interscapular back pain in descending aortic dissection and pleuritic chest pain with retrograde invasion of the pericardial sac. This can progress to cardiac tamponade. Chest pain is an important presentation. Consideration of the diagnosis of aortic dissection is the reason a chest X-ray should be performed in patients presenting with chest pain. Thrombolysis in such patients in contraindicated. Other presentations of aortic dissection include those of aortic insufficiency, including shock, hypotension, neurological symptoms (syncope, stroke, ischaemic peripheral neuropathy, paraplegia), cardiological symptoms (myocardial infarction, heart failure) and abdominal symptoms (renal artery hypoperfusion, mesenteric ischaemia).

Other examination findings of aortic dissection may include asymmetrical pulses (radio-radial or radio-femoral delay), heart murmurs and arterial bruits. The most important predisposing factor in aortic dissection is hypertension, which is present in 70–80% of patients with aortic dissection. Other predisposing factors include connective tissue disorders (Marfan's syndrome, Ehlos–Danlos syndrome), vasculitides (tertiary syphilitic aortitis and large-vessel vasculitides such as Takayasu's arteritis), cardiovascular abnormalities (bicuspid aortic valve, aortic coarctation, aortic root dilatation in Turner's syndrome), cocaine use, pregnancy and chest trauma (iatrogenic or deceleration injury). Granulomatosis with polyangiitis is a small- to medium-vessel ANCA-positive vasculitis, which used to be called Wegener's granulomatosis.

2.56

D – Radioactive iodine

Radioactive iodine (^{131}I) is a radioactive isotope which, in comparison to the stable form of iodine (^{127}I), has four extra nuclear neutrons (78 instead of 74). Like other forms of iodine, ^{131}I is actively taken up into the thyroid gland (particularly in overactive thyroid glands) where it undergoes beta-radiation (release of an electron), which disrupts the function of surrounding cells. ^{131}I is therefore used, over months/years, to ablate the thyroid in hyperthyroidism (e.g. Graves' disease, toxic multinodular goitre, solitary toxic adenoma).

However, because ^{131}I aims to induce total hypothyroidism (and therefore requires lifelong thyroxine therapy), it is reserved for refractory disease (after a period of failed medical therapy with carbimazole/propyluracil) or when these therapies are contraindicated. ^{131}I also has relative and absolute complications. Due to the theoretical risk to the unborn foetus (beta-radiation is carcinogenic), an absolute contraindication is pregnancy. A relative contraindication is the presence of Graves' ophthalmopathy because, through unknown mechanisms, Graves' eye disease has been found to worsen in some patients treated with radioactive iodine. This is the most likely scenario in this patient, and therefore total thyroidectomy should have been the next management option instead.

Propranolol is a beta-adrenoreceptor antagonist which is used for symptomatic relief in hyperthyroidism to counter the thyroid hormone-induced increase in the sensitivity of the adrenoreceptors to circulating catecholamines, which causes some of the symptoms of hyperthyroidism (sweating, tremor, tachycardia, anxiety, etc.). Once a euthyroid state is achieved they can be stopped. Interestingly, at the initiation of ^{131}I therapy, the symptoms of hyperthyroidism can become acutely worse due to release of thyroid hormone from the damaged tissue. In this scenario propranolol should also be given. The first-line medical therapy of hyperthyroidism is propylthiouracil and/or carbimazole, which both inhibit thyroid peroxidase, the enzyme which iodinates tyrosine residues on thyroglobulin. These drugs therefore decrease the production of thyroxine (T_4) and triiodothyronine (T_3). An important side effect of these two medications is neutropaenia. Therefore patients are asked to return for a full blood count if they develop symptoms of infections.

2.57

B – Eisenmenger's syndrome

This patient has developed Eisenmenger's syndrome, which is the combination of cyanosis and pulmonary hypertension as the end result of a shunt between the left (systemic) and right (pulmonary) sides of the circulation. *In utero*, normal breathing is not feasible and therefore oxygen is sourced from the mother's circulation via the placenta. This is achieved by a right-to-left shunt, in which venous return from the foetal systemic circulation is shunted away from the foetal lungs by three mechanisms:

- Some venous return is redirected from the right atrium into the left atrium through the foramen ovale
- Most of the remaining right ventricular output is redirected from the pulmonary artery into the descending aorta via the ductus arteriosus
- Hypoxia-induced pulmonary vasoconstriction further reduces pulmonary blood flow to an absolute minimum.

Right-to-left shunting is only sustainable when blood can be reoxygenated elsewhere. *In utero*, this is achieved in the placenta, into which a fraction of cardiac output is redirected (via the umbilical arteries) for oxygenation in the placenta and removal of waste products. On return from the placenta, the umbilical vein supplies the ductus venosus, which connects to the proximal inferior vena cava to mix oxygenated blood with the deoxygenated venous blood, before it returns to the heart.

During childbirth, the three mechanisms above should reverse in order to enable oxygenation via the lungs and to allow for removal of the placenta from the umbilical cord. The first breath expands the lungs, reducing pulmonary vascular resistance, increasing pulmonary venous return and increasing the pressures in the right atrium, which initiates closure of the foramen ovale (a flap valve between the left and right atrium). The improved oxygenation inhibits prostaglandin production in the ductus arteriosus, resulting in closure of the ductus (normally by 48 hours) and initiation of the normal adult circulation; the pulmonary and the systemic circulations working in series with identical cardiac outputs but different blood pressures.

However, as a result of various congenital cardiac defects (e.g. patent ductus arteriosus, atrial septal defect, ventricular septal defect), shunts between the left and right circulations can persist. The pulmonary pressures are normally around one-fifth that of systolic, and therefore a shunt is initially a left-to-right shunt. Over time this results in compensatory remodelling and fibrosis of the fragile pulmonary vasculature, which begins to even out the pressures between the left and right side. During this time, the shunting of blood (and the murmurs associated with them) reduce; however, continued pulmonary vascular remodelling increasingly impairs gas exchange and pulmonary vascular resistance, which results in right ventricular hypertrophy and worsening pulmonary hypertension.

At around 10–15 years of age, Eisenmenger's syndrome results, whereby pulmonary hypertension is so severe that blood is shunted from right to left (as *in utero*, but without the placenta) such that the patient becomes increasingly cyanotic, short of breath, fatigued and syncopal, and develops a compensatory secondary polycythaemia (to improve the oxygen-carrying capacity of the blood) which can progress to hyperviscosity syndrome (thrombophilia, spontaneous bleeding from mucous membranes, retinopathy, blurred vision, gout, chest pain from pulmonary infarction, haemoptysis and/or neurological symptoms).

Another feature of cyanotic heart disease is clubbing, of which the other cardiovascular causes are subacute bacterial endocarditis and atrial myxoma. However, these two conditions present differently. Tetralogy of Fallot does not result in Eisenmenger's syndrome because the right-to-left shunt (and therefore cyanosis) is present from birth (unless the ductus arteriosus remains patent) due to pulmonary artery stenosis and a ventricular septal defect (i.e. not due to pulmonary vascular remodelling and pulmonary hypertension). By definition, uncomplicated patent ductus arteriosus also does not result in Eisenmenger's syndrome. Finally, once pulmonary hypertension has developed, the only definitive management option for patients with Eisenmenger's syndrome is either heart-lung transplant, or lung transplant and heart surgery.

2.58

D – Plaque psoriasis

Plaque psoriasis is a skin condition in which there is an increased turnover of keratinocytes, the celltype that forms the very outer layer of the skin (the epidermis). This hyperproliferation results in a thickening of the epidermis and the build up of keratin, which forms the classical silvery-white scaly plaques. Beneath these plaques inflammatory cell infiltrate results in an erythematous, painful, salmon-pink base that can become haemorrhagic if the plaques come loose and break off. The skin lesions classically involve the extensor surfaces, including the elbows, knees, scalp, hair margin, umbilicus, sacrum or behind the ears. This differs from inverse or flexural psoriasis, in which smoother, glazed-looking lesions affect the folds, recesses and flexor surfaces of the skin such as the axillae, submammary areas, groin, the overweight abdomen and between the buttocks. Precipitating factors in plaque psoriasis include Koebnerisation (where lesions occur at sites of trauma), infection, drugs and psychological stress. Typically patients experience significant improvement in the sunlight. Psoriasis treatments are directed towards avoiding precipitating factors (e.g. drugs and psychological stress), applying moisturisers (e.g. emollients, bath oils), topical inhibition of keratinocyte hyperproliferation (e.g. coal tar, vitamin D analogues, dithranol), ultraviolet therapy (e.g. sunlight, ultraviolet-B, or psoralen and ultraviolet-A) and finally immunosuppression (e.g. retinoids, steroid-sparing agents and anti-tissue necrosis factor biological agents). Twenty-five percent of patients with psoriasis experience nail changes, including thimble pitting, onycholysis (a raised distal nail bed), transverse nail ridges and subungual keratosis. Upwards of 50% of patients with psoriasis have an associated inflammatory arthritis. Nail pitting is more than twice as common in patients with psoriatic arthritis (90%) than in those with psoriasis alone (40%). Psoriatic arthritis can take one of five forms (below) and can predate the skin lesions.

- I: Oligoarthritis
- II: Symmetrical polyarthritis resembling rheumatoid arthritis
- III: A pattern resembling osteoarthritis with Heberden's and Bouchard's nodes
- IV: Sacroiliitis (usually unilateral) resembling ankylosing spondylitis
- V: A destructive pattern termed arthritis mutilans.

2.59

B – Hyperkalaemia

The findings from this young patient's history and ECG suggest the diagnosis of hyperkalaemia. The most likely underlying diagnosis is hyperkalaemic periodic paralysis. This is an autosomal dominant inherited mutation of the SCN4A sodium channel, which is present in muscle cells and also regulates potassium levels in the bloodstream. The dysfunctional channels fail to regulate serum potassium and, in the presence of hyperkalaemia, they fail to activate properly, resulting in episodes of paralysis. Patients present in childhood with episodes of muscle weakness lasting less than 2 hours. Some patients experience myotonia. These attacks typically occur during transient periods of hyperkalaemia;

however, some patients are normokalaemic during attacks. Common precipitants include exercise, stress, cold, large meals, fasting and fatigue. Between attacks patients are often asymptomatic. The ECG changes seen in hyperkalaemia are flattening of P waves, widening of the QRS complex and peaked T waves. Hypercalcaemia can also cause peaked T waves; however, this is unlikely in this scenario. Hypocalcaemia and hypomagnesaemia are associated with flattened T waves. T wave inversion may also occur in hypocalcaemia.

2.60

E – Verapamil and warfarin

The irregularly irregular heartbeat and absent P waves found on this patient's ECG are diagnostic of atrial fibrillation. As his symptoms have been present for more than 48 hours, rate control is the best option as successful cardioversion is less likely. A calcium channel blocker (e.g. verapamil) or a beta-adrenoreceptor antagonist (e.g. atenolol) is the most appropriate agent in this scenario. Digoxin is used as first-line treatment for patients with heart failure who have atrial fibrillation or as an addition to a calcium channel blocker or a beta-adrenoreceptor antagonist if patients remain poorly controlled. Flecainide and sotalol are agents used to maintain sinus rhythm or cardiovert the heart back into sinus rhythm.

Atrial fibrillation increases the risk of atrial emboli formation. Emboli can then enter the systemic circulation and cause an infarct (e.g. cerebral arteries or mesenteric arteries). As a result, patients should have their risk of developing emboli assessed using the $CHADS_2$ scoring criteria. The $CHADS_2$ score is calculated as follows:

Feature	Score
Congestive heart failure	One point
Hypertension	One point
Age greater than 75	One point
Diabetes mellitus	One point
Previous Stroke or transient ischaemic attack	Two points

This patient's $CHADS_2$ score is two and therefore warfarin is a more appropriate anticoagulant than aspirin. Patients with a $CHADS_2$ score of less than two can be given aspirin alternatively. Patients with a $CHADS_2$ score of zero or one should be further risk stratified using the $CHA2DS_2$-VASc scoring system, which includes further modifiable stroke risk factors. The $CHA2DS_2$-VASc scoring system is calculated as follows:

Feature	Score
Congestive heart failure	One point
Hypertension	One point
Age greater than 75 years	Two points
Diabetes mellitus	One point
Previous Stroke or transient ischaemic attack	Two points
Vascular disease (previous myocardial infarction, peripheral vascular disease, mesenteric ischaemia)	One point
Age between 65 and 74 years	One point
Sex (female)	One point

Patients with a $CHA2DS_2$-VASc of one should be treated with either low-dose aspirin or an oral anticoagulant such as warfarin (oral anticoagulant is preferred to aspirin). Patients with a score of zero are very low risk and can therefore be treated with either low-dose aspirin or no antithrombotic therapy (no antithrombotic therapy is preferred).

Paper 3

Paper 3: Questions

3.1 A 33-year-old male presents with fever, shortness of breath and a new-onset pansystolic murmur heard loudest in inspiration at the lower left sternal edge. On further questioning he is found to be an intravenous drug user.

Which one of the following is the most likely diagnosis in this patient?

A Aortic valve regurgitation
B Mitral valve regurgitation
C Pulmonary valve regurgitation
D Tricuspid valve regurgitation
E Tricuspid valve stenosis

3.2 A 53-year-old female with systemic lupus erythematosus is admitted to hospital and has an initial ECG, which shows peaked T waves and an absence of P waves. Her blood results are as follows:

Serum creatinine	489 µmol/L
Serum potassium	6.7 mmol/L
Serum urea	34.3 mmol/L

Which one of the following is most appropriate in the initial management of this patient?

A Calcium chloride, insulin and dextrose
B Calcium Resonium®
C Dietary restriction of potassium and amino acids
D Furosemide
E Salbutamol

3.3 A 47-year-old female presents to the Emergency Department with dyspnoea. A chest X-ray confirms a large right-sided pleural effusion. Fluid is then aspirated from the right lung under ultrasound guidance. Clinical chemistry analysis shows a pleural fluid lactate dehydrogenase: serum lactate dehydrogenase ratio of 0.76.

Which one of the following is the most likely cause of this patient's pleural effusion?

A Constrictive pericarditis
B Hypothyroidism
C Meigs' syndrome
D Nephrotic syndrome
E Rheumatoid arthritis

3.4 An 18-year-old female with cystic fibrosis presents with a productive cough of green sputum. She feels generally unwell and has a temperature of 38.1 °C.

Which one of the following organisms is most likely to be implicated in this patient?

A *Burkholderia cepacia*
B *Chlamydia pneumoniae*
C *Klebsiella pneumoniae*
D *Legionella pneumophila*
E *Moraxella catarrhalis*

3.5 A 68-year-old female presents with a six-month history of exertional breathlessness and wheeze. The patient also has a cough with regular sputum production, which is worse in the winter months. She is a smoker with a 40-pack year history.

Which one of the following pathological features is most likely to be found in this patient?

A Mucous gland hyperplasia, goblet cell hyperplasia and ciliated respiratory epithelium hyperplasia
B Mucous gland hyperplasia, goblet cell hyperplasia and columnar metaplasia of respiratory epithelium

C Mucous gland hyperplasia, goblet cell hypoplasia and squamous dysplasia of respiratory epithelium
D Mucous gland hypertrophy, goblet cell hyperplasia and squamous dysplasia of respiratory epithelium
E Mucous gland hypertrophy, goblet cell hyperplasia and squamous metaplasia of respiratory epithelium

3.6 A 24-year-old male presents to his General Practitioner with increasing exertional shortness of breath, chest pain and syncope. Further questioning reveals that his father died suddenly when he was 33 years old. On examination the patient is afebrile and there is an ejection systolic murmur heard best in the fourth left intercostal space that increases in intensity when the patient is asked to perform the Valsalva manoeuvre. The General Practitioner requests a transthoracic echocardiogram.

Which one of the following is the most likely echocardiographic finding?

A Asymmetric septal enlargement
B Bicuspid aortic valve
C Coarctation of the aorta
D Concentric left ventricular hypertrophy
E Mobile echodense valvular vegetations

3.7 A 68-year-old male presents with a two-day history of fever, productive cough and dyspnoea. On examination the patient has cool peripheries, dry mucous membranes and decreased skin turgor, increased tactile vocal fremitus and dullness to percussion at the right lung base. His observations are as follows:

Blood pressure	96/55 mmHg
Oxygen saturations on room air	90%
Respiratory rate	28 breaths per minute
Temperature	38.3 °C

An arterial blood gas taken with the patient breathing room air is as follows:

PaO$_2$ 7.3 kPa
PaCO$_2$ 5.3 kPa
Haemoglobin   15.5 g/dL

Which one of the following is the most effective immediate way to improve oxygen delivery in this patient?

A Amoxicillin
B Amoxicillin and erythromycin
C Fluid resuscitation using 0.9% sodium chloride
D High-flow oxygen using a non-rebreathe mask with a reservoir bag
E Intubation and administration of 100% oxygen

3.8 A 33-year-old female with a 20-year history of asthma presents with severe shortness of breath, cough and chest tightness. On examination, she has a widespread wheeze auscultated throughout the chest. Her observations are as follows:

Heart rate   117 beats per minute
Oxygen saturations on room air   93%
Respiratory rate   26 breaths per minute

An arterial blood gas taken with the patient breathing room air is as follows:

PaO$_2$ 8.1 kPa
PaCO$_2$ 5.1 kPa

The patient is commenced on a combined salbutamol and ipratropium nebuliser that is driven by oxygen and is given oral prednisolone. Despite these measures, the patient does not improve.

Which one of the following is the most appropriate subsequent treatment option for this patient?

A Intravenous amoxicillin and oral clarithromycin
B Intravenous magnesium sulphate

C Nebulised furosemide
D Oral monteleukast
E Oral sodium cromoglycate

3.9 A 37-year-old male presents to his General Practitioner with increasing fatigue. He is subsequently found to be anti-smooth muscle antibody positive.

Which one of the following diseases is most associated with anti-smooth muscle antibodies?

A Autoimmune hepatitis type I
B Autoimmune hepatitis type II
C Dermatomyositis
D Polymyositis
E Primary biliary cirrhosis

3.10 A 56-year-old male with longstanding type II diabetes mellitus controlled by an oral biguanide undergoes coronary angiography to investigate his worsening angina. Angiography reveals severe stenosis of the left anterior descending coronary artery into which a stent is inserted. Following the procedure, the patient develops deep and rapid breathing and arterial blood gas analysis reveals a pH of 7.26 and a blood lactate level of 7 mmol/L. The patient is noted to have an anion gap of 40 mmol/L.

Which one of the following is most likely to worsen this patient's condition?

A Consideration of haemodialysis
B Further angiography and stenting of coronary vessels
C Rehydration with intravenous fluids
D Stopping oral biguanide therapy
E Taking blood for serum urea and electrolytes

3.11 A 76-year-old female presents to the Emergency Department with cognitive impairment. A Mini Mental State Examination reveals a score of 19/30. On examination she is found to have periorbital oedema, alopecia and slow-relaxing reflexes.

Which one of the following is the most likely cause of her symptoms?

A Chemotherapy toxicity
B Coeliac disease
C Hypothyroidism
D Systemic lupus erythematosus
E Vitamin B_{12} deficiency

3.12 A 64-year-old male is diagnosed with multiple myeloma and is due to undergo his first cycle of chemotherapy.

Which one of the following medications is it most appropriate to commence him on prior to chemotherapy?

A Allopurinol
B Colchicine
C Dexamethasone
D Hydroxychloroquine
E Naproxen

3.13 A 71-year-old female with metastatic colorectal cancer on the ward is found to be bleeding from her cannula site. She has the following blood test results:

Haemoglobin	8.8 g/dL
Platelets	76×10^9/L
Prothrombin time	28 seconds
Activated partial thromboplastin time	53 seconds
Thrombin time	42 seconds
Fibrinogen	1.3 g/L.

Which one of the following is the single most appropriate initial treatment option?

A Blood transfusion
B Fibrinogen concentrate
C Fresh frozen plasma
D Platelet infusion
E Prothrombin complex concentrate

3.14 A 73-year-old male with poorly controlled type II diabetes mellitus presents to his General Practitioner as he has felt increasingly lethargic over the last two months. A blood test reveals that he has a haemoglobin of 10.1 g/dL and an estimated glomerular filtration rate of 17 mL/min/1.73 m^2.

Which one of the following metabolic abnormalities is most likely in this patient?

A Hypercalcaemia
B Hyperphosphataemia
C Hypokalaemia
D Hypoparathyroidism
E Metabolic alkalosis

3.15 A 26-year-old male presents to the Emergency Department with periorbital oedema, ascites and bilateral pitting oedema to the knees. A urine dipstick reveals 4+ protein and blood tests reveal an albumin of 23 g/L and low-density lipoprotein level of 5 mmol/L. Renal biopsy is undertaken and reveals the presence of normal glomerular appearance on light microscopy with podocyte effacement on electron microscopy.

Which one of the following should be avoided in the initial management of this patient?

A Antibiotics
B Corticosteroids
C Cyclo-oxygenase inhibitors
D Factor Xa inhibtors
E HMG-CoA reductase inhibitors

3.16 A 45-year-old male presents to the Emergency Department with a one-day history of right-sided facial pain and weakness. On examination, the following movements can be performed on the left side only: wrinkling his brow, closing his eyes tightly, blowing out his cheeks and showing his teeth.

Which one of the following is the most appropriate immediate step in the management of this patient?

A Aciclovir
B Examination of the tympanic membrane
C Eye lubrication ointment and eye patch
D Prednisolone
E Referral to otolaryngology

3.17 A 58-year-old male is found to have fractured his left tibia following a minor fall at home. X-ray reveals the presence of a well-circumscribed, hypolucent area on the left tibia. The orthopaedic surgeon takes a bone biopsy during surgery. The pathologist's report is as follows:

'Multiple areas of cystic degeneration are seen. The stroma is fibrous. Numerous giant cells are present.'

Which one of the following is the most likely underlying diagnosis?

A Metastatic disease
B Multiple myeloma
C Osteopetrosis
D Osteoporosis
E Primary hyperparathyroidism

3.18 A 78-year-old man presents with a one-month history of generalised bony pain and deafness. He is still able to mobilise fully. A skull X-ray reveals bony enlargement with patchy sclerotic lesions.

Which one of the following blood biochemistry profiles is most likely to be found in this patient?

	Serum calcium	Serum phosphate	Serum alkaline phosphatase
A	Normal	Normal	Normal
B	Normal	Normal	Raised
C	Raised	Reduced	Raised

D	Reduced	Raised	Normal
E	Reduced	Reduced	Raised

3.19 A 67-year-old male with gastro-oesophageal reflux disease presents with an acutely painful swollen right metatarsophalangeal joint. Joint aspiration reveals the presence of needle-shaped crystals that are negatively birefringent when viewed under polarised light.

Which one of the following is the most appropriate initial treatment option in this patient?

A Allopurinol
B Colchicine
C Febuxostat
D Indomethacin
E Steroids

3.20 A 58-year-old male presents with a cough and general malaise. Target lesions are present on his arms and legs. His chest X-ray shows bilateral consolidation and *Mycoplasma* serology is positive. His past medical history is unremarkable except for hypercholesterolaemia, for which the patient is taking high-dose simvastatin. He is allergic to macrolide antibiotics.

Which one of the following is the most appropriate antibiotic to prescribe this patient?

A Amoxicillin
B Ceftriaxone
C Clarithromycin
D Levofloxacin
E Vancomycin

3.21 A 38-year-old female with multiple telangiectasia, skin tightening, Raynaud's phenomenon and sclerodactyly presents with progressive difficulty in swallowing that is worse with solid food than liquids.

Which one of the following is the single most appropriate investigation?

A Barium follow through
B Barium swallow
C Dental radiograph
D Oesophageal manometry
E Upper gastrointestinal endoscopy

3.22 A 56-year-old male presents with a four-month history of progressively worsening ability to grip objects in his hands. He has also recently noticed difficulty getting up from a chair and climbing the stairs. Investigations are as follows:

Serum creatine kinase   5000 IU/L
Electromyography   Low amplitude, short duration
                               potentials
Muscle biopsy   Basophilic intracellular vacuoles
                               on microscopy

Which one of the following is the most likely diagnosis?

A Becker's muscular dystrophy
B Dermatomyositis
C Inclusion body myositis
D Polymyalgia rheumatica
E Polymyositis

3.23 A 20-year-old female who returned two weeks ago from a holiday in Malawi presents with fever, an urticarial rash and cough. On clinical examination there is a widespread polyphonic wheeze and hepatosplenomegaly.

Which one of the following is the most appropriate initial treatment?

A Amphotericin
B Co-amoxiclav
C Metronidazole
D Praziquantel
E Sodium stibogluconate

3.24 A 43-year-old male presents to his General Practitioner with a painless ulcer on his penis. *Treponema pallidum* enzyme immunoassay and Venereal Disease Reference Laboratory tests are both positive. The patient is treated with a single dose of intramuscular benzathine penicillin. Five hours after the injection the patient develops fever, flu-like symptoms and notices that the ulcer on his penis has got bigger.

Which one of the following best describes this patient's symptoms?

A Allergy to penicillin
B Erythema multiforme
C Jarisch–Herxheimer reaction
D Patient has EBV and is reacting to penicillin
E Stevens–Johnson syndrome

3.25 A 67-year-old male with lung cancer presents with abdominal pain, polyuria and confusion. His blood tests are as follows:

Serum calcium   2.9 mmol/L
Serum albumin   35 g/L

Which one of the following lung tumours is most likely to be associated with this clinical scenario?

A Adenocarcinoma
B Alveolar cell carcinoma
C Large cell carcinoma
D Small cell carcinoma
E Squamous cell carcinoma

3.26 A 45-year-old female presents to the Emergency Department after taking an overdose of a medication she was recently prescribed. An ECG is performed and reveals a ventricular tachycardia. The patient has no history of underlying cardiac abnormalities.

Which one of the following medications is this patient most likely to have overdosed on?

A Fluoxetine
B Imipramine

C Levothyroxine
D Metoprolol
E Naproxen

3.27 A 32-year-old female presented to her General Practitioner with headaches. She was noted to have a blood pressure of 162/102 mmHg. She was started on lisinopril and two weeks later has a blood test, which reveals a serum creatinine of 164 μmol/L. The General Practitioner stopped the lisinopril and referred the patient for further investigation. A CT angiogram of the renal arteries is performed and reveals a 'string of beads' appearance bilaterally.

Which one of the following is the most appropriate treatment option for this patient?

A Commence the patient on amlodipine
B Commence the patient on irbesartan
C Percutaneous angioplasty of the renal arteries
D Stenting of the renal arteries
E Surgical revascularisation of the renal arteries

3.28 A 25-year-old female attends the Emergency Department with acute-onset generalised abdominal tenderness. There is no vomiting or diarrhoea. Initial investigations are unremarkable and a diagnostic laparoscopy is performed, the results of which are as follows:

'Normal architecture of the colon with an abnormal appearance of the proximal ileum.'

Which one of the following is the most appropriate next step in the management of this patient?

A Commence prednisolone
B Faecal calprotectin levels
C Radio-labelled white cell scan
D Small bowel follow through
E Urgent colonoscopy

3.29 A 70-year-old male with a 60-pack year history of cigarette smoking attends the Emergency Department via ambulance with a two-hour history of crushing central chest pain. An ECG reveals marked ST elevation in leads V_5, V_6, I and AvL.

Which one of the following coronary vessels is most likely to have been affected in this patient?

A Left anterior descending artery
B Left circumflex artery
C Left main stem
D Right coronary artery
E Right posterior descending artery

3.30 A 65-year-old male with metastatic bronchial carcinoma presents to the emergency department with an 18-hour history of pleuritic chest pain and increasing shortness of breath. He is noted to have the following observations:

Blood pressure	96/55 mmHg
Heart rate	112 beats per minute
Oxygen saturations on room air	88%
Respiratory rate	24 breaths per minute
Temperature	37.1 °C

Which one of the following is the most appropriate investigation to aid the management of this patient?

A Chest X-ray
B CT pulmonary angiography
C D-dimer
D Transthoracic echocardiogram
E Ventilation-perfusion scan

3.31 A 39-year-old male with known liver cirrhosis presents with increasing shortness of breath on exertion. On examination he is noticed to have a barrel-shaped chest and the lung fields are hyper-resonant. His peak flow is 420 L/minute and his FEV_1:FVC ratio is 0.55. A lung biopsy is performed.

Which one of the following is the most likely histological finding on biopsy?

A Centriacinar emphysema
B Charcot–Leyden crystals
C Interstitial lung fibrosis
D Non-caseating granuloma
E Panacinar emphysema

3.32 A 40-year-old male with Crohn's disease presents with perianal pain and pruritus. He also reports a malodorous rectal discharge. On examination there is evidence of a perianal fistula, which has a single external opening on the left buttock and is surrounded by granulated tissue. Internal examination of the anus reveals an opening in the anal canal and evidence of an anorectal abscess.

Which one of the following is the most appropriate management for this patient?

A Intravenous infliximab infusion
B Oral metronidazole
C Surgical referral
D Topical diltiazem
E Topical nitroglycerin

3.33 A 35-year-old male presents with a three-month history of lethargy and weight loss. He has the following blood test results:

Total white cell count	$13 \times 10^9/L$
Lymphocyte count	$2.8 \times 10^9/L$
Neutrophil count	$5.6 \times 10^9/L$
Eosinophil count	$0.8 \times 10^9/L$

Which one of the following is the most likely diagnosis in this patient?

A Addison's disease
B Amoebiasis
C Giardiasis

D Granulomatosis with polyangiitis
E Type I diabetes mellitus

3.34 A 58-year-old male with poorly controlled type II diabetes mellitus presents with a three-day history of severe right thigh pain. Over the past day the patient also describes weakness and wasting in this region.

Which one of the following is the most likely diagnosis in this patient?

A Diabetic amyotrophy
B Diabetic sensorimotor polyneuropathy
C Meralgia paraesthetica
D Obturator nerve palsy
E Polymyalgia rheumatica

3.35 A 65-year-old male presents to his General Practitioner with polyuria and polydipsia. The fasting blood glucose is 5.9 mmol/L. A subsequent water deprivation test reveals the following results:

Urine osmolality after fluid deprivation   270 mOsm/kg
Urine osmolality after desmopressin bolus   285 mOsm/kg

Which one of the following is the most likely diagnosis in this patient?

A Craniopharyngioma
B Hypercalcaemia
C Hyperkalaemia
D Impaired glucose tolerance
E Pituitary macroadenoma

3.36 A 24-year-old male presents to his General Practitioner due to several episodes of sudden onset of flushing, headache and palpitations, which usually last for around 40 minutes. He also states that he has become increasingly unstable on his feet in the last three months and was treated for a deep vein thrombosis six weeks previously. A full neurological examination reveals horizontal nystagmus maximal to the right, a right-sided intention tremor and an ataxic gait. He is noted to have a blood pressure of 155/102 mmHg. A full blood count shows a haemoglobin of 18.2 g/dL.

Which one of the following is the most likely underlying diagnosis in this patient?

A Birt–Hogg–Dubé syndrome
B Multiple endocrine neoplasia type II
C Neurofibromatosis type I
D Phaeochromocytoma
E Von Hippel–Lindau syndrome

3.37 An 87-year-old female presents to her General Practitioner complaining of increasing forgetfulness and inability to concentrate for prolonged periods of time. She also reports that she frequently sees young children sitting at the end of her bed.

Which one of the following is the most likely neuropathological finding in this patient?

A Accumulation of cytoplasmic tau protein
B Aggregation of cytoplasmic alpha-synuclein
C Aggregation of cytoplasmic SOD1
D Aggregation of cytoplasmic TDP-43
E Extracellular accumulation of beta amyloid

3.38 A 45-year-old male presents to the Emergency Department with a headache. On examination his right pupil is dilated and unresponsive to light. There is a normal range of eye movements without any ptosis and at rest there is no deviation of the right eye.

Which one of the following is the most likely diagnosis in this patient?

A Cavernous sinus thrombosis
B Diabetic oculomotor nerve palsy
C Pituitary adenoma

D Posterior communicating artery aneurysm
E Weber's syndrome

3.39 A 28-year-old female presents to the Emergency Department with severe epigastric pain that has lasted for two days. She also has some weakness in her left arm and a history of depression, for which she takes fluoxetine. On examination, there is fever, mild tachycardia and generalised abdominal tenderness. The patient's blood pressure was recorded at 130/84 mmHg. Neurological examination reveals hypotonia and absent reflexes in the left arm. Initial blood tests were unremarkable apart from a serum sodium of 130 mmol/L.

Which one of the following is the most likely diagnosis in this patient?

A Acute intermittent porphyria
B Acute pancreatitis
C Appendicitis
D Cholecystitis
E Guillain–Barré syndrome

3.40 A 65-year-old male presents to his General Practitioner with increasing unsteadiness on his feet and several episodes of urinary incontinence. His wife states that she feels that his short-term memory has worsened on the previous 18 months. A head CT scan is ordered and reveals enlarged ventricles and absent sulci.

Which one of the following is the most likely diagnosis in this patient?

A Alzheimer's disease
B Creutzfeldt–Jakob disease
C Lewy body dementia
D Normal pressure hydrocephalus
E Parkinson's disease

3.41 A 43-year-old female with secondary progressive multiple sclerosis presents with several episodes of urinary urge incontinence; they are now causing her to limit her social activities.

Which one of the following medications is most likely to improve symptom control in this patient?

A Clonidine
B Desmopressin
C Fluoxetine
D Rivastigmine
E Tolterodine

3.42 A 52-year-old male who is currently taking azathioprine for Crohn's disease develops a tender and inflamed first right metatarsal.

Which one of the following medications should be avoided in this patient?

A Allopurinol
B Colchicine
C Indomethacin
D Naproxen
E Paracetamol

3.43 A 53-year-old male presents to the Emergency Department with sudden-onset central chest pain that radiates down the left arm. An initial ECG shows ST elevation in leads V1, V2 and V3 and therefore thrombolytic therapy is administered in the Emergency Department. Forty-eight hours later he begins complaining of the same central chest pain.

Which one of the following is the most appropriate test to confirm myocardial reinfarction?

A B-type natriuretic peptide
B Creatine kinase MB
C Lactate
D Procalcitonin
E Troponin I

3.44 A General Practitioner refers a 54-year-old male with type II diabetes mellitus to the ophthalmologist after his regular check up. The General Practitioner explains to the patient that she has observed changes that are the result of insufficient blood flow to the retina.

Which one of the following is most likely to have been observed on fundoscopy of this patient?

A Cotton wool spots
B 'Dots and blots'
C Flame-shaped haemorrhages
D Microaneurysms
E Silver wiring

3.45 A 43-year-old male with type II diabetes mellitus is started on a new medication. After the patient enquires, the General Practitioner assures the patient that the new medication does not increase the risk of hypoglycaemia.

Which one of the following classes of drugs has the patient most likely been started on?

A Beta-adrenoreceptor antagonist
B Biguanide
C Glinide
D Insulin analogue
E Sulphonylurea

3.46 A 52-year-old male with a history of ulcerative colitis presents to his General Practitioner with episodic fever and rigors. On examination he is jaundiced and has evidence of excoriations on his upper arms.

Which one of the following is the most likely diagnosis in this patient?

A Acute cholecystitis
B Chronic autoimmune hepatitis
C Pancreatic cancer

D Primary biliary cirrhosis
E Primary sclerosing cholangitis

3.47 A 68-year-old female is started on alendronic acid and Calcichew D3 Forte® following a fractured neck of femur. A dual-energy X-ray absorptiometry scan had revealed a T-score of −3.9.

Which one of the following is it most important to communicate to the patient?

A A six-month course of alendronic acid should suffice
B Alendronic acid is best taken at night
C Alendronic acid should be taken at the same time as Calcichew D3 Forte®
D Alendronic acid should be taken with food
E Remain upright for 30 minutes after each dose of alendronic acid and eat and drink nothing except water

3.48 A 34-year-old male presents to the Emergency Department with a febrile flu-like illness and a sharp central chest pain. The pain is worsened by inhalation and on lying flat. On inspection he appears sweaty and unwell, stating that 'something is catching his breath'. On auscultation of the chest there is a friction rub and normal breath sounds.

Which one of the following is the most likely diagnosis in this patient?

A Gastro-oesophageal reflux
B Myocardial infarction
C Pancreatitis
D Pericarditis
E Pneumonia

3.49 A 63-year-old female presents to the Emergency Department after experiencing repeated episodes of haematemesis. She has a history of alcohol abuse and on examination she is confused. She is resuscitated and is awaiting urgent endoscopy.

Which one of the following is the most appropriate medication to initiate?

A Ciprofloxacin
B Octreotide
C Propranolol
D Terlipressin
E Vasopressin

3.50 A 36-year-old female is admitted to hospital with acute liver failure following a paracetamol overdose the previous evening.

Which one of the following individual test results indicates a poor prognosis and therefore justifies placing the patient on the liver transplant list?

A Arterial pH less than 7.3
B Aspartate transaminase greater than 100 IU/L
C Bilirubin greater than 60 µmol/l
D International normalised ratio greater than 2.5
E Serum creatinine greater than 150 µmol/L

3.51 A 46-year-old male is brought into the Emergency Department by ambulance after feeling faint and collapsing at home. He is breathless and pale. On examination his lungs are clear, his jugular venous pressure cannot be visualised and there is no ankle oedema. He is noted to have the following observations:

Blood pressure (lying)	95/65 mmHg
Heart rate	105 beats per minute
Capillary refill time	4 seconds
Respiratory rate	18 breaths per minute
Temperature	37.0 °C

Investigations reveal the following:

Serum sodium	128 mmol/L
Urinary sodium	17 mmol/L

Which one of the following is the most likely cause of this clinical scenario?

A Bendroflumethiazide
B Congestive cardiac failure
C Nephrotic syndrome
D Severe gastroenteritis
E Small cell lung cancer

3.52 A 45-year-old female smoker with numerous co-morbidities presents to her General Practitioner after feeling lethargic for two months. Her blood tests reveal the following:

Haemoglobin	7.9 g/dl
Mean corpuscular volume	112 fL
Blood film	Multiple hypersegmented poly-morphonuclear leukocytes

Which of the following is the most likely underlying cause of this clinical scenario?

A Chronic kidney disease
B COPD
C Menorrhagia
D Previous ileal resection for Crohn's disease
E Splenectomy secondary to trauma

3.53 A 73-year-old male is admitted to hospital with an exacerbation of COPD. Whilst on the ward he complains of palpitations and dizziness during which his blood pressure falls to 100/70 mmHg. The patient has no previous cardiac history. A 12-lead ECG is recorded and reveals the following:

Rate	150 beats per minute
Rhythm	Regular
Axis	Normal
P waves	Two large irregularly shaped P waves precede every QRS complex
PR interval	160 milliseconds
QRS complexes	80 milliseconds
ST segment	Isoelectric

Which one of the following is the most likely diagnosis?

A Atrial fibrillation
B Atrial flutter
C Atrial tachycardia
D Sinus tachycardia
E Ventricular tachycardia

3.54 A 64-year-old male is seen in the respiratory outpatients department. Over the last ten years he has suffered 9 kg unintentional weight loss and has a persistent wet cough, which is productive of large quantities of purulent sputum. On examination there is digital clubbing, an inspiratory click, as well as coarse crackles that localise well to the left lower zone and change in character when the patient is asked to cough.

Which one of the following is the most appropriate investigation?

A Bronchoscopy
B High-resolution CT chest
C Lung biopsy
D Sweat test
E Ventilation-perfusion scan

3.55 A 17-year-old female presents to her General Practitioner with fatigue and muscle cramps. Examination is normal. Blood pressure is 110/60 mmHg. The patient is referred to secondary care. Investigations are performed and yield the following results:

Serum sodium	131 mmol/L
Serum potassium	2.9 mmol/L
Serum chloride	88 mmol/L
Serum bicarbonate	32 mmol/L
Serum urea	4 mmol/L
Serum creatinine	68 µmol/L
24-hour urine sodium	65 mmol
24-hour urine potassium	58 mmol
24-hour urine calcium	1.3 mmol

Which one of the following is the most likely diagnosis?

A Conn's syndrome
B Gitelman's syndrome
C Laxative abuse
D Liddle's syndrome
E Villous adenoma

3.56 A 42-year-old male with known alcohol dependence is brought to the Emergency Department with confusion. On examination he appears sweaty and has a marked tremor that worsens when he is given a cup of water to hold. The cranial nerve examination reveals that eye movements are abnormal in all directions; his ophthalmo-plegia doesn't seem to fit into any recognisable neuromuscular pattern of pathology. A fingertip glucose measurement reveals a blood glucose level of 2.4 mmol/L.

Which one of the following is the single most appropriate initial management?

A Hypostop® oral glucose gel
B Intravenous 5% dextrose
C Intravenous cyclizine
D Intravenous Pabrinex®
E Oral thiamine supplementation

3.57 A 57-year-old male presents to the Emergency Department with weight loss, diarrhoea and chronic epigastric pain relieved by leaning forward. On examination of the abdomen there are multiple interlacing, reticulated, hyperpigmented, macular patches overlying the painful area. A social history reveals he is dependent on alcohol and illicit drugs.

Which one of the following is the most likely diagnosis?

A Acute hepatitis
B Acute pericarditis
C Chronic pancreatitis
D Gastro-oesophageal reflux

E Hiatus hernia

3.58 A 32-year-old female presents to her General Practitioner with fatigue and lethargy. On further questioning she reveals that she has recently developed tingling in her feet. She has the following blood test results:

Haemoglobin	10.1 g/dL
Mean corpuscular volume	110 fL
Serum vitamin B_{12}	0.05 nmol/L
Serum folate	2 nmol/L
Serum ferritin	125 μg/L
Serum iron	19 μmol/L

Which one of the following initial treatment options is most appropriate in this patient?

A Intramuscular hydroxocobalamin every two days
B Oral folate supplements
C Oral folate supplements and three monthly intramuscular hydroxocobalamin
D Oral iron supplements
E Three monthly intramuscular hydroxocobalamin

3.59 A 29-year-old female with brittle asthma presents to the Emergency Department with palpitations. She does not have any chest pain and is not short of breath. She has the following observations:

Blood pressure	130/82 mmHg
Heart rate	147 beats per minute
Temperature	37.1 °C
Oxygen saturations on room air	97%
Respiratory rate	16 breaths per minute

An ECG is performed and reveals the presence of a regular narrow complex tachycardia with absent P waves. A subsequent carotid massage is unsuccessful.

Which one of the following is the most appropriate management for this patient?

A DC cardioversion
B Intravenous adenosine
C Intravenous amiodarone
D Intravenous metoprolol
E Intravenous verapamil

3.60 A 65-year-old female is admitted to hospital for an exacerbation of COPD. During her inpatient stay she is catheterised to monitor her urine output. After seven days in hospital she begins to develop cloudy urine and rigors. Blood cultures are taken which reveal the presence of an extended-spectrum beta-lactamase-producing organism.

Which one of the following antibiotics is most appropriate to initiate in this patient?

A Ciprofloxacin
B Co-amoxiclav
C Meropenem
D Piperacillin-tazobactam
E Trimethoprim

Paper 3: Answers

3.1

D – Tricuspid valve regurgitation

This patient clinically displays signs of infective endocarditis causing tricuspid valve regurgitation. Intravenous drug users have an increased risk of developing infective endocarditis of the tricuspid valve as bacteria injected using a non-sterile needle will arrive at the right side of the heart before the left. Tricuspid valve regurgitation classically causes a pansystolic murmur heard loudest in inspiration at the lower left sternal edge between the third and sixth intercostal spaces.

Mitral valve regurgitation also causes a pansystolic murmur. However, it is heard loudest in expiration over the apex (fifth intercostal space, mid-clavicular line). In addition, this murmur will radiate to the axilla. By contrast, aortic and pulmonary valve regurgitation both present with an early-diastolic murmur. In aortic valve regurgitation the murmur is heard loudest in expiration over the aortic region (second right intercostal space) with the patient sitting forward. In contrast, the murmur of pulmonary valve regurgitation is heard loudest in inspiration over the pulmonary region (second left intercostal space). Left-sided murmurs are louder in expiration because the higher intrathoracic pressure increases venous return to the left side of the heart. The reverse is true of right-sided murmurs. Inspiration reduces intrathoracic pressure, drawing blood into the lungs, increasing venous return to the right side of the heart and increasing the volume of right-sided murmurs. Tricuspid valve stenosis is rare and presents with a mid-diastolic murmur heard loudest at the lower left sternal edge in inspiration; it is associated with carcinoid syndrome.

3.2

A – Calcium chloride, insulin and dextrose

This patient has developed hyperkalaemia due to acute kidney injury. Worrying ECG features of hyperkalaemia are present; peaked T waves and prolonged or absent P waves. Therefore, this patient needs to be given calcium chloride to acutely stabilise the myocardium. The patient also requires insulin and dextrose infusions to reduce the serum potassium concentration. Without treatment to stabilise the myocardium, further hyperkalaemic ECG changes may occur, including small R waves and widening of the QRS complex. These may subsequently progress to form a 'sine wave' pattern, followed by ventricular fibrillation and finally asystolic cardiac arrest.

Calcium chloride is an essential cardioprotective agent that is used to antagonise the membrane effects of hyperkalaemia. It is important to note that it does not reduce serum potassium levels. Insulin, in binding to its cellular receptor, increases Na^+-K^+-ATPase activity, and drives potassium ions into cells. An infusion of dextrose is given simultaneously in order to prevent hypoglycaemia and to decrease serum potassium levels further by stimulating endogenous insulin release. Nebulised salbutamol can also be used in the acute setting to drive potassium ions into cells. However, as this patient is displaying ECG changes it is essential to administer a cardioprotective agent. To reduce the total body potassium in the long term, other measures such as loop diuretics, cation exchange resins, dialysis and dietary restriction of potassium can be used. Loop diuretics, such as furosemide, increase urinary excretion of potassium ions and are only of use if the patient has a urine output. Cation exchange resins, such as calcium polystyrene sulphonate (Calcium Resonium®) exchange calcium or sodium ions for potassium ions in the gut. This increases gut potassium ion excretion. Cation exchange resins are most effective when given rectally.

3.3

E – Rheumatoid arthritis

Rheumatoid arthritis causes an exudative pleural effusion, whereas the four other options cause transudative pleural effusions. Pleural fluid is defined as an exudate by Light's criteria.

Light's criteria for pleural fluid (exudates will meet one of these three criteria):

- Effusion protein more than 0.5 serum protein
- Effusion lactate dehydrogenase more than 0.6 serum lactate dehydrogenase
- Effusion lactate dehydrogenase more than two thirds of the upper limit of normal serum lactate dehydrogenase.

Exudative pleural effusions occur due to increased pleural capillary permeability secondary to increased release of cytokines. This occurs in infection, malignancy or inflammatory disorders, such as rheumatoid arthritis. Transudative pleural effusions occur as a result of increased venous pressure (e.g. cardiac failure, constrictive pericarditis) or hypoproteinaemia (e.g. nephrotic syndrome). Transudates are also found in hypothyroidism and Meigs' syndrome (a benign ovarian fibroma in conjunction with a right-sided pleural effusion).

3.4

A – *Burkholderia cepacia*

Cystic fibrosis is an autosomal recessive condition characterised by mutations in the cystic fibrosis transmembrane regulator gene found on chromosome 7. The most common form is caused by the deletion of the codon for the amino acid phenylalanine. In exocrine glands the cystic fibrosis transmembrane regulator protein is responsible for the transport of chloride from the inside to the outside of the cell in order to form secretions. Mutations cause an increased concentration of intracellular chloride, and subsequently other positively charged ions and water enter the cells. As a consequence, pulmonary, pancreatic and intestinal secretions are thickened. In the lungs,the excessive production of a thick and viscid mucous provides a fertile breeding ground for bacteria. Initially, patients become infected with *Staphylococcus aureus* before subsequent colonisation with Gram-negative bacteria. The most commonly implicated Gram-negative bacteria are *Burkholderia cepacia* and *Pseudomonas aeruginosa*.

Legionella pneumophila is a Gram-negative bacterium associated with contaminated water used in air conditioning and swimming pools. It causes a pneumonia associated with myalgia, fever and a dry cough. *Chlamydia pneumoniae* is an obligate intracellular bacterium that initially causes a sore throat, which is then followed by pneumonia. *Klebsiella pneumoniae* is another Gram-negative bacteria; it is associated with pneumonias in alcoholics. *Moraxella catarrhalis* is also a Gram-negative bacterium that can cause community-acquired pneumonia.

3.5

E – Mucous gland hypertrophy, goblet cell hyperplasia and squamous metaplasia of respiratory epithelium

This patient has COPD, which is predominantly caused by smoking and is characterised by progressive airflow obstruction that is not fully reversible. The main pathological features of COPD are those of:

- Mucous gland hypertrophy, which causes bronchial wall thickening and reduction in luminal diameter
- Goblet cell hyperplasia, which leads to increased mucin production (and therefore increased sputum production)
- Squamous metaplasia of the respiratory epithelium (replacing the normal ciliated respiratory epithelium)
- Loss of cilia, causing impaired clearance of foreign particles.

Columnar metaplasia is not found in respiratory epithelium; it is commonly found in Barrett's oesophagus as the normal squamous epithelium is replaced with columnar epithelium due to prolonged exposure to acid. Squamous dysplasia is indicative of a neoplastic process and in a respiratory setting is associated with squamous cell carcinoma of the lung.

3.6

A – Asymmetric septal enlargement

This patient's symptoms and signs are highly suggestive of aortic tract outflow obstruction. In a young patient with a family history of sudden cardiac death the most likely diagnosis is hypertrophic obstructive cardiomyopathy. Hypertrophic cardiomyopathy is an autosomal dominant condition caused by mutations in 1 of over 200 different genes that code for proteins in the muscle sarcomere. The condition has a prevalence of about 0.2% and is well known as the leading cause of sudden cardiac death in young athletes. Fifty percent of cases are inherited and 50% are sporadic. In contrast to the symmetrical concentric left ventricular hypertrophy (the free ventricular wall and interventricular septum hypertrophy equally) caused by conditions of cardiac pressure overload (e.g. aortic stenosis, systemic hypertension), hypertrophic cardiomyopathy is associated with an additional disproportionate enlargement of the septum known as asymmetric hypertrophy. For the 25% of patients who experience a resting aortic outflow tract obstruction, the term 'hypertrophic obstructive cardiomyopathy' is applicable. Otherwise the term 'hypertrophic cardiomyopathy' is more appropriate. The enlarged septum causes a sub-valvular aortic outflow obstruction and a dynamic aortic outflow gradient worse when the early systolic volume is low (e.g. with the Valsalva manoeuvre) or the heart rate is high (e.g. during exercise). The outflow gradient is further exacerbated by anterior movement of the mitral valve; the valve is drawn closer to the enlarged septum during systole due to the increased systolic ejection velocity (known as the Venturi effect).

Coarctation of the aorta and bicuspid aortic valve are both important congenital cardiac conditions. Bicuspid aortic valve is the commonest congenital cardiac anomaly in young adults and does cause
a left ventricular outflow obstruction (aortic valve stenosis).
However, it tends to present in the fourth and fifth decade.
Coarctation of the aorta is a cause of supravalvular aortic outflow
tract obstruction, whereby the most common site for coarctation is
distal to the left subclavian artery, causing radio-femoral delay.
Radio-radial delay occurs if the coarctation is between the right
brachiocephalic and the left common carotid or left subclavian
artery. However, the murmurs of coarctation and aortic stenosis
both decrease in intensity with the Valsalva manoeuvre, due to the
reduced flow across the obstruction. Finally, as with any cause of
disrupted cardiac blood flow and/or cardiac epithelial disruption,
hypertrophic obstructive cardiomyopathy is associated with an
increased risk of infective endocarditis and septic valvular vegetations. However, in this afebrile patient this is an unlikely finding.

3.7

C – Fluid resuscitation using 0.9% sodium chloride

This patient is clinically dehydrated and hypoxic, which is most
likely as a result of a bacterial respiratory tract infection. He therefore requires improved delivery of oxygen to the tissues. Oxygen
delivery (ml/minute) is calculated by the following equation:

> Cardiac output (L/minute) × 1.34 (ml of oxygen
> carried per gram of haemoglobin) × haemoglobin
> concentration (g/L) × oxygen saturation (%).

From this equation it is apparent that the most effective way of
delivering oxygen to the tissues of this dehydrated patient is by
increasing the cardiac output (e.g. from 4 L/minute to 5 L/minute)
rather than oxygen saturations (e.g. from 90% to 100%):

- Cardiac output at 4L/minute and oxygen saturations at
  90%: $4 \times 1.34 \times 155 \times 0.9 = $ **747.72 ml/minute**

- Increasing cardiac output from 4 L/minute to 5 L/minute:
  $5 \times 1.34 \times 155 \times 0.9 = $ **934.65 ml/minute**
- Increasing oxygen saturations from 90% to 100%: $4 \times 1.34 \times 155 \times 1 = $ **830.8 ml/minute**.

Antibiotics such as amoxicillin (a penicillin) and erythromycin (a macrolide) play an important role in treating bacterial respiratory tract infections. However, they take time to work and would not play an important role in the initial improvement of oxygen delivery in this patient.

3.8

B – Intravenous magnesium sulphate

This patient is having an acute severe asthma attack that has not responded to initial therapy and so treatment with intravenous magnesium sulphate is the most appropriate option. Features of an acute severe asthma attack include:

- Heart rate greater than 110 beats per minute
- PEFR 33–50% of predicted
- Respiratory rate of greater than 25 breaths per minute
- An inability to complete sentences in one breath.

Magnesium sulphate relaxes the smooth muscle in the airways and has been shown to have a bronchodilator effect in adults. Intravenous magnesium sulphate can be given in acute severe asthma where patients have not had a good response to inhaled bronchodilator therapy, and in life-threatening or near-fatal asthma. Alongside magnesium sulphate, referral to an intensive care unit and early involvement of an anaesthetist is necessary in this instance as the patient is at a high risk of deteriorating.

Intravenous amoxicillin (a penicillin) and oral clarithromycin (a macrolide) are not indicated routinely for acute asthma, as infectious exacerbations are most likely to be viral. Nebulised furosemide has been shown to theoretically produce bronchodilation; however, clinical trials have failed to show any significant benefit compared to inhaledbeta-2-adrenoreceptor agonists. Montelukast is a leukotriene receptor antagonist and sodium cromoglycate is a mast cell stabiliser. There is no clear evidence for their use in the management of acute asthma.

3.9

A – Autoimmune hepatitis type I

Anti-smooth muscle antibodies are most associated with autoimmune hepatitis type I. Anti-liver/kidney microsomal type I antibodies are most associated with autoimmune hepatitis type II. Type I autoimmune hepatitis can affect both adults and children, whereas type II affects predominantly children and is more likely to progress to cirrhosis.

The following conditions are paired with their associated autoantibodies:

- Dermatomyositis and polymyositis: anti-Jo1 antibodies
- Primary biliary cirrhosis: anti-mitochondrial antibodies.

3.10

B – Further angiography and stenting of coronary vessels

This patient has developed a high anion gap lactic acidosis as a result of being maintained on metformin, an anti-diabetic agent of the biguanide category, whilst undergoing angiography. Administration of contrast, such as in angiography, can induce an acute kidney injury. As metformin is excreted renally, levels in the blood can rise and precipitate lactic acidosis. Administering the patient further contrast is likely to worsen this problem and hence should be avoided in this scenario. Metformin should also be stopped in order to ensure that the lactic acidosis does not worsen any further.

Metformin should be avoided if the creatinine is greater than 150 µmol/l, and in patients with heart failure and those prone to dehydration. It should ideally either be withheld 48 hours before contrast administration, or be combined with adequate intravenous rehydration with isotonic bicarbonate to maintain renal perfusion. Some use intravenous N-acetylcysteine instead, which also reduces the incidence of contrast-induced nephropathy. Accumulation of lactate occurs for two reasons. First, lactate is a substrate for hepatic gluconeogenesis and this process is inhibited by metformin, resulting in an increase in serum lactate. Secondly, metformin is cleared renally, as is 25% of serum lactate (the other 75% is metabolized by the liver). Therefore contrast-induced renal impairment results in impaired clearance of both compounds and subsequently their levels increase. Blood for serum urea and electrolytes should be taken in order to assess renal function, and if there is severe renal impairment, haemodialysis should be considered.

3.11

C – Hypothyroidism

Hypothyroidism causes many symptoms including fatigue, weight gain, cold intolerance, dry skin, menorrhagia and constipation. Additionally, patients with hypothyroidism are also known to develop cognitive impairment, periorbital oedema, alopecia and slow-relaxing reflexes. The constellation of symptoms found in this scenario is virtually diagnostic of hypothyroidism. Patients with impaired cognitive function must undergo a blood test for thyroid dysfunction as correction of any thyroid abnormalities can improve mental function.

Patients with cognitive impairment should also be investigated for other causes of a reversible dementia. Therefore in addition to thyroid function the following blood tests should also be considered:

- Bone profile for hypercalcaemia or hypocalcaemia
- Liver function tests for hepatic failure

- Full blood count, ESR and C-reactive protein for anaemia and vasculitis
- Levels of serum vitamin B_{12} and serum folate
- Serum caeruloplasmin levels for Wilson's disease
- Serum glucose for hypo/hyperglycaemia
- Serum urea and serum creatinine for chronic kidney disease
- Syphilis and HIV serology.

All patients with cognitive impairment should have CT or MRI scan of the head to rule out an underlying structural abnormality, e.g. space-occupying lesion.

Although vitamin B_{12} deficiency can present with cognitive impairment it is unlikely to produce the other features present in this patient. Chemotherapy toxicity can cause alopecia and neurological problems; however, it is likely that patients on chemotherapy would complain of nausea and vomiting in addition to these symptoms. Patients with coeliac disease and systemic lupus erythematosus are very unlikely to present with a triad of alopecia, periorbital oedema and slow-relaxing reflexes, although both can cause cognitive impairment.

3.12

A – Allopurinol

Patients with multiple myeloma and other haematological malignancies should be given allopurinol prior to chemotherapy in order to reduce the risk of tumour lysis syndrome. This phenomenon occurs in patients soon after their first dose of chemotherapy as large numbers of rapidly dividing malignant cells die and release their intracellular contents. This can result in hyperkalaemia, hyperuricaemia and renal failure. Allopurinol inhibits xanthine oxidase, the enzyme which catalyses the breakdown of purines to uric acid. These patients should also be given large volumes of fluid prior to chemotherapy in order to minimise the risk of renal failure.

Colchicine (an anti-mitotic), dexamethasone (a potent synthetic steroid) and naproxen (an NSAID) play an important role in the management of gout, a crystal arthropathy characterised by hyper-uricaemia and the formation of negatively birefringent, needle-shaped uric acid crystals. However, these agents play no role in the prevention of tumour lysis syndrome. Hydroxychloroquine is also used as a disease-modifying agent in rheumatoid arthritis and sys-temic lupus erythematosus.

3.13

C – Fresh frozen plasma

This patient has developed disseminated intravascular coagulation secondary to her malignancy and should be given fresh frozen plasma. Mucin-secreting adenocarcinomas, such as colon cancer, secrete procoagulant factors into the circulation and are the most common solid organ tumours to be associated with disseminated intravascular coagulation. In disseminated intravascular coagula-tion, there is an overwhelming increase in the activity of circulating thrombin, either due to release of procoagulant factors (as in malig-nancy) or as a result of endothelial damage, such as in a vasculitic process or meningococcal sepsis. This results in widespread activa-tion of coagulation factors, generalised platelet aggregation and fibrinolysis. Due to consumption of platelets and coagulation fac-tors, patients are prone to haemorrhage. The clinical feature of dis-seminated intravascular coagulation is predominantly bleeding, especially from venepuncture sites and surgical wounds. Laboratory findings classically reveal a low platelet count, prolonged pro-thrombin time and activated partial thromboplastin time, grossly prolonged thrombin time and depleted fibrinogen. While the key to the management of disseminated intravascular coagulation is treat-ment of the underlying condition, in this case additional supportive treatment is required. Fresh frozen plasma is most appropriate in this patient as they have evidence of ongoing bleeding that requires rapid treatment. Fresh frozen plasma refers to the liquid portion (the platelets and red cells are removed) of leucodepleted blood that has been stored at under −30 °C. It is mostly used to replace coagulation factors.

Blood transfusion would not be appropriate in this case as packed red cells do not provide the necessary coagulation factors required to replace bleeding in disseminated intravascular coagulation. Fibrinogen concentrate is derived from fresh frozen plasma; however, its role is reserved for patients with disseminated intravascular coagulation who have fibrinogen levels less than 1 g/L despite treatment with fresh frozen plasma. Prothrombin complex concentrate lacks essential factors, such as factor V, and is only recommended if transfusion of fresh frozen plasma is not possible (e.g. the patient is fluid overloaded). Platelet transfusion should only be considered in patients with disseminated intravascular coagulation who are bleeding or are at a high risk of bleeding and have a platelet count of less than 50×10^9/L.

3.14

B – Hyperphosphataemia

This patient has stage IV chronic kidney disease (estimated glomerular filtration rate of 15–29 mL/min/1.73 m^2) and the anaemia is likely to be due to impaired synthesis of erythropoietin by the kidneys. In patients with chronic kidney disease, hyperphosphataemia is a common finding as the kidneys are unable to excrete phosphate efficiently. The same is true of sulphate.

Patients with chronic kidney disease have hypocalcaemia as the kidneys are less efficient at converting 25-hydroxyvitamin D_3 to 1,25-dihydroxyvitamin D_3 (active vitamin D). Hypocalcaemia and hyperphosphataemia leads to increased secretion of parathyroid hormone via a negative feedback loop; secondary hyperparathyroidism, not hypoparathyroidism. Hyperparathyroidism leads to a rise in serum calcium levels through increased renal reabsorption of calcium and increased bone turnover. Furthermore, it decreases serum phosphate by increasing its excretion in the kidney although this is impaired in patients with chronic kidney disease. Patients with chronic kidney disease are at risk of developing a metabolic acidosis, hyperkalaemia and uraemia due to impaired excretion of hydrogen ions, potassium ions and urea, respectively.

3.15

C – Cyclo-oxygenase inhibitors

Podocyte effacement on electron microscopy and normal glomerular appearance on light microscopy is characteristic of minimal change glomerulonephritis. This patient has nephrotic syndrome as a result of the glomerulonephritis. Nephrotic syndrome is a triad of:

- Proteinuria greater than 3.5 g per 24 hours
- Oedema
- Hypoalbuminaemia.

The oedema occurs as a result of hypoalbuminaemia, which reduces oncotic pressure and enables fluid to extravasate from blood vessels.

Patients with nephrotic syndrome should not be given cyclo-oxygenase inhibitors as they prevent the synthesis of prostaglandins from arachidonic acid. In nephrotic syndrome and other situations where acute kidney injury is present, prostaglandins are vital for the maintenance of glomerular perfusion as they cause dilatation of the afferent arteriole, increasing theglomerular filtration rate. Therefore, cyclo-oxygenase inhibitors must not be given in acute kidney injury.

To compensate for a low oncotic pressure in nephrotic syndrome, the liver increases the synthesis of low-density lipoproteins and cholesterol. Therefore, serum lipid levels are raised in nephrotic syndrome and so patients should be commenced on HMG-CoA reductase inhibtors (statins) in order to reduce the risk of developing cardiovascular complications such as atherosclerosis. Factor Xa inhibitors such as enoxaparin and dalteparin should be given in nephrotic syndrome. This is because there is glomerular loss of the protein antithrombin III, which results in the development of a prothrombotic state. Antibiotics should also be given, as there is glomerular loss of complement and immunoglobulins. This leaves the patient at risk of infection, especially from encapsulated bacteria. Corticosteroids are used to induce remission in minimal change glomerulonephritis and should therefore be given in this patient.

3.16

B – Examination of the tympanic membrane

This patient has an acute-onset, unilateral, lower motor neuron lesion of their facial nerve. There are many causes of lower motor neuron facial nerve palsies, with (idiopathic) Bell's palsy being the most common (80%). However, it is essential to exclude Ramsay Hunt syndrome by examining the tympanic membrane for the presence of vesicles. Ramsay Hunt syndrome is caused by infection of the facial nerve (which provides motor and sensory fibres to the ear) by VZV.

In Bell's palsy, prednisolone has been shown to be of benefit in patients who present within 72 hours of the onset of symptoms. Aciclovir is often co-prescribed but continuing evidence of its additional benefit is lacking. Eye lubrication ointment and an eye patch should be offered to patients who cannot close their eye to prevent development of a corneal ulcer. Referral to otolaryngology (the ear, nose and throat specialists) is only indicated if symptoms do not improve within one month, or if the facial nerve palsy is recurrent or bilateral.

3.17

E – Primary hyperparathyroidism

The bone biopsy in this scenario is consistent with osteitis fibrosa cystica, a rare but well-recognised complication of longstanding primary hyperparathyroidism. Raised levels of parathyroid hormone leads to osteoclast activation and increased bone turnover. During this process, collagen fibres are laid down within the bone marrow. If levels of parathyroid hormone remain raised for an elongated period of time, more bone is reabsorbed, and fibrous tissue, macrophages, areas of haemorrhage and reactive woven bone replace the marrow. Eventually cystic degeneration occurs and osteoclast giant cells can be visualised. This type of lesion is also called a brown tumour, which is a misnomer as the tissue is not malignant.

Metastatic bone disease most commonly occurs in breast, prostate, thyroid, lung and renal malignancies. Biopsy of the bone in metastatic disease would show cells from the primary site of the cancer. Multiple myeloma is associated with an increase in osteoclastic bone resorption and a reduction in bone formation. Osteopetrosis is a congenital disorder associated with reduced osteoclast function and bone remodelling. Bone density is increased. Osteoporosis is defined as a bone mineral density of 2.5 or more standard deviation below the mean peak bone mass. Pathological findings include thinly trabeculated, discontinuous lamellar bone.

3.18

B – Normal serum calcium, normal serum phosphate and raised serum alkaline phosphatase

This patient has Paget's disease of bone, a disease characterised by an increase in bone turnover with subsequent bone enlargement, deformation (bowing of the long bones), bone pain and stress fractures. The blood biochemistry of these patients reveals a normal serum calcium, normal serum phosphate and raised serum alkaline phosphatase. The raised serum alkaline phosphatase reflects increased osteoblastic activity. Increased osteoblastic activity causes sclerosis of the bones, which is seen as increased density on X-rays. Patients with Paget's disease can develop deafness as the vestibulocochlear nerve calcifies as it leaves the cranial cavity through the internal auditory meatus. Other complications associated with

Paget's disease include high-output cardiac failure (secondary to arteriovenous connections in the bones) and osteosarcoma. Patients with Paget's disease can very rarely develop hypercalcaemia; this only occurs when patients have had prolonged immobility.

The table below highlights the bone profiles of several different conditions:

	Serum calcium	Serum phosphate	Serum alkaline phosphatase
Osteoporosis	Normal	Normal	Normal
Paget's disease	Normal	Normal	Raised
Primary hyperparathyroidism	Raised	Reduced	Raised
Chronic renal failure	Reduced	Raised	Normal
Osteomalacia and rickets	Reduced	Reduced	Raised

3.19

B – Colchicine

This patient has an acute episode of gout and should initially be commenced on colchicine, an anti-mitotic agent that inhibits micro-tubule formation. Gout is a condition characterised by hyperuri-caemia and formation of negatively birefringent, needle-shaped uric acid crystals when viewed under polarised light.

Indomethacin is a potent NSAID that can also be used in the initial treatment of gout. However, it should not be used in patients with gastro-oesophageal reflux disease because it can worsen symptoms. Steroids can play a role in the management of acute gout. However, their use isn't as widespread as that of colchicine and NSAIDs as their true justification remains to be proven. Xanthine oxidase is a cellular enzyme that catalyses the formation of uric acid from purines. Allopurinol and febuxostat are xanthine oxidase inhibitors that play an important role in reducing serum uric acid in the long term. However, they are contraindicated in the management of acute gout as they initially increase serum urate levels and worsen symptoms before they improve them. Therefore, xanthine oxidase inhibitors should not be introduced until at least three weeks after an acute episode.

3.20

D – Levofloxacin

As this patient is allergic to macrolide antibiotics, clarithromycin should not be prescribed. Therefore the most appropriate treatment is levofloxacin. This antibiotic is a member of the quinolone family of antibiotics and acts by inhibiting bacterial DNA gyrase. Most macrolides (except azithromycin) inhibit the cytochrome P450 isoenzyme CYP3A4, which is the route by which most statins are metabolised. Therefore, the concurrent use of macrolides and statins raises the level of statins to potentially toxic levels, which can cause a myopathy, and in severe cases, rhabdomyolysis. Macrolides must therefore not be co-prescribed to patients with a statin. The most obvious way of avoiding this is by either stopping the statin for the duration of treatment with a macrolide antibiotic or by prescribing an alternative clinically effective antibiotic. In the case of *Mycoplasma pneumoniae* levofloxacin has proven efficacy and is a good alternative to a macrolide antibiotic. *Mycoplasma pneumoniae* is a member of the Mollicute class of bacteria. All members of the Mollicute class of bacteria lack a peptidoglycan cell wall and hence will be unaffected by antibiotics whose mechanism of action occurs at this site.

Amoxicillin (a penicillin) and ceftriaxone (a cephalosporin) are members of the beta-lactam group of antibiotics. They act by inhibiting penicillin-binding proteins, a group of proteins involved in the final stage of cell wall transpeptidation. Vancomycin is a glycopeptide antibiotic that inhibits cell wall synthesis at an earlier stage, by inhibiting polymerisation of the peptides *N*-acetylmuramic acid and *N*-acetylglucosamine.

3.21

E – Upper gastrointestinal endoscopy

This patient's history of multiple telangiectasia, skin tightening, Raynaud's phenomenon and sclerodactyly is highly suggestive of limited cutaneous scleroderma. This patient's dysphagia, which is worse for solids than liquids, suggests she has developed an oesophageal stricture secondary to the scleroderma. Therefore, the most appropriate investigation for this patient is an upper gastro-intestinal endoscopy, which will allow dilatation of the stricture.

Limited cutaneous scleroderma is also known as 'CREST' syndrome, which stands for:

- **C**alcinosis
- **R**aynaud's phenomenon
- o**E**sophageal dysfunction
- **S**clerodactyly
- **T**elangiectasia.

The gastrointestinal tract is the most commonly involved organ system in scleroderma. Patients can develop small bowel dysmotility for which investigation with a barium follow through and treatment with metoclopramide (a prokinetic and antiemetic) is most appropriate. Over 90% of patients with limited cutaneous scleroderma develop oesophageal dysmotility, which is best investigated with a barium swallow and treated with metoclopramide. There is an increased incidence of sicca syndrome and dental caries in scleroderma. Therefore, patients should be investigated with dental radiographs and be given artificial saliva and/or sugar-free chewing gum to reduce dental problems. Oesophageal manometry may be useful if patients complain of gastro-oesophageal reflux. However, treatment with a high-dose proton pump inhibitor without the need for investigation is usually sufficient.

3.22

C – Inclusion body myositis

This patient has inclusion body myositis, which differs from the other inflammatory myopathies (polymyositis and dermatomyositis) because patients present with both proximal and distal muscle weakness, rather than just proximal muscle weakness alone.

The presence of basophilic intracellular vacuoles on muscle biopsy is specific for inclusion body myositis, whereas the markedly increased creatine kinase and characteristic electromyographic changes (low-amplitude, short-duration potentials) are also found in polymyositis and dermatomyositis. Becker's muscular dystrophy occurs due to a mutation on the short arm of the X chromosome, which results in a reduction in production of the muscle protein dystrophin. This is in contrast to the more severe Duchenne's muscular dystrophy, where a frame shift mutation results in an absence in production of dystrophin. Patients with Becker's muscular dystrophy develop a proximal myopathy at a later stage than in Duchenne's muscular dystrophy (as a teenager rather than as a young child). The age of this patient makes the diagnosis of Becker's muscular dystrophy unlikely. Patients with polymyalgia rheumatica present with shoulder and hip girdle pain but do not have any true muscle weakness. It is important to note that any apparent muscle weakness found on testing occurs secondary to pain rather than intrinsic muscle disease.

3.23

D – Praziquantel

This patient has developed acute schistosomiasis, also known as Katayama's fever, following her holiday in Malawi. Common presenting features of acute schistosomiasis include:

- Cough
- Diarrhoea

- Fever
- Fatigue
- Hepatosplenomegaly
- Urticarial rash and eosinophilia.

Patients with acute schistosomiasis should initially be treated with praziquantel, an anti-helminthic agent that is effective against schistosomes. Schistosomes are trematodes that infect fresh water snails and are commonly found in Africa, the Middle East, Southeast Asia, South America and the Caribbean.

Amphotericin is used to treat fungal infections. Co-amoxiclav is used to treat bacterial infections. Metronidazole is a nitroimidazole antibiotic used to treat anaerobic bacterial and protozoal infections. Sodium stibogluconate is a chemotherapeutic agent used to treat leishmaniasis, a protozoal infection.

3.24

C – Jarisch–Herxheimer reaction

This patient has syphilis, due to infection with the spirochaete *Treponema pallidum*. He has developed the Jarisch–Herxheimer reaction as a result of treatment with intramuscular benzathine penicillin, an antibiotic active against treponemes. The Jarisch–Herxheimer reaction describes a combination of fever, myalgia and headache due to an immunologically mediated reaction against endotoxins released from killed bacteria. Occasionally, the primary syphilitic chancre enlarges as part of this reaction. It is usually self-limiting and does not last for more than 24 hours before symptoms recede. However, if symptoms during this period are severe, steroids should be considered. It is important to warn patients about this phenomenon before treatment is commenced.

This reaction is clearly different from allergic reactions as it is not associated with oedema or an erythematous, pruritic rash. Erythema multiforme describes target lesions, which are usually present over the palms, soles and arms. A target lesion consists of three concentric zones of colour change: a central erythematous area surrounded by a pale, oedematous ring, followed by a peripheral ring of erythema. Stevens–Johnson syndrome describes a rare, severe variant of erythema multiforme with fever and mucosal involvement. Patients with EBV do not develop a hypersensitivity reaction following benzathine penicillin administration. This hypersensitivity reaction only occurs with amoxicillin or ampicillin and is characterised by a diffuse maculopapular rash.

3.25

E – Squamous cell carcinoma

This patient has symptoms suggestive of hypercalcaemia and he has a corrected serum calcium of 3.0 mmol/L. This is calculated using the following formula:

$$\text{Corrected serum calcium} = \text{measured serum calcium} + 0.02 (40 - \text{serum albumin}).$$

Squamous cell carcinoma of the lung is associated with the production of parathyroid hormone-related peptide. Increased parathyroid hormone-related peptide leads to a rise in serum calcium levels through increased renal reabsorption of calcium ions and increased bone turnover. The presenting complaint of patients with hypercalcaemia is usually one or more of:

- Stones (renal or biliary colic)
- Bones (bone pain)
- Groans (abdominal pain, nausea and vomiting)
- Moans (fatigue, confusion and depression).

Small cell carcinomas can secrete ectopic adrenocorticotropic hormone and adrenocorticotropic hormone-like substances, which leads to Cushing's syndrome. Unlike most Cushingoid patients, these patients do not gain weight, but instead have a cachectic appearance as malignant cells have a highenergy demand. Small cell carcinoma is also associated with the syndrome of inappropriate antidiuretic hormone and neurological paraneoplastic syndromes such as the Lambert–Eaton myasthenic syndrome. Large cell carcinoma, adenocarcinoma and alveolar cell carcinoma are less associated with paraneoplastic syndromes.

3.26

B – Imipramine

Tricyclic antidepressants such as imipramine can cause ventricular tachycardia and this is the major cause of mortality when taken in overdose. Tricyclic antidepressants inhibit fast sodium channels, which slows depolarisation in the His-Purkinje fibres. This manifests as a reduction in the ventricular conduction rate with resultant prolongation of the QRS complex. This predisposes the patient to the development of re-entry arrhythmias such as ventricular tachycardia, ventricular fibrillation and torsade de pointes. Intravenous sodium bicarbonate is the single most effective intervention for the management of cardiovascular complications of tricyclic antidepressents as it can reverse QRS prolongation, ventricular arrhythmias and hypotension.

The initial symptoms and signs of tricyclic antidepressant overdose are associated with the anticholinergic properties of tricyclics. These include:

- Hyperthermia
- Flushing
- Dilated pupils
- Intestinal ileus
- Urinary retention
- Sinus tachycardia.

Central nervous system involvement is also common and early signs such as confusion, delirium and hallucinations typically occur before the onset of seizures or coma.

Serotonin selective reuptake inhibitors such as fluoxetine, which are also used to treat depression, inhibit CYP450 enzymes important in the metabolism of tricyclic antidepressants. Thus, concurrent use of serotonin selective reuptake inhibitors and tricyclic antidepressants can increase the likelihood of developing cardiac complications associated with tricyclic antidepressants. However, when used on their own, serotonin selective reuptake inhibitors are unlikely to predispose to ventricular arrhythmias. Instead, the major complication of overdosing on serotonin selective reuptake inhibitors is the potential to develop the serotonin syndrome, due to excess serotonin activity. Features include:

- Mental status change (anxiety, delirium)
- Autonomic manifestations (tachycardia, hyperthermia, hypertension, vomiting)
- Neuromuscular hyperactivity (tremor, rigidity, myoclonus, hyperreflexia).

Levothyroxine overdose will result in signs and symptoms of thyrotoxicosis. The cardiac abnormalities associated with thyrotoxicosis include sinus tachycardia, atrial fibrillation and ventricular arrhythmias. However, unlike this patient, ventricular arrhythmias associated with levothyroxine usually occur in patients with underlying cardiac abnormalities. Beta-adrenoreceptor antagonists such as metoprolol will cause bradyarrhythmias and complete heart block if taken in overdose as they reduce the sympathetic drive to the myocardium. NSAIDs such as naproxen are unlikely to cause ventricular arrhythmias in overdose. Overdose of NSAIDs commonly manifests with gastrointestinal disturbances such as diarrhoea, vomiting and heartburn. They also increase the risk of gastrointestinal haemorrhage since they inhibit prostaglandin production in the stomach.

3.27

C – Percutaneous angioplasty of the renal arteries

This patient's history is highly suggestive of fibromuscular dysplasia, an autosomal dominant disorder that mainly affects females aged 15–50 years. It is characterised by arterial stenosis predominantly in the renal arteries, carotid arteries and less commonly the mesenteric arteries. The stenosis occurs due to an abnormal proliferation of vascular endothelial cells and results in the classical 'string of beads' appearance on angiography of the renal arteries. Fibromuscular dysplasia is a cause of secondary hypertension due to distal renal artery stenosis. In comparison, renal artery stenosis secondary to atherosclerosis usually affects the proximal arterioles. The primary aim in the management of renal artery fibromuscular dysplasia is to prevent hypertension. In patients with new-onset hypertension secondary to renal artery fibromuscular dysplasia, percutaneous balloon angioplasty is the preferred initial treatment. This is because the chance of curing patients so that they no longer need to take anti-hypertensive medications is highest when the patient is young and the duration of hypertension is short.

Hypertension secondary to renal artery fibromuscular dysplasia is often successfully treated with balloon angioplasty alone and consequently there is often no need for stent implantation. Percutaneous angioplasty has supplanted surgical revascularisation as the preferred treatment of renal artery fibromuscular dysplasia as it is less invasive, has a markedly shorter recovery time, has fewer complications and can frequently be performed electively onan outpatient basis.

Anti-hypertensives such as amlodipine (a dihydropyridine calcium channel antagonist) can be used to maintain optimal blood pressure control in patients with fibromuscular dysplasia who were not diagnosed at anearly age or who have longstanding hypertension. Irbesartan (an angiotensin II receptor antagonist) is contraindicated in patients with renal artery stenosis. Angiotensin II is a potent vasoconstrictor of the efferent arteriole and irbesartan will reduce this effect. Consequently, when a patient is started on irbesartan there is efferent arteriolar dilation. In normal patients, the afferent arteriole would also dilate to maintain glomerular filtration. However, in patients with renal artery stenosis there is limited afferent arteriole dilation. Patients with renal artery stenosis who commence on irbesartan can therefore develop acute kidney injury within 24 hours of starting the medication.

3.28

B – Faecal calprotectin levels

Diagnostic laparoscopy is indicated in patients with non-specific acute abdominal pain forless than seven days where the diagnosis remains uncertain even after examination and investigation. In this scenario, although the abnormal appearance of the proximal ileum is suggestive of inflammation, further investigations are required to confirm this suspicion. The most appropriate investigation is therefore a faecal calprotectin level. This is a relatively new, simple and uninvasive biochemical test for intestinal inflammation. Raised faecal calprotectin levels may eliminate the need for further invasive investigations such as colonoscopy or radio-labelled white cell scanning. Increased neutrophils are seen at the site of intestinal inflammation and consequently the gold standard measurement of intestinal inflammation is a radio-labelled white cell scan using 111-indium-labelled leukocytes. However, there is a strong correlation between the findings of radio-labelled white cell scanning and faecal calprotectin levels. The main causes of an increased excretion of faecal calprotectin are:

- Infectious colitis
- Crohn's disease
- Ulcerative colitis
- Gastrointestinal malignancy.

In this young patient with abnormal architecture of the proximal ileum, raised faecal calprotectin levels would be highly suggestive of Crohn's disease rather than ulcerative colitis (which only affects the colon). Small bowel follow through is indicated in patients with evidence of Crohn's disease to examine the location and extent of disease in the small bowel. Oral prednisolone is used to induce remission in patients with a known inflammatory bowel disease; however, as corticosteroids do not prevent relapses they are not appropriate for the long-term management of inflammatory bowel disease.

3.29

B – Left circumflex artery

This patient's history and ECG is highly suggestive of an ST elevation myocardial infarction, which is most likely to be as a result of occlusion to the left circumflex artery. A standard ECG has 12 leads which each cover the electrical conduction of the myocardium from a different perspective. These also correlate to different anatomical areas of the heart. The major anatomical territories are anterolateral, anteroseptal, inferior, lateral and posterior. Anatomical territories are important in acute coronary ischaemia as each territory is supplied by a different coronary artery and represented by different leads on the ECG. The table below shows which leads correspond to which anatomical location and the coronary artery affected:

Anatomical location	ECG changes	Coronary artery affected
Anterolateral	I, aVL, V_4–V_6	Left main stem
Anteroseptal	V_1–V_4	Left anterior descending
Inferior	II, III and aVF	Right coronary
Lateral	I, aVL, +/– V_5 and V_6	Left circumflex
Posterior	Tall R waves in V_1 and V_2	Usually left circumflex but can be right coronary

3.30

D – Transthoracic echocardiogram

Patients with metastatic cancer are prothrombotic and as a result this patient is likely to have suffered from a pulmonary embolism.

The patient's observations in this scenario are suggestive of haemo-dynamic instability and the most appropriate investigation to perform is an urgent transthoracic echocardiogram. In patients with a suspected pulmonary embolism presenting with shock or hypotension, the absence of echocardiographic signs of right ventricular dysfunction excludes a pulmonary embolism as a cause of haemo-dynamic instability. Conversely, in a patient with likely pulmonary embolism and haemodynamically instability, the presence of right ventricular dysfunction is highly suggestive of a pulmonary embolism and may therefore justify the need for urgent thrombolysis. Furthermore, echocardiography is quick, can be performed at the bedside of an acutely unwell patient and may help in the differential diagnosis of the cause of shock (e.g. by detecting cardiac tamponade or acute myocardial infarction).

The gold standard investigation used to confirm the diagnosis of a pulmonary embolism is CT pulmonary angiography. It will typically show filling defects in the pulmonary vessels when contrast is injected. Although CT pulmonary angiography could be used in this patient, the practicalities make echocardiography more appropriate. Unlike a CT pulmonary angiography, echocardiography can be performed urgently at the patient's bedside. Furthermore, placing a haemodynamically unstable patient in a CT scanner is high risk as the patient may deteriorate during the scan.

CT pulmonary angiography is generally avoided during pregnancy due to the high doses of radiation to the mother's breast tissue. It is also contraindicated in patients who are allergic to contrast or have impaired renal function. In these situations a ventilation-perfusion scan is the preferred choice of investigation. A ventilation-perfusion scan is as accurate as a CT pulmonary angiography but is often used less due to the widespread availability of CT scanners.

A D-dimer may be performed in patients who have a low likelihood of having a pulmonary embolism based on history and examination. This is because D-dimer is highly sensitive for a thrombotic event as it is a fibrin degradation product. As a result, a negative D-dimer will essentially rule out the presence of thrombosis. However, D-dimer is not a very specific test and is raised in many other conditions (e.g. malignancy). Therefore, a positive result is not necessarily indicative of thrombosis. As a diagnostic test for pulmonary embolism, chest X-ray is neither sensitive nor specific. The main use of a chest X-ray is to exclude other causes of shortness of breath and pleuritic chest pain when the diagnosis was uncertain (e.g. malignancy, pneumothorax).

3.31

E – Panacinar emphysema

This patient with obstructive lung disease and history of liver cirrhosis is most likely to have alpha 1-antitrypsin deficiency. The characteristic histological finding on lung biopsyis panacinar emphysema. Alpha 1-antitrypsin deficiency is an autosomal recessive disorder caused by defective production of alpha 1-antitrypsin, leading to decreased antitrypsin activity in the lungs, and deposition of excessive abnormal antitrypsin protein in liver cells.

Trypsins are digestive enzymes that break down elastase, which is needed for the elastic recoil of the lung. Therefore, inhibition of trypsin (by anti-trypsin) is required to maintain elastase within the lung. Antitrypsin deficiency results in loss of trypsin inhibition and excess elastase breakdown. Causes of antitrypsin deficiency can be genetic (e.g. alpha 1-antitrypsin deficiency) or environmental (e.g. cigarette smoke). The reduction in elastase decreases the ability of the lungs to recoil and as a result there is air trapping in the terminal bronchioles/alveoli (referred to as emphysema). In alpha 1-antitrypsin deficiency there is destruction of all parts of the acinus — referred to as panacinar emphysema. Centrilobular emphysema refers to destruction of the respiratory bronchioles.

The genotype of patients with alpha 1-antitrypsin deficiency will determine the severity of the disease. Patients with the PiSS, PiMZ and PiSZ genotypes of alpha 1-antitrypsin have approximately 50% of normal enzyme levels and this is usually sufficient to protect the lungs from the effects of trypsin in people who do not smoke. However, in patients with the more severe PiZZ genotype, antitrypsin levels are only 15% of normal. These patients will develop emphysema in their thirties and forties even in the absence of cigarette smoking.

Interstitial lung fibrosis typically causes a restrictive pattern on spirometry. This is because the interstitium (tissue surrounding the alveoli) is fibrotic and the alveoli cannot fully expand. Interstitial lung fibrosis is thought to be as a result of chronic interstitial inflammation, of which there are multiple causes. This inflammation then leads to fibroblast activation and proliferation. Finally, this progresses to the common endpoint of pulmonary fibrosis and tissue destruction.

Charcot–Leyden crystals are microscopic crystals consisting of lysophospholipase, an enzyme synthesised by eosinophils. Consequently, Charcot–Leyden crystals are found in people who have bronchial eosinophilia such as in asthma, parasitic infections or rarely eosinophilic granulomatosis with polyangiitis.

Non-caseating granulomas are a collection of macrophages surrounding a non-necrotised centre and can be seen in a variety of inflammatory conditions. The classical example of a non-caseating granuloma affecting the lungs is sarcoidosis. Caseating granulomas are collections of macrophages with a necrotic core and are typically seen in patients with tuberculosis.

3.32

C – Surgical referral

This patient has a perianal abscess complicating their Crohn's disease. A fistula is defined as an abnormal communication between two epithelial surfaces. In this patient the fistula has occurred between the skin and the anus. Fistulae can also occur between the anus or rectum and other organs, including the vagina, bladder or small bowel. Roughly 30 to 50% of patients with Crohn's disease will develop perianal fistulae. One of the major complications of a perianal fistula is the development of a perianal abscess, which typically presents with acute perianal pain, pruritus and discharge from the fistula. Occasionally, systemic symptoms may be present. There is no role for medical management in patients with a perianal abscess. The most appropriate management for this patient is urgent surgical referral to eliminate perineal sepsis and treat fistula tracts, with the least possible risk to the patient's continence.

Once acute sepsis has been eliminated, fistulae may be medically treated, especially if proctitis (inflammation of the anus and rectal lining) is present. Proctitis results in poor wound healing and therefore medical management should be initiated. Patients with Crohn's disease who have asymptomatic fistulae can be managed conservatively. Medical management is indicated when patients develop symptoms but do not have a perianal abscess or severe infection. Antibiotics such as metronidazole (a nitroimidazole) and ciprofloxacin (a quinolone) often represent the first-line medical treatment for Crohn's fistulae. It is unclear whether antibiotics are effective due to their anti-microbial action or whether they also have an ability to cause immunosuppression. In addition to antibiotics, many immunosuppressive agents have proven efficacy in the treatment of Crohn's fistulae. Infliximab (a TNF alpha antagonist) can be commenced once the fistula is controlled with surgery and antibiotics. Topical nitroglycerin (a nitrate) and topical diltiazem (calcium channel antagonist) are not used in the management of fistulae. Instead they are used in the management of idiopathic fissures (tears or splits in the distal anal canal).

3.33

A – Addison's disease

Addison's disease occurs as a result of adrenal insufficiency of cortisol and aldosterone and is associated with a mild eosinophilia in 10% of patients. In the United Kingdom, the most common cause of Addison's disease is autoimmune destruction of the adrenal cortex. Addison's disease often presents with non-specific clinical features including excessive fatigue, weight loss, abdominal pain and weakness. On examination there may be areas of hyperpigmentation. This is most prominent in the palmar creases, the buccal mucosa and underneath bra-strap lines in females. Hyperpigmentation occurs because melanocyte-stimulating hormone and adrenocorticotropic hormone share the same precursor molecule. This precursor is known as pro-opiomelanocortin, which gets cleaved in the anterior pituitary gland to produce adrenocorticotropic hormone and gamma melanocyte-stimulating hormone (which induces skin pigmentation). In Addison's disease there is increased production of adrenocorticotropic hormone in an attempt to stimulate the adrenal glands and therefore increased cleavage of pro-opiomelanocortin.

Patients with Addison's disease tend to develop a hyperkalaemic, hyponatraemic metabolic acidosis. This is because low levels of aldosterone result in increased excretion of sodium ions from the collecting ducts and increased reabsorption of potassium and hydrogen ions. The hyponatraemia results in increased water loss due to a direct osmotic effect in the kidneys. This increased water loss leads to the development of postural hypotension in these patients. Additionally, Addisonian patients may suffer from hypoglycaemia, as cortisol antagonises the actions of insulin.

Several other causes of eosinophilia are known, with two of the most common being allergy or multicellular parasitic infections. Giardia and amoeba are both unicellular protozoa and therefore do not result in an eosinophilia. Granulomatosis with polyangiitis (Wegener's granulomatosis) is a small- to medium-vessel necrotising, granulomatous vasculitis and is not associated with eosinophilia. Eosinophilic granulomatosis with polyangiitis (Churg–Strauss syndrome) is another small- to medium-vessel vasculitis, which is associated with an eosinophilia. Type I diabetes mellitus can present with lethargy and weight loss but patients will often also present with polydipsia and polyuria. Type I diabetes mellitus is not associated with an eosinophilia.

3.34

A – Diabetic amyotrophy

This patient with type II diabetes mellitus is most likely to have developed diabetic amyotrophy as a result of his poor glycaemic control. Diabetic amyotrophy is characterised by pain followed by marked, usually asymmetrical wasting of the quadriceps. The painful, wasted area is usually exquisitely tender to palpation. Improvement of glycaemic control often results in resolution of symptoms.

Diabetic sensorimotor polyneuropathy is predominantly sensory in nature; early signs include loss of vibration sensation, which is followed by loss of pain and temperature sensation. The longest nerves are affected first, which means that sensation is impaired distally to start with, before being affected proximally. Motor neuropathy occurs later, and results in wasting of the small muscles of the feet. This, combined with traction by the long flexor muscles, leads to clawing of the toes and a high arch. This abnormal foot shape alters the pressure points on the sole and results in callus formation and perforating neuropathic ulceration. Meralgia paraesthetica is a mononeuropathy of the lateral femoral cutaneous nerve that is more common in patients who experience rapid increase (nerve compression from tight clothing) or decrease in weight (loss of protection from subcutaneous fat). They present with pain, tingling or numbness in the anterolateral thigh, most commonly due to entrapment of the nerve as it passes through the inguinal ligament. Prolonged standing and strenuous leg exercises are also risk factors, due to increased tension of the inguinal ligament. As the lateral femoral cutaneous nerve is a pure sensory nerve it is not associated with muscle wasting. Obturator nerve palsy rarely occurs in isolation and most commonly occurs secondary to pelvic trauma and associated fractures, during childbirth or as a result of compression by a pelvic tumour. Patients develop medial thigh pain and wasting of the adductor muscles. Patients with polymyalgia rheumatica present with shoulder and hip girdle pain but do not have any true muscle weakness; any apparent muscle weakness found on examination occurs secondary to pain not intrinsic muscle disease.

3.35

B – Hypercalcaemia

This patient's history of polyuria and polydipsia in the absence of hyperglycaemia is highly suggestive of diabetes insipidus, of which the most likely cause in this patient is hypercalcaemia-induced nephrogenic diabetes insipidus. Patients with diabetes insipidus are unable to concentrate their urine and this can be due to either a lack of antidiuretic hormone release from the posterior pituitary gland (cranial diabetes insipidus) or an inability for the kidneys to respond to antidiuretic hormone (nephrogenic diabetes insipidus). To distinguish between the two, patients undergo a fluid deprivation test, which involves restricting fluid intake and monitoring urine osmolality. In patients with diabetes insipidus, urine osmolality will remain low despite lack of fluid intake (i.e. urine remains paradoxically dilute). Patients are then given a bolus of synthetic antidiuretic hormone (desmopressin). Patients with nephrogenic diabetes insipidus cannot respond to antidiuretic hormone, and therefore this will have little effect on urine osmolality. Patients with cranial diabetes insipidus will respond, and therefore the urine osmolality will increase after the desmopressin bolus. The table below highlights the results of the fluid deprivation test in patients with cranial andnephrogenic diabetes insipidus.

Type of diabetes insipidus	Urine osmolality in mOsm/kg, after fluid deprivation	Urine osmolality in mOsm/kg, after desmopressin bolus
Cranial	<300	>800
Nephrogenic	<300	<300

This patient has a low urine osmolality after both fluid deprivation and the desmopressin bolus, which suggests a diagnosis of nephrogenic diabetes insipidus. There are many causes of nephrogenic diabetes insipidus with acquired causes accounting for the vast majority of cases. Hypercalcaemia is a well-recognised cause and is the most likely diagnosis in this patient. Hypokalaemia (not hyperkalaemia) is also another electrolyte imbalance that can result in nephrogenic diabetes insipidus. Other important causes of acquired nephrogenic diabetes insipidus include lithium administration, amyloidosis and polycystic kidney disease.

Patients with a pituitary macroadenoma or craniopharyngioma may develop cranial rather than nephrogenic diabetes insipidus. A craniopharyngioma is a benign slow-growing tumour that arises from remnants of Rathke's pouch (an embryonic precursor of the anterior pituitary gland). A large pituitary mass may compress the infundibulum (pituitary stalk), which connects the hypothalamus with the pituitary gland. Compression of the infundibulum will stop antidiuretic hormone produced in the supra-optic nucleus of the hypothalamus from reaching the posterior pituitary. It is the posterior pituitary from which antidiuretic hormone enters the bloodstream to exert its effects on the kidneys.

Patients with diabetes mellitus may present with polyuria and polydipsia. However, this patient is unlikely to have diabetes mellitus as the fasting blood glucose of 5.9 mmol/L is within normal limits.

3.36

E – Von Hippel–Lindau syndrome

This patient has cerebellar signs, adrenergic symptoms and polycythaemia. The most likely diagnosis is von Hippel–Lindau syndrome. This is an autosomal dominant condition due to mutations in the *VHL* gene on chromosome 3. It results in the development of haemangioblastomas, which are central nervous system tumours that originate from the vascular system. Haemangioblastomas usually show a preference for the cerebellum, accounting for this patient's right-sided cerebellar signs. Ectopic erythropoietin production is a known complication of haemangioblastomas and can result in polycythaemia (a risk factor for arterial and venous thrombosis). This patient's history of intermittent flushing, headache and palpitations is suggestive of episodic sympathetic overactivation. The most likely cause is phaeochromocytoma, which is one of the recognised features of von Hippel–Lindau syndrome. Phaeochromocytoma is a neuroendocrine tumour of the adrenal medulla that oversecretes catecholamines (e.g. adrenaline). Patients with von Hippel–Lindau syndrome can also develop renal cell carcinoma and cysts in the liver, kidney and pancreas.

Neurofibromatosis type I is caused by a mutation in the gene which encodes the protein neurofibromin. Patients with neurofibromatosis type I typically develop neurocutaneous signs including more than six café au lait spots and axillary/inguinal freckling. They can also develop Lisch nodules in the eye, which are pigmented hamartomatous nodular aggregates of dendritic melanocytes in the iris. Other features of neurofibromatosis type I include phaeochromocytomas and neurofibromas (benign tumours that arise from non-myelinating-type Schwann cells).

Multiple endocrine neoplasia type II is a genetic cancer syndrome characterised by phaeochromocytoma and medullary cell carcinoma of the thyroid. It is subdivided into multiple endocrine neoplasia type IIa (where there is also hyperparathyroidism) and type IIb (where there is also a marfanoid habitus and submucosal neurofibromata of the tongue, eyelids and lips).

Birt–Hogg–Dubé syndrome is a rare autosomal dominant disorder caused by mutations in the flocculin gene. It presents with a classical triad of:

- Benign growths of hair follicles particularly on the face, neck and chest
- Pulmonary cysts and spontaneous pneumothorax
- Bilateral renal tumours.

3.37

B – Aggregation of cytoplasmic alpha-synuclein

This patient has the classical features of Lewy body dementia: new-onset inattentiveness and visual hallucinations. This type of dementia is characterised histologically by the formation of Lewy bodies, which are cytoplasmic aggregations of the protein alpha-synuclein within the cytoplasm of neurons and glia. These aggregations are also associated with Parkinson's disease, a disease which is itself associated with Lewy body dementia.

A common feature of all neurodegenerative diseases is the accumulation of misfolded proteins either intracellularly (nucleus and cytoplasm) or extracellularly. Cytoplasmic TDP-43 is associated with non-hereditary and hereditary motor neuron disease. In contrast to TDP-43, aggregation of cytoplasmic SOD1 is associated almost invariably with hereditary forms of motor neuron disease. Aggregation of cytoplasmic tau protein (fibrils) and extracellular beta amyloid (plaques) are the neuropathological hallmarks of Alzheimer's disease.

3.38

D – Posterior communicating artery aneurysm

This patient has a surgical oculomotor nerve palsy and the most likely diagnosis is a posterior communicating artery aneurysm. The oculomotor nerve has a motor and parasympathetic component, which arise from the brainstem oculomotor nuclear and Edinger–Westphal nucleus, respectively. The somatic fibres control the striated muscle in levator palpebrae superioris along with all the extraocular muscles except for the superior oblique muscle and the lateral rectus muscle. The parasympathetic fibres responsible for pupillary constriction travel with the somatic fibres. Importantly, the parasympathetic fibres are superficial to the somatic fibres along the course of the oculomotor nerve.

Broadly speaking, oculomotor nerve palsies are either surgical or medical. Surgical causes of oculomotor nerve palsies are due to compressive lesions along the path of the nerve. Medical oculomotor nerve palsies occur as a consequence of a systemic disease that can cause a peripheral neuropathy. Surgical oculomotor nerve palsies commonly present with parasympathetic dysfunction (seen clinically as a dilated pupil) whereas medical causes more frequently present with failure of the somatic fibres. This is because parasympathetic fibres are most superficial and compressive lesions will initially impinge on these. Posterior communicating artery aneurysms are the most common cause of a surgical oculomotor nerve palsy because when the oculomotor nerve emerges from the brain it passes in close proximity to the posterior communicating artery.

In medical causes of an oculomotor nerve palsy, the blood vessels that supply the somatic fibres (the vasa nervorum) are affected by a systemic disease such as diabetes. The superficial parasympathetic fibres have a different blood supply and are not affected. Consequently, these patients present with extraocular and levator palpebrae muscle paralysis due to loss of somatic fibres. The most common cause of a medical oculomotor nerve palsy is diabetes mellitus. Other causes include systemic lupus erythematosus and vasculitis.

The oculomotor nerve runs along the lateral wall of the cavernous sinus, together with the trochlear nerve and the ophthalmic division of the trigeminal nerve (cranial nerve V_1). The abducens nerve and internal carotid artery run free in the cavernous sinus. The cavernous sinuses run bilateral to the pituitary fossa. Lesions of the cavernous sinus such as a cavernous sinus thrombosis, or very rarely pituitary apoplexy (infarction of an existing pituitary adenoma), may produce an oculomotor nerve palsy. However, this is unlikely to occur in isolation and, as a result, cavernous sinus lesions tend to cause a complex ophthalmoplegia.

Weber's syndrome is a cause of a complete unilateral third nerve palsy with a contralateral hemiparesis. It is due to a midbrain infarction as a result of occlusion of the paramedian branches of the posterior cerebral artery.

3.39

A – Acute intermittent porphyria

The most likely diagnosis in this patient is acute intermittent porphyria, a metabolic disorder that affects the production of haem. It is caused by porphobilinogen deaminase deficiency, an enzyme usually required for the synthesis of haem. Without porphobilinogen deaminase, the precursors porphobilinogen and amino-laevulinic acid accumulate in the cytoplasm. These metabolites are neurotoxic. Features of acute intermittent porphyria include peripheral and autonomic neuropathies, as well as psychiatric symptoms. Unlike other porphyrias, a photosensitive rash is not a typical feature of acute intermittent porphyria. Acute intermittent porphyria usually manifests with episodic attacks of symptoms. Patients are symptom free between attacks. Chemicals or situations that increase the rate of haem synthesis can precipitate attacks. This includes fasting and many medications such as sulphonamides, barbiturates and phenytoin. One of the main features of an attack is the presence of neurovisceral symptoms, which occur predominantly due to autonomic neuropathies. The neurovisceral symptoms consist of constipation, colicky abdominal pain, vomiting and hypertension. Acute intermittent porphyria is a well-recognised cause of the acute medical abdomen, for which the differential diagnosis includes acute pancreatitis, appendicitis and cholecystitis. However, peripheral neuropathy would not be associated with surgical causes of the acute abdomen.

The peripheral neuropathy in patients with acute intermittent porphyria usually occurs in the upper limbs. It is episodic in nature and acute in onset, and predominantly affects motor fibres. Although the neuropathies usually occur in the upper limbs, they can be observed in any nerve distribution and may mimic Guillain–Barré syndrome (an acute inflammatory demyelinating polyneuropathy which presents with ascending weakness).

Psychiatric symptoms are common in patients with acute intermittent porphyria. Patients may present with episodes of depression although other psychiatric symptoms can occur (e.g. anxiety, agitation, hallucinations, hysteria or delirium).

Acute intermittent porphyria is a known cause of the syndrome of inappropriate antidiuretic hormone and patients may therefore have hyponatraemia. The most important investigation to perform in patients with suspected acute intermittent porphyria is a urinary porphyrin screen. However, it is important to remember that porphobilinogen (a porphyrin precursor) is usually not included in a urine porphyrin screen and must be ordered specially.

3.40

D – Normal pressure hydrocephalus

The most likely diagnosis in this patient is normal pressure hydrocephalus, which occurs due to abnormal accumulation of cerebrospinal fluid in the ventricles. Affected patients have a normal intracranial pressure and therefore do not present with the classical symptoms of raised intracranial pressure (e.g. headache, nausea, vomiting, altered consciousness). Instead, the enlarged ventricles put increased pressure on the adjacent cortical tissue and result in a triad of:

- Gait disturbance
- Urinary incontinence
- Dementia.

Gait disturbance is the most prominent initial feature, and occurs because of ventricular compression of the corticospinal tract as it travels from the motor cortex to the spinal cord. The disturbance is sometimes referred to as magnetic gait in which the feet appear to be stuck to the ground. Urinary incontinence occurs late in the disease and is associated with urgency. It occurs due to decreased bladder inhibition by autonomic fibres, which results in detrusor muscle instability. The dementia is predominantly frontal lobe and subcortical in nature, presenting with apathy, forgetfulness, inertia, inattention and decreased speed of complex information processing. It is thought to be due to compression on frontal and limbic fibres that run in the periventricular region. Normal pressure hydrocephalus can be treated surgically with a ventriculoperitoneal shunt to drain excess cerebrospinal fluid; around 20% of patients show an improvement after the procedure.

The progressive cognitive decline seen in patients with normal pressure hydrocephalus is often mistaken for other more common forms of dementia like Alzheimer's disease, vascular dementia, Lewy body dementia and fronto-temporal lobe dementia. Alzheimer's disease is the most common form of non-reversible dementia with the most common early symptom being an inability to remember recent events. As the disease progresses symptoms can include confusion, irritability, mood swings, progressive aphasia and long-term memory loss. Gait disturbance and incontinence are less typical features of the early stages of Alzheimer's disease. A CT scan of patients with Alzheimer's disease may reveal enlarged ventricles (due to atrophied cerebral hemispheres); however, for the same reason the sulci are usually prominent. In this patient, the sulci are absent because the increased cerebrospinal fluid in the ventricles is causing them to be compressed.

The major features of Lewy body dementia include visual hallucinations, REM sleep disorders, fluctuating cognition and variations in attentiveness.It is associated with Parkinson's disease but is distinguished from the dementia that occurs in Parkinson's disease by the time frame in which dementia symptoms appear relative to Parkinson symptoms. Lewy body dementia is diagnosed when the cognitive symptoms occur at the same time or within a year of Parkinson's disease whereas if the diagnosis of dementia occurs more than one year after the onset of Parkinson's disease it is referred to as Parkinson's disease with dementia.

Creutzfeldt–Jakob disease causes a rapidly progressive dementia, which leads to memory loss, personality changes and hallucinations. This is also accompanied by physical symptoms including myoclonus and speech impairment. It occurs due to an aggregation of an abnormal variant of the prion protein throughout the brain. The abnormal variant of the prion protein is infectious and can be transmitted from human to human via contaminated human brain products, immunoglobulins, corneal grafts and contaminated blood products. Creutzfeldt–Jakob disease is usually fatal within six months to two years of onset.

3.41

E – Tolterodine

This patient has developed a spastic, hypercontractile bladder secondary to multiple sclerosis. The most appropriate medication is tolterodine, an anticholinergic medication that inhibits detrusor muscle activity, and so improves bladder capacity and retention of urine.

Clonidine is an alpha-2-adrenoreceptor agonist, which is very rarely used to treat hypertension. Desmopressin is an antidiuretic hormone analogue that acts to reduce urine production and can be used in the shortterm to reduce urge incontinence symptoms. Desmopressin can also be used in:

- Patients with cranial diabetes insipidus
- Children with nocturnal enuresis
- Patients with factor VIII deficiency.

Fluoxetine is a selective serotonin reuptake inhibitor used to treat depression. Rivastigmine is an acetylcholinesterase inhibitor used in the treatment of mild to moderate dementia. As it is a cholinergic agent, it acts to increase detrusor muscle activity and therefore would worsen urge incontinence.

3.42

A – Allopurinol

This patient has developed an acute episode of gout and allopurinol should not be prescribed. This is because in acute attacks allopurinol can actually cause a transient rise in uric acid levels and consequently prolong the length of an acute attack. The patient is also taking azathioprine (see below).

Patients are usually prescribed a strong NSAID (e.g. indomethacin or naproxen) during an acute attack to reduce the inflammation of the affected joint. If NSAIDs are contraindicated, e.g. the patient has cardiac failure or a history of peptic ulcer disease, then colchicine can be prescribed. Colchicine is an anti-mitotic agent that inhibits microtubule formation. Anti-mitotic medications such as colchicine affect rapidly dividing cells and can therefore cause:

- Gastrointestinal disturbances, e.g. diarrhoea
- Bone marrow suppression
- Hair loss
- Rashes.

These side effects are more likely to occur at higher doses, in overdose or in patients on long-term colchicine therapy.

Paracetamol is rarely useful in acute gout, as it has no anti-inflammatory properties.

In patients with repeated attacks of gout, allopurinol can be prescribed. It inhibits xanthine oxidase and consequently reduces uric acid production. However, caution should be taken whenco-prescribing allopurinoland azathioprine. Azathioprine is metabolised by two enzymes, xanthine oxidase and thiopurine methyltransferase. If the activity of either of these enzymes is reduced by drugs or by various genetic polymorphisms, then patients are at risk of developing azathioprine toxicity. Consequently, allopurinol is best avoided in patients taking azathioprine. Thiopurine methyltransferase levels should also be measured before commencing a patient on azathioprine as 10% of the population has reduced activity of this enzyme.

3.43

B – Creatine kinase MB

Creatine kinase, the enzyme that catalyses the phosphorylation of creatine to creatine phosphate, is made of two polypeptide chains. Each can be a B or an M chain. There are therefore three different creatine kinase isoenzyme combinations: MM, BB and MB. Although many tissues contain different levels of each, cardiac muscle is the only tissue to contain over 5% creatine kinase MB isoenzyme (20–30%). Creatine kinase MB is therefore a more specific indicator for cardiac muscle damage than other isoenzymes. Following a myocardial infarction creatine kinase MB is detectable at 4–6 hours and remains elevated until 24–36 hours. On the other hand, troponin I has a longer half-life; it remains elevated for 3–10 days. This gives troponinI a wider diagnostic window (they can diagnose patients who present late) but the shorter half-life makes creatine kinase MB more appropriate for detecting re-infarction, as has occurred in this scenario.

B-type natriuretic peptide is a protein secreted from the ventricular cardiomyocytes in response to stretch, and results in natriuresis, reduced vascular resistance and reduced central venous pressure. It is a specific biomarker of acute congestive heart failure. Serum lactate levels increase when there is increased production (any cause of tissue hypoxia) or impaired hepatic metabolism (liver impairment). Procalcitonin is a precursor to calcitonin that is produced in the parafollicular C-cells of the thyroid. Levels are high in medullary thyroid carcinoma; however, procalcitonin is also secreted from pulmonary and gastrointestinal neuroendocrine tissue in response to bacterial inflammation. Levels do not seem to increase in response to viral infection or non-infectious inflammatory stimuli such as autoimmune and chronic inflammatory conditions. Although research is ongoing, serum procalcitonin may be useful to risk stratify patients with bacterial sepsis, to distinguish bacterial from viral infections (e.g. meningitis), to monitor response to antibiotic therapy and to aid diagnosis of infection in previously non-infective necrosis (e.g. acute pancreatitis). It has no use in the diagnosis of myocardial infarction.

3.44

A – Cotton wool spots

Retinal ischaemia results in formation of cotton wool spots, venous looping and new vessel formation (neovascularisation). Cotton wool spots are fluffy white retinal patches that are due to accumulation of axonoplasmic material within the nerve fibre layer as a consequence of ischaemia. Diabetes mellitus and hypertension are the two commonest causes of cotton wool spots.

'Dots' are retinal venous microaneurysms. If these microaneurysms rupture in the deeper layers of the retina then 'blots' form. If they rupture in the superficial layers then flame-shaped haemorrhages form. Silver wiring is due to arteriosclerosis secondary to hypertension.

3.45

B – Biguanide

Metformin is the most widely used biguanide, and acts to increase sensitivity of the peripheral tissues to insulin and inhibit hepatic gluconeogenesis. It has no effect on insulin secretion and is therefore not associated with a significant risk of hypoglycaemia. It is for this reason it is preferentially used in obese patients because it does not increase insulin release and therefore does not cause weight gain (insulin is an anabolic hormone). Sulphonylureas and glinides increase insulin release by binding to and closing the ATP-sensitive potassium channel in the pancreatic beta islet cell, just as ATP does in response to a physiological increase in blood glucose. Therefore, much like insulin analogues, sulphonylureas and glinides do increase the risk of hypoglycaemia and do cause weight gain. Beta-adrenoreceptor-antagonists can be dangerous in diabetes mellitus as they can antagonise the hyperglycaemic effects of adrenaline, contributing to hypoglycaemia. They can also mask the adrenergic symptoms of hypoglycaemia.

3.46

E – Primary sclerosing cholangitis

Five percent of patients with ulcerative colitis have co-existing primary sclerosing cholangitis and 70% of patients with primary sclerosing cholangitis have ulcerative colitis. Primary sclerosing cholangitis is a rare autoimmune condition that causes inflammation and progressive sclerosis of both the intra- and extra-hepatic bile ducts, leading to a characteristic 'beads on a string' appearance on endoscopic retrograde cholangiopancreatography. The typical patient is a middle-aged male, and pANCA is present in 80% of cases. Ultimately, primary sclerosing cholangitis can progress to portal tract fibrosis, portal hypertension and liver failure.

In this patient, progressive sclerosis has caused cholestasis (jaundice and pruritus) and cholangitis (fever and rigors). In the presence of conjugated hyperbilirubinaemia, patients develop pale stools and dark urine. In addition, malabsorption of lipids in primary sclerosing cholangitis can lead to deficiencies in the fat-soluble vitamins (vitamins A, D, E and K). The patient needs urgent admission for broad-spectrum intravenous antibiotics, as well asurgent imaging of the biliary system to confirm the diagnosis and exclude other causes of obstructive jaundice. There is no proven treatment that slows down the progression of primary sclerosing cholangitis. Liver transplantation is the definitive treatment of choice.

3.47

E – Remain upright for 30 minutes after each dose of alendronic acidand eat and drink nothing except water

Alendronic acid is a bisphosphonate and acts to reduce osteoclast activity. It is used first-line in the treatment of osteoporosis and is taken as a once-weekly medication. One of the adverse effects of bisphosphonates isoesophageal irritation, inflammation and ulceration, and therefore as a precautionthe patient should be told to remain upright for 30 minutes after taking each dose. Other adverse effects of bisphosphonates include atrial fibrillation, osteonecrosis of the jaw and unusual femoral fractures. These so-called bisphosphonate fractures occur in the diaphysis or sub-trochanteric region and are thought to be due to over-suppression of bone turnover, impaired bone repair and subsequent propagation of microfractures.

Bisphosphonates should be taken 30 minutes before a meal (usually breakfast) because their absorption is affected by food, especially milk and dairy products, and other medications, most notably those containing polyvalent cations, such as calcium (e.g. Calcichew D3 Forte®), magnesium, iron and aluminium. Most experts advise that bisphosphonates should be taken for five years before reassessing osteoporotic fragility fracture risk.

3.48

D – Pericarditis

Pericarditis is inflammation of the pericardial sac usually caused by viral infection; pericardial inflammation initially reduces the amount of pericardial fluid, allowing the heart to rub against the pericardium, causing a characteristic sharp (similar to pleuritic) chest pain and a rustling on auscultation (pericardial friction rub). As the condition progresses, there is an overproduction of serous fluid, which accumulates and can reduce the ability of the heart to expand, causing cardiac tamponade.

Pneumonia can cause pleuritic chest pain and a pleural rub; however, in pneumonia it would be unlikely for the pain to be central and for breath sounds to be normal. Pancreatitis and gastro-oesophageal reflux are also more symptomatic on lying flat but do not cause a friction rub. Finally, it is always important to exclude myocardial infarction as the cause of acute-onset central chest pain;

however, the pain associated with a myocardial infarction is typically neither sharp nor pleuritic in nature.

3.49

D – Terlipressin

This patient has an acute variceal bleed. After acute resuscitation and endoscopy, the next priority is terlipressin, a fast-acting vasopressin analogue.

Most oesophageal venous blood is drained from the oesophageal veins, via the azygous vein into the superior vena cava. However, some blood drains into the superficial submucosal veins that in turn drain, via the left gastric vein, into the portal vein. Increased portal pressures (such as those that occur in liver cirrhosis) are therefore transmitted into the superficial veins, which become engorged. These veins cannot cope with the high pressures, leaving them prone to rupture. Other collateral circulations in the abdominal wall, stomach, duodenum and rectum can also dilate in patients with portal hypertension. In patients who are suspected to have oesophageal variceal haemorrhage, immediate resuscitation is vital because their risk of bleeding is compounded by their impaired ability to synthesise hepatic clotting factors. After resuscitation and repletion of circulating volume an upper gastrointestinal endoscopy should be ordered immediately for attempted band ligation or sclerotherapy. If endoscopy is not immediately available then the most appropriate medical management is terlipressin, a prodrug that is slowly metabolised to lypressin, an antidiuretic hormone (vasopressin) analogue. In comparison to vasopressin, terlipressin is longer acting and can therefore be given as a bolus rather than an infusion. Terlipressin also produces fewer side effects of systemic vasoconstriction, an important physiologic effect of ADH to compensate for hypovolaemia. ADH analogues act to constrict the splanchnic circulation, reducing portal flow and therefore portal venous pressures. This results in lower levels of variceal bleeding.

Somatostatin and octreotide (a somatostatin analogue) also act to reduce portal venous pressures; however, the evidence for terlipressin is more convincing. Propranolol is a non-selective beta-adrenoreceptor antagonist and splanchnic vasoconstrictor, which in addition to isosorbide mononitrate can be given to reduce portal venous pressures and therefore reduce the risk of re-bleeding in patients with known oesophageal varices. They are, however, not given in the acute management of oesophageal variceal haemorrhage. Finally, although the routine administration of short-term prophylactic broad-spectrum antibiotics (e.g. ciprofloxacin or a third-generation cephalosporin) over 'on demand' antibiotics does improve mortality and reduce the risk of bacterial infection (e.g. spontaneous bacterial peritonitis) in patients with acute variceal haemorrhage, reducing the bleeding with terlipressin takes priority.

Note: In patients with established portal hypertension who present with haematemesis, 50% of cases are due to a peptic ulcer or gastritis.

3.50

A – Arterial pH less than 7.3

The prognosis of patients with acute liver failure (and therefore the necessity to place them on the liver transplant list) is assessed using the King's College Criteria:

If liver failure is due to paracetamol overdose, the presence of the following is associated with a poor prognosis:

1. Arterial pH result of less than 7.3 or
2. All three of:
    *   INR greater than 6.5
    *   Creatinine greater than 300 µmol/L
    *   Hepatic encephalopathy stage III or IV.

If liver failure is due to something other than paracetamol, the presence of the following is associated with a poor prognosis:

1. INR greater than 6.5 or
2. Three out of five of:
   - Age less than 11 or greater than 40
   - Bilirubin greater than 300 µmol/L
   - Jaundice of more than seven days before the onset of encephalopathy
   - INR greater than 3.5
   - Non-A/B hepatitis, halothane hepatitis, idiosyncratic drug reactions.

3.51

D – Severe gastroenteritis

This patient has hypovolaemic hyponatraemia. In this scenario diarrhoea due to gastroenteritis is a recognised cause. His urine sodium is low as sodium is lost through the gut.

The differential diagnosis of hyponatraemia is wide and although there can be specific clues elsewhere (e.g. drug history, other blood results, urine osmolality) the pivotal differentiating point is the assessment of the patient's fluid status. Patients can be classified as hypovolaemic, euvolaemic or hypervolaemic. This patient clearly has hypovolaemic hyponatraemia and this can be classified according to the urinary sodium concentration. The table below shows the causes of a hypovolaemic hyponatraemia:

Urinary sodium concentration <20 mmol/L	Urinary sodium concentration >20 mmol/L
Diarrhoea	Addison's disease
Large burns	Diuretic overuse
High-output stoma	Salt-wasting nephropathy
Excessive sweating	Severe vomiting

Small cell lung cancer can be associated with the development of a paraneoplastic syndrome of inappropriate antidiuretic hormone production. This results in a euvolaemic hyponatraemia. Nephrotic syndrome and congestive cardiac failure are both causes of a hypervolaemic hyponatraemia due to fluid retention.

3.52

D – Previous ileal resection for Crohn's disease

This patient has a macrocytic anaemia. A sub-population of macrocytic anaemias are due to impaired DNA synthesis and are known as a megaloblastic anaemia. The main causes of a macrocytic megaloblastic anaemia are:

- Vitamin B_{12} deficiency
- Folate deficiency
- Cytotoxic drugs (e.g. azathioprine and methotrexate).

This patient is most likely to have a macrocytic megaloblastic anaemia secondary to B_{12} deficiency. B_{12} is absorbed in the terminal ileum after it has been conjugated with intrinsic factor, which is produced by the parietal cells of the stomach. Therefore a terminal ileal resection is the most likely underlying cause of this patient's macrocytic megaloblastic anaemia.

In megaloblastic anaemia there is insufficient DNA synthesis during erythropoiesis. As a result erythroblastic nuclei are immature and cell division is impaired. The combination of normal cytoplasmic growth with impaired cell division results in the production of unusually large erythroblasts, as well as nuclear-cytoplasmic asynchrony. The resultant erythrocytes have a large mean corpuscular volume (macrocytosis), low mean cell haemoglobin concentration (anaemia) and a reduced lifespan (less than 120 days). The increased breakdown of erythrocytes may result in haemolysis, raised lactate dehydrogenase, raised unconjugated bilirubin and jaundice. Because all haematopoietic stem cells are affected, there may also be thrombocytopaenia and leukopaenia.

An important feature of megaloblastic anaemia is the presence of hypersegmented polymorphonuclear leukocytes (neutrophils with more than five segments to their nucleus). Neutrophils normally have a lifespan of five to six days and throughout their lifespan the nucleus divides into more segments. In megaloblastic anaemia, there is thought to be a compensatory increase in their lifespan to compensate for their reduced numbers and thus an increase in the number of segments.

Iron deficiency can cause neutrophil hypersegmentation; however, iron is absorbed in the jejunum and deficiency causes a hypochromic microcytic anaemia. In young women the most common cause of iron deficiency is menorrhagia. Chronic kidney disease typically results in a normocytic normochronic anaemia due to reduced production of erythropoietin by the kidneys. Patients without a spleen are not typically anaemic. However, asplenic patients are unable to remove nuclear remnants from erythrocytes. Such remnants can be seen on the blood film, and are known as Howell–Jolly bodies. Patients with COPD are chronically hypoxic and, in order to compensate, increase the production of erythropoietin, resulting in increased haemoglobin synthesis. Patients with COPD can therefore develop a secondary polycythaemia; however, as with all patients with polycythaemia the red cell mass should be analysed to exclude a 'relative polycythaemia', polycythaemia due to reduced levels of plasma (e.g. dehydration).

3.53

B – Atrial flutter

This patient has a narrow complex tachycardia (QRS complex less than 120 milliseconds), which is therefore most likely to be supraventricular in origin. Once this is determined, the location of the accelerated depolarisation can be determined based on the P waves, the QRS complexes and the rate. This patient has a regular rhythm with abnormal P waves and a ventricular rate of exactly 150 bpm. This is suggestive of atrial flutter with an associated 2:1 type II second-degree heart block. In atrial flutter there is a re-entry rhythm in the atria that produces atrial depolarisations at 300 beats per minute, giving a sawtooth appearance to the ECG baseline. However, as the atrioventricular node will not usually conduct this fast, there is often an associated 2:1 (150 bpm), 3:1 (100 bpm) or 4:1 (75 bpm) type II second-degree atrioventricular block, which reduces the ventricular rate accordingly. Atrial flutter is often an unstable rhythm and many patients will subsequently develop atrial fibrillation.

In atrial fibrillation (which becomes a tachycardia once the rate rises to more than 100 bpm and bradycardia once it falls below 60 bpm) the atrial depolarisation is fibrillatory and is conducted to the ventricles at an irregularly irregular rate. Discretely identifiable P waves are absent; however, the fibrillating atria may produce a wavy isoelectric line. In sinus tachycardia (where the source of the heart rhythm is the sinoatrial node) the rhythm is normal, there are normal P waves and a normal, narrow QRS complex precedes each P wave. In atrial tachycardia there is either one (unifocal atrial tachycardia) or multiple (multifocal atrial tachycardia) sources of atrial depolarisation. Unifocal atrial tachycardias have a regular rate and rhythm with abnormal P waves of regular morphology. This represents a single ectopic atrial focus. In multifocal atrial tachycardia there is an irregular rhythm and multiple different P wave morphologies because there are multiple sources of ectopic depolarisation. In ventricular tachycardia there is a broad QRS complex (more than 120 milliseconds); it must be treated promptly as it can quickly degenerate to life-threatening ventricular fibrillation.

3.54

B – High-resolution CT chest

This patient's history is characteristic of bronchiectasis and the most appropriate investigation is high-resolution CT chest. High-resolution

CT chest offers thinner cross-sectional images with improved spatial resolution when compared to standard CT. Bronchiectatic imaging findings include visualisation of dilated bronchi ('tram lines') that are wider than their adjacent blood vessels. This combination gives the appearance of a signet ring on high-resolution CT chest (the 'signet ring' sign).

Bronchiectasis is a chronic, localised, necrotising, transmural inflammation of the bronchial and bronchiolar walls, which destroys their elasticity resulting in abnormal, permanent airway dilation and obstructive airways disease. It occurs due to a persistent cycle of two insults: infection or airway inflammation (immune over activity or under activity) and airway obstruction. Which comes first depends on the cause:

Infection:

- Viral: measles
- Bacterial: tuberculosis, *Bordetella pertussis* (whooping cough).

Immune over activity:

- Allergic bronchopulmonary aspergillosis
- Autoimmune disease (e.g. rheumatoid arthritis, Sjögren's syndrome, inflammatory bowel disease).

Immune under activity:

- AIDS
- Panhypoglobulinaemia
- Selective immunoglobulin deficiency.

Obstruction:

- Congenital mucociliary clearance disorders:
  o Kartagener's syndrome
  o Young's syndrome
  o Cystic fibrosis (for which a screening test is the sweat test).

- Mechanical obstruction:
  - o Endobronchial malignancy
  - o Chronic aspiration of gastric contents (e.g. gastro-oesophageal reflux disease, alcoholism)
  - o Inhaled foreign body
  - o Obstruction by lymph nodes/granulomas (e.g. sarcoid and tuberculosis).

The characteristic features of bronchiectasis are recurrent chest infections, chronic cough with excessive purulent sputum production and digital clubbing. The differential diagnosis for coarse crackles, digital clubbing and cough also includes lung cancer (which may be diagnosed with lung biopsy) and lung abscess. Unlike bronchiectasis these conditions are not associated with a chronic history. Pulmonary fibrosis can also produce this triad; however, the crackles tend to be bilateral and fine, and do not change or move with coughing. Bronchiectasis is a chronic inflammatory condition and is arecognised cause of weight loss and other constitutional symptoms, as well as AA amyloidosis.

3.55

B – Gitelman's syndrome

Gitelman's syndrome is an autosomal recessive condition associated with reduced sodium and chloride reabsorption. This occurs as a result of a defect in the sodium/chloride transporter in the distal convoluted tubule and, as a result, gives a similar biochemical picture to that caused by thiazide diuretics:

- Low serum sodium
- Low serum chloride
- High urine sodium
- Low urine calcium.

In addition, to compensate for the sodium loss in this group of patients, there is overactivation of the renin-angiotensin-aldosterone system. Aldosterone acts at the distal tubule to reabsorb sodium in exchange for excretion of either a potassium or a hydrogen ion. As a consequence, patients present with weakness, fatigue and muscle cramps and are found to have a profound hypokalaemic metabolic alkalosis and raised urinary potassium.

Gitelman's syndrome is similar to another autosomal recessive tubulopathy, Bartter's syndrome, which is caused by mutations in the sodium/potassium/chloride transporter in the thick ascending limb of the loop of Henle. These patients also have hyperaldosteronism and a similar biochemical picture to that caused by loop diuretics. The urinary calcium in Bartter's syndrome is either normal or high, however.

As there is constant tubular sodium loss, patients remain normotensive despite hyperaldosteronism. This is unlike Conn's syndrome, where the hyperaldosteronism occurs as a result of a solitary aldosterone-producing adenoma, rendering the patient hypertensive, hypokalaemic and alkalotic.

Laxative abuse and a villous adenoma, a secretory polyp that can occur throughout the gastrointestinal tract, also form part of the differential diagnosis for a hypokalaemic, metabolic alkalosis. However, in these cases the patient would experience diarrhoea and, as the potassium loss is from the gastrointestinal tract, one would expect a low urinary potassium.

Liddle's syndrome is an exceptionally rare autosomal dominant disorder associated with mutations in the epithelial sodium channel that results in severe hypertension, low aldosterone levels and a hypokalaemic metabolic alkalosis.

3.56
D – Intravenous Pabrinex®

This patient with acute alcohol withdrawal has developed Wernicke's encephalopathy due to thiamine deficiency. Without resolution there is a 20% chance of mortality and significant risk of progression to the irreversible Korsakoff's syndrome, which itself has an 85%

mortality if left untreated. The most appropriate initial treatment is parenteral thiamine in the form of intravenous Pabrinex®. This is a branded nutritional supplement that comes in two types; type I contains thiamine (vitamin B_1), riboflavin (vitamin B_2) and pyridoxine (vitamin B_6) and type II contains ascorbic acid (vitamin C), nicotinamide (an amide of nicotonic acid, vitamin B_3) and glucose. They are commonly prescribed in pairs (comprising one 5 ml ampoule of type I and one 5 ml ampoule of type II) and are added to 50–100 ml of infusion fluid and given over 30 minutes.

Although patients with alcoholism or Wernicke's encephalopathy are malnourished and often dehydrated, carbohydrates (in the form of a nutritious meal, glucose gel of an intravenous dextrose infusion) must not be given prior to thiamine supplementation. This is because thiamine pyrophosphate (the metabolically active form of thiamine) is an important co-factor for many of the Krebs cycle enzymes that are involved in carbohydrate metabolism. Anything that encourages glucose metabolism will only serve to exacerbate existing thiamine deficiency. This can worsen overt Wernicke's encephalopathy (perhaps initiating its progression to the irreversible Korsakoff's syndrome) or reveal covert thiamine deficiency (perhaps initiating its progression to Wernicke's encephalopathy). This must be considered when managing all patients who are at risk of thiamine deficiency. Other causes of thiamine deficiency include AIDS, dialysis, advanced malignancy and severe malnutrition of any cause (e.g. anorexia, hyperemesis gravidarum).

Patients with alcoholism become thiamine deficient for many reasons:

- Poor dietary intake
- Alcohol metabolism utilises thiamine
- Hepatic thiamine storage is impaired
- Alcohol inhibits gastrointestinal absorption of oral thiamine.

Oral bioavailability of thiamine is relatively poor. Therefore, although oral thiamine is satisfactory for maintenance of thiamine sufficiency, it is not appropriate in the acute setting for management of patients with overt thiamine deficiency.

Other important considerations in the management of acute alcohol withdrawal are a reducing regimen of a long-acting benzodiazepine (e.g. chlordiazepoxide, regular and as required), an antiemetic (e.g. intravenous cyclizine), adequate rehydration (e.g. intravenous 0.9% saline) and preventative measures, such as referral to alcohol liaison services.

3.57

C – Chronic pancreatitis

This patient is suffering from weight loss, diarrhoea and chronic epigastric pain that is relieved by leaning forward. The most likely diagnosis is chronic pancreatitis. It typically produces a gnawing epigastric pain that radiates to the back and is relieved by leaning forward, consuming opiates and applying heat (e.g. a hot water bottle). This may produce the characteristic heat rash known as erythema ab igne. Although the discomfort associated with acute hepatitis is not relieved by leaning forward, the pain in acute pericarditis, gastro-oesophageal reflux and hiatus hernia may be. However, these diagnoses would not fit with the patient's other complaints. Chronic pancreatitis usually occurs secondary to recurrent bouts of acute pancreatitis, with cycles of inflammation and fibrosis. Fibrotic tissue gradually replaces the functional pancreatic exocrine tissue resulting in gastrointestinal malabsorption and steatorrhoea. This fibrotic tissue can become calcified and therefore easily visualised on CT scans or abdominal X-rays. In advanced cases, replacement of endocrine tissue can cause secondary type II diabetes mellitus. Weight loss is also common due to poor dietary intake, post-prandial pain and/or diabetes mellitus. Alcohol and gallstones are the two most common causes of acute pancreatitis in the UK.

3.58

A – Intramuscular hydroxocobalamin every two days

This patient has a macrocytic anaemia secondary to both folate and vitamin B_{12} deficiency. Folic acid is used to make active tetrahydrofolate, which is subsequently used in the synthesis of nucleotides. If there is no folic acid nucleotide synthesis cannot occur. There is also a storage form of folate called methyl tetrahydrofolate. Vitamin B_{12} is necessary to convert methyl tetrahydrofolate into the active tetrahydrofolate that is used for nucleotide synthesis. Giving supplemental folic acid will regenerate the folate stores and allow increased conversion of methyl tetrahydrofolate to tetrahydrofolate. Since this process requires vitamin B_{12}, this will reduce vitamin B_{12} levels further and can precipitate subacute combined degeneration of the spinal cord(if vitamin B_{12} levels are already low). Therefore, before commencing a patient on folate supplements it is essential to check their serum vitamin B_{12} levels. Vitamin B_{12} is required in neurons to convert methylmalonyl coenzyme A to succinyl coenzyme A. Deficiency of vitamin B_{12} therefore results in accumulation of methylmalonyl coenzyme A that is neurotoxic and causes demyelination.

Patients with vitamin B_{12} defiency and neurological symptoms initially require intramuscular hydroxocobalamin (vitamin B_{12}) on alternate days until there is no further neurological improvement. They should then have intramuscular hydroxocobalamin every two to three months. In patients with vitamin B_{12} deficiency folate supplements should never be started prior to intramuscular hydroxocobalamin due to the risk of precipitating subacute combined degeneration of the spinal cord.

3.59

E – Intravenous verapamil

This patient has a narrow complex tachycardia (QRS complex less than 120 milliseconds), which is therefore most likely to be supraventricular in origin. Initially, it is important to assess whether a patient is haemodynamically compromised, as these patients will require immediate DC cardioversion (for example, shock myocardial infarction, syncope or heart failure). In haemodynamically stable patients, the first step in management should be to perform vagal manoeuvres (Valsalva manoeuvre, carotid massage). If these are unsuccessful, intravenous adenosine should be administered. Adenosine has a short half-life and should therefore be administered quickly and flushed through a large, proximal vein while the arm is raised above the head. However, adenosine can induce bronchospasm. It is therefore contraindicated in this patient with brittle asthma. Other contraindications of adenosine include second/third-degree heart block and sinoatrial disease. Patients should always be warned of the side effects of adenosine prior to administration. These include transient chest tightness, dyspnoea, headache, flushing and a 'feeling of impending doom'. In patients with a contraindication to adenosine (such as this patient) or if adenosine fails, verapamil (a non-dihydropyridine calcium channel blocker) is the drug of choice. Verapamil should not be used in patients already on a beta-blocker as this can precipitate third-degree heart block. Beta-blockers (metoprolol) can be used in the management of an acute episode of supraventricular tachycardia. However, they cannot be patients with brittle asthma due to the risk of inducing bronchospasm. Amiodarone has no role in the management of acute attacks of supraventricular tachycardia. It is used in individuals with haemodynamically stable monomorphic ventricular tachycardia, but is contraindicated in polymorphic ventricular tachycardia (torsades de pointes) as it prolongs the QT interval.

3.60

C – Meropenem

Extended-spectrum beta-lactamase–producing organisms are also referred to collectively as problem Gram-negative organisms. They produce extended-spectrum beta-lactamases that hydrolyse third-generation cephalosporins. Extended-spectrum beta-lactamases were first described in the 1980s and were initially found in *Klebsiella* species, mostly in intensive care units. Recently, a new class of extended-spectrum beta-lactamases has emerged and these have been widely detected among *Escherichia coli* species. These extended-spectrum beta-lactamase-producing *Escherichia coli* are able to resist penicillins and cephalosporins and are found most often in urinary tract infections (though not simple cystitis). Fifty percent of extended-spectrum beta-lactamase-producing organisms are now resistant to gentamicin and piperacillin-tazobactam (tazocin), 80% to ciprofloxacin and 100% to trimethoprim. The main options to treat these infections are the carbapenems such as meropenem and amikacin (an aminoglycoside). In addition to being effective against extended-spectrum beta-lactamase-producing organisms, the carbapenems are effective against Gram-positive organisms, Gram-negative organisms, pseudomonas and anaerobes. They are not effective against problem Gram-positive organisms such as methicillin-resistant *Staphylococcus aureus*. Ertapenem is not effective against pseudomonas and therefore meropenem is the carbapenem of choice in patients with a suspected pseudomonal infection. There is now a small amount of carbapenem resistance (carbapenemases), in which case the drug of choice is colistin (a polymyxin antibiotic).

Paper 4

Paper A

Paper 4: Questions

4.1 A 33-year-old male presents with fever, shortness of breath and a new-onset pansystolic murmur, which is best heard at the lower left sternal edge on inspiration. On further questioning he is found to be an intravenous drug user.

Which one of the following organisms is most likely to be implicated in this patient?

A *Coxiella burnetii*
B *Enterococcus faecalis*
C HACEK organisms
D *Staphylococcus aureus*
E *Streptococcus viridans*

4.2 A 59-year-old male develops progressively worsening shortness of breath and a dry cough over the period of a year. On examination the patient has digital clubbing and bibasal, fine, late inspiratory crepitations. The chest X-ray shows reticular interstitial shadowing in both lower zones. The FEV_1 is 2.7 L and the FVC is 3.1 L.

Which one of the following is the most likely diagnosis?

A Ankylosing spondylitis
B Berylliosis
C Extrinsic allergic alveolitis
D Idiopathic pulmonary fibrosis
E Sarcoidosis

4.3 A 69-year-old male presents with a one-year history of worsening exertional breathlessness and wheeze. The patient also has a three-year history of cough with regular sputum production, which is worse during the winter months. He is a smoker with a 45-pack year smoking history. His doctor organises some investigations to help confirm the diagnosis.

Which one of the following result profiles would help confirm your clinical diagnosis?

A FEV_1:FVC ratio of 0.58, FEV_1 57% of predicted, haemoglobin 18.5 g/dL

B FEV_1:FVC ratio of 0.72, FEV_1 77% of predicted, haemoglobin 17.3 g/dL

C FEV_1:FVC ratio of 0.88, FEV_1 57% of predicted, haemoglobin 15.5 g/dL

D Post-bronchodilator FEV_1:FVC ratio of 0.58, FEV_1 57% of predicted, haemoglobin 18.5g/dL

E Post-bronchodilator FEV_1:FVC ratio of 0.8, FEV_1 83% of predicted, haemoglobin 16.5g/dL

4.4 A 36-year-old female with longstanding asthma develops a cough and fever with expectoration of dark mucous plugs. This is associated with increasing shortness of breath and wheeze. Investigations reveal the following:

IgG precipitins to *Aspergillus fumigatus*

Eosinophils	4×10^9/L
Total serum IgE	650 kU/L
Skin prick testing	Type I hypersensitivity reaction to *Aspergillus fumigatus*

Which one of the following is the single most appropriate treatment option for this patient?

A Amphotericin B
B Flucytosine
C Prednisolone
D Salbutamol
E Salmeterol

4.5 A 43-year-old male is brought into the Emergency Department with a thoracic stab wound. Examination reveals a raised jugular venous pressure, a trachea deviated to the right, and reduced air entry and hyperresonance of the left lung. He is noted to have the following observations:

Blood pressure   93/46 mmHg
Heart rate   128 beats per minute
Oxygen saturations   85% on room air
Respiratory rate   33 breaths per minute
Temperature   37.2 °C

The patient is sitting up and has been given 15 L/minute of oxygen using a non-rebreathe mask.

Which one of the following is the most appropriate immediate management?

A 1 L 0.9% sodium chloride STAT
B 10 ml adrenaline 1:10000
C Chest X-ray
D Insert a left-sided chest drain
E Insert a 14-gauge cannula above the left third rib

4.6 A 53-year-old male with known alcoholic liver disease and negative hepatitis viral serology undergoes liver biopsy. The biopsy shows eosinophilic 'twisted rope' inclusions in the hepatocyte cytoplasm.

Which one of the following terms is most likely to be included in the histopathology report?

A Councilman body
B Feathery degeneration
C Ground glass hepatocyte
D Kayser–Fleischer ring
E Mallory body

4.7 A 67-year-old male presents with weight loss, easy bruising and fever. The results of his full blood count are as follows:

Haemoglobin   7. 9 g/dL
Total white cell count 65×10^9/L
Platelets 42×10^9/L

A bone marrow biopsy is performed and subsequent cytogenetic testing reveals a translocation involving the long arms of chromosomes 15 and 17. The patient is then treated with a vitamin A derivative, which induces complete remission.

Which one of the following leukaemias has this patient most likely been diagnosed with?

A Acute lymphoblastic leukaemia
B Acute myelomonocytic leukaemia
C Acute promyelocytic leukaemia
D Chronic lymphocytic leukaemia
E Chronic myeloid leukaemia

4.8 A 42-year-old female presents to her General Practitioner with dry eyes, dry mouth and joint pain. She undergoes Schirmer's test, which reveals a tear absorption rate of 3mm in 5 minutes.

Which one of following statements is most correct with regards to this clinical scenario?

A Patients are at an increased risk of non-Hodgkin's lymphoma
B Rheumatoid factor is positive in 20% of patients
C The peak age of onset is in the second decade of life
D This disease is associated with anti-mitochondrial antibodies
E Women are three times more likely to be affected than men

4.9 A 72-year-old female presents with a two-year history of right hip pain. She can now walk less than 200 yards without severe pain in the right groin that radiates to the right knee. A hip X-ray shows loss of joint space, subchondral sclerosis and bone cysts.

Which one of the following is the most effective treatment for this lady?

A Glucosamine and chondroitin sulphate
B Joint replacement
C NSAIDs
D Physiotherapy
E Weight loss

4.10 A 34-year-old female who has recently started taking isonia-zid for prophylactic treatment of *Mycobacterium tuberculosis* presents to her General Practitioner with lethargy, myalgia and pleuritic chest pain.

Which one of the following antibodies is most likely to be present in this patient?

A Anti-Ro
B Anti-La
C Anti-centromere
D Anti-histone
E Anti-dsDNA

4.11 A 72-year-old male is noted to have renal impairment by his General Practitioner and is referred to a nephrologist. Ultrasound shows kidneys of 6cm bilaterally.

Which one of the following is most likely to be the cause of this patient's chronic kidney disease?

A Autosomal dominant polycystic kidney disease
B Bilateral hydronephrosis
C Hypertensive nephropathy
D Renal amyloidosis
E Renal cell carcinoma

4.12 A 52-year-old male presents to the Emergency Department with confusion. He has a past medical history of bipolar disorder, angina and hypertension. He is taking lithium for bipolar disorder and several other medications for his angina and hypertension. On examination he is disorientated, ataxic and has slurred speech.

Which one of the following medications that the patient is taking is most likely to have interacted with lithium?

A Amlodipine
B Bendroflumethiazide
C Bisoprolol
D Clopidogrel
E Simvastatin

4.13 A 68-year-old male presents to the Emergency Department with reduced consciousness and sudden-onset left-sided motor weakness and sensory loss that began 1 hour ago. On examination of his visual fields there is a left-sided hemianopia.

Which one of the following is the most likely diagnosis in this patient?

A Left posterior cerebral artery infarct
B Left posterior inferior cerebellar artery infarct
C Right anterior cerebral artery infarct
D Right lacunar infarct
E Right middle cerebral artery infarct

4.14 A 36-year-old female with newly diagnosed rheumatoid arthritis presents with acute-onset shortness of breath, dry cough, headache and fever. She has recently been commenced on methotrexate, hydroxychloroquine and a short course of corticosteroids for her rheumatoid arthritis. Investigations are as follows:

PaO$_2$ 7 kPa on room air
Chest X-ray   Diffuse bilateral interstitial shadowing

Which one of the following is the most appropriate immediate management plan?

A Commence folinic acid
B Commence high-dose intravenous prednisolone
C Commence sulphasalazine
D Perform bronchoalveolar lavage
E Stop methotrexate and perform blood cultures

4.15 A 37-year-old pregnant female presents with increasing fatigue and shortness of breath. Her past medical history is unremarkable, except for recently diagnosed hypertension for which she is being treated. She has the following blood test results:

Haemoglobin   9.7 g/dL
Mean corpuscular volume   84 fL
Reticulocyte count   7%

Serum bilirubin	44 µmol/L
Serum unconjugated bilirubin	34 µmol/L
Serum conjugated bilirubin	10 µmol/L

Which one of the following is the likely cause of this clinical scenario?

A Cold autoimmune haemolytic anaemia
B Folate deficiency anaemia
C Iron deficiency anaemia
D Sideroblastic anaemia
E Warm autoimmune haemolytic anaemia

4.16 A 36-year-old male presents with a three-day history of fever, widespread joint pain and raised, painful, purple nodules on his shins. His temperature is 38.6 °C and chest X-ray shows the presence of bilateral hilar lymphadenopathy.

Which one of the following is the most likely diagnosis?

A Crohn's disease
B Lymphoma
C Polyarteritis nodosa
D Sarcoidosis
E Tuberculosis

4.17 An 84-year-old female presents with a painful, swollen right shoulder. On examination of her shoulder active range of movement is restricted in all directions; passive mobility is painful but largely unrestricted. A shoulder X-ray shows destruction of the humeral head. Joint fluid aspirate reveals the presence of a haemorrhagic effusion. Gram stain, culture and polarised light microscopy of the joint are all negative. Alizarin red staining of the synovial fluid identifies the presence of hydroxyapatite crystals.

Which one of the following is the most likely underlying diagnosis in this patient?

A Adhesive capsulitis
B Gonococcal arthritis

C Milwaukee shoulder
D Pseudogout
E Trauma

4.18 A 73-year-old female with persistent atrial fibrillation is commenced on amiodarone. She is currently taking warfarin. Her past medical history is notable for congestive heart failure, thromboembolic stroke and asthma.

Which one of the following is the most appropriate management option?

A Change warfarin to aspirin
B Increase current warfarin dose by 50%
C Maintain current warfarin dose
D Reduce current warfarin dose by 50%
E Stop warfarin

4.19 A 34-year-old HIV-positive male presents with increasing confusion. Lumbar puncture is performed and staining of the cerebrospinal fluid with India ink reveals the presence of spherical organisms, surrounded by a transparent 'halo'.

Which one of the following is the most likely causative organism in this patient?

A *Candida albicans*
B *Cryptococcus neoformans*
C *Mycobacterium tuberculosis*
D *Pneumocystis jiroveci*
E *Toxoplasma gondii*

4.20 A 40-year-old male under the care of the infectious disease team is found to be anti-phospholipid antibody positive.

Which one of the following infections is most likely to yield a positive antiphospholipid antibody result?

A *Borrelia burgdorferi*
B *Brucella melitensis*

C *Leptospira interrogans*
D *Treponema pallidum*
E *Yersinia pestis*

4.21 A 59-year-old male presents to his General Practitioner with a three-month history of cough, haemoptysis and weight loss. On examination, the General Practitioner notices generalised hyperpigmentation and that the patient has difficulty rising from the chair to the examination couch.

Which one of the following is most associated with this clinical scenario?

A Inability to suppress cortisol levels after a high-dose dexamethasone bolus
B Loss of temporal visual fields bilaterally
C Raised serum potassium levels
D Reduced arterial pH and reduced $PaCO_2$
E Reduced serum sodium levels

4.22 A 47-year-old female is diagnosed with Addison's disease. She is subsequently commenced on hydrocortisone twice daily and fludrocortisone once daily. Investigations are as follows:

Adrenal cortex autoantibodies	Negative
21-hydroxylase autoantibodies	Negative
Adrenal CT	Adrenal calcification suggestive of tuberculosis

Standard quadruple therapy for tuberculosis is initiated.

Which one of the following management options is most appropriate in this patient?

A Change the fludrocortisone to midodrine
B Continue anti-tuberculosis medications for 24 months
C Increase steroid replacement doses
D Random serum cortisol
E Thyroid function tests

4.23 A 53-year-old female with multiple myeloma presents with increasing shortness of breath and lethargy. On examination, there is marked ankle oedema and a raised jugular venous pressure. A transthoracic echocardiogram reveals non-hypertrophied, non-dilated ventricles with preserved systolic function and dilated atria. A subsequent endomyocardial biopsy stained with Congo red displays apple-green birefringence when viewed under polarised light.

Which one of the following medications should be avoided in this patient?

A Digoxin
B Furosemide
C Low-molecular-weight heparin
D Midodrine
E Spironolactone

4.24 A 12-year-old boy who has recently migrated from Western Africa presents to the Emergency Department with a three-day history of muscle weakness and jerky arm movements. His mother also reports that in the last three days he has episodically had difficulty talking. On examination, he has a clumsy gait and his tongue is noted to pop in and out when he is asked to hold it out. Further questioning reveals that six months previously he had a sore throat for about two weeks. There is no family history of any movement disorder. His baseline blood tests are normal and he has a negative anti-nuclear antibody.

Which one of the following is the most likely diagnosis in this patient?

A Juvenile Huntington's disease
B Polycythaemia rubra vera
C Sydenham's chorea
D Systemic lupus erythematosus
E Wilson's disease

4.25 A 55-year-old male presents to the Emergency Department with severe muscle pain and weakness. On further questioning it is noted that the patient is currently being treated for a community-acquired pneumonia. The only medications he is taking are the antibiotic prescribed by his General Practitioner and simvastatin for hypercholesterolaemia. A blood test reveals a creatine kinase of 5285 IU/L.

Which one of the following antibiotics is this patient most likely to have been prescribed?

A Amoxicillin
B Ceftriaxone
C Cephalexin
D Clarithromycin
E Penicillin V

4.26 A 54-year-old female with hereditary haemochromatosis presents with a two-day history of bilateral acutely painful and swollen knee joints. Microscopic examination of the joint aspirate reveals positively birefringent rhomboid-shaped crystals.

Which one of the following is the most likely compound to have been deposited in the knee joints of this patient?

A AA amyloid
B Calcium pyrophosphate
C Haemosiderin
D Hydroxyapatite
E Uric acid

4.27 A 36-year-old male with ulcerative colitis presents with his wife as they have had difficulty conceiving for 15 months. Both the patient and his wife have had a child in a previous relationship. The wife is referred for a gynaecological assessment, which is unremarkable. The patient has a semen analysis that reveals a sperm count of 4 million spermatozoa/ml.

Which one of the following medications is the most likely cause of this result?

A Ciclosporin
B Infliximab

C Loperamide
D Metronidazole
E Sulphasalazine

4.28 A 35-year-old male presents due to excessive sweating and hair loss. Further questioning reveals that over the last six months he has had increasing difficulty in sleeping. On examination there is a fine tremor of the hands and moderate exophthalmos. His thyroid function tests are:

Free T$_3$	12 nmol/L
Free T$_4$	41 nmol/L
Thyroid-stimulating hormone	Undetectable

Which type of autoimmune condition (Gell and Coombs reaction) is responsible for this patient's symptoms?

A Type I
B Type II
C Type III
D Type IV
E Type V

4.29 A 32-year-old male presents with fatigue, renal colic and depression. A systemic review reveals the patient has also recently experienced dyspepsia and impotence. On examination, the patient has expressible galactorrhoea. Selected investigations reveal the following:

Serum calcium	3.12 mmol/L
Prolactin	4000 U/L
Fasting gastrin	350 ng/L

Which one of the following is the most likely unifying diagnosis in this patient?

A McCune–Albright syndrome
B Multiple endocrine neoplasia type I
C Multiple endocrine neoplasia type IIa

D Multiple endocrine neoplasia type IIb
E Zollinger–Ellison syndrome

4.30 A 22-year-old female presents to the General Practitioner with menorrhagia and recurrent nose bleeds. She is otherwise well and her examination is unremarkable. She has the following blood test results:

Haemoglobin	13.5×10^9/L
Total white cell count	7×10^9/L
Platelets	225×10^9/L
Activated partial thromboplastin time	47 seconds
Prothrombin time	14 seconds

Which one of the following is most likely to confirm the diagnosis in this patient?

A Bone marrow biopsy
B Factor IX assay
C Factor VIII assay
D Measurement of serum vitamin K levels
E Von Willebrand factor antigen assay

4.31 A 42-year-old HIV-positive male is found to have proteinuria of 300 mg/dL and microhaematuria on routine urinalysis.

Which one of the following investigations would be of most diagnostic value in this patient?

A Abdominal CT
B $CD4^+$ T lymphocyte levels
C Renal biopsy
D Renal ultrasound
E Urea:creatinine ratio

4.32 A 32-year-old female patient with a long-term catheter presents to her General Practitioner as she has begun to feel unwell over the last two days. On examination the patient has a temperature of 38.3 °C and there is marked tenderness in the left loin.

Which one of the following organisms is most likely to be responsible for this patient's symptoms?

A *Escherichia coli*
B *Klebsiella pneumoniae*
C *Proteus mirabilis*
D *Pseudomonas aeruginosa*
E *Staphylococcus aureus*

4.33 A 28-year-old male presents with a headache, nuchal rigidity and photophobia. On examination, he has a temperature of 38.8 °C and there are multiple target lesions over the upper limbs. He has a serum glucose of 6.5 mmol/L. A lumbar puncture is performed and the results of his cerebrospinal fluid analysis are:

Appearance	Clear
Predominant cell type	Mononuclear
Glucose	5.3 mmol/L
Total protein	0.35 g/L
Total cell count	280/ml

Which one of the following is the most appropriate treatment for this patient?

A Intramuscular benzylpenicillin
B Intravenous aciclovir
C Intravenous amphotericin
D Intravenous ceftriaxone and dexamethasone
E Oral izoniazid, ethambutol, rifampicin and pyrazinamide

4.34 A 35-year-old male presents to the Emergency Department with a sudden onset of pain in his neck accompanied by visual loss in the right eye. Further questioning reveals that he has also developed pulsatile tinnitus in his right ear. On examination it is noted that there is a right ptosis and his right pupil is smaller than the left. A neurological examination of both arms is unremarkable.

Which one of the following is the most likely diagnosis in this patient?

A Internal carotid artery dissection
B Klumpke's syndrome
C Pancoast tumour
D Posterior communicating artery aneurysm
E Posterior inferior cerebellar artery infarction

4.35 A 45-year-old male presents with bilateral ptosis and fatigability on exertion. A blood test reveals that the patient has antibodies against the acetylcholine receptor.

Which one of the following medications is most likely to worsen his weakness?

A Amoxicillin
B Ceftriaxone
C Doxycycline
D Erythromycin
E Gentamicin

4.36 A 42-year-old male attends the Emergency Department after experiencing two episodes of right arm weakness, which both resolved spontaneously after a few minutes. His previous medical history is unremarkable apart from recurrent episodes of oral candidiasis. A contrast-enhanced CT head scan reveals the presence of multiple ring-enhancing lesions in the left parietal lobe.

Which one of the following is the most appropriate next step in the management of this patient?

A Commence intravenous aciclovir
B Commence intravenous sulphadiazine and pyrimethamine
C Perform a lumbar puncture
D Referral to neurosurgeon
E Request an HIV test

4.37 A 45-year-old male is admitted to the Emergency Department with a sudden-onset severe headache, which he described as like 'being hit over the head with a cricket bat'. He is in a dimly lit room and is complaining of some neck stiffness. Over the course of the next 30 minutes he becomes increasingly drowsy and his blood pressure is recorded at 125/82 mmHg. The patient only opens his eyes in response to pain and appears to be making incomprehensible sounds. When pressure is applied to the nailbed of his index finger there is extension of his arm.

Which one of the following is the most appropriate initial step in this patient's management?

A Commence intravenous nimodipine
B Contact the anaesthetist for intubation
C Perform an urgent lumbar puncture
D Refer the patient to a neurosurgical unit
E Request an urgent head CT scan

4.38 A 35-year-old male presents to the Emergency Department with a fever and multiple target lesions. On further examination it is apparent that there is blistering and erosion of the skin over the trunk. It is also noted that there is blistering of the oral mucous membranes. The patient reveals that he has recently been given a diagnosis of granulomatosis with polyangiitis (Wegener's granulomatosis) and has been commenced on a medication to reduce exacerbations of this disease.

Which one of the following medications is this patient most likely to be taking?

A Co-trimoxazole
B Ibuprofen
C Indomethacin
D Lorazepam
E Trimethoprim

4.39 A 45-year-old male is admitted to the Emergency Department and is started on an intravenous medication. This is the first time that the patient has received this medication. Immediately after starting the medication, the patient develops shortness of breath, angioedema and is noted to have an audible wheeze. The patient's blood pressure is recorded as 99/68 mmHg.

Which one of the following medications is most associated with an anaphylactoid reaction?

A Cephalexin
B Co-amoxiclav
C Insulin
D *N*-acetylcysteine
E Protamine sulphate

4.40 A 69-year-old male presents with a one-year history of a generalised decrease in his mobility accompanied by multiple episodes of falling. His wife states that he has also developed some personality changes and that his memory has deteriorated. On examination, there is a masked facial appearance, widespread rigidity and a lack of downwards gaze.

Which one of the following is the most likely diagnosis in this patient?

A Corticobasal degeneration
B Idiopathic Parkinson's disease
C Multi-system atrophy
D Progressive supranuclear palsy
E Wilson's disease

4.41 A 35-year-old female with type I diabetes mellitus attends the Emergency Department with a three-day history of nausea and vomiting. She is currently on a basal-bolus insulin regimen. She recently returned from a holiday abroad and gastroenteritis is suspected. The patient is unable to tolerate a normal diet.

Which one of the following is the most appropriate course of action with regards to this patient's insulin regime?

A Change her to a twice-daily regimen of Novomix 30
B Continue her normal four times daily insulin regimen

C Stop her insulin regime completely
D Stop her long-acting evening dose of insulin only
E Stop her short-acting pre-meal doses of insulin only

4.42 A 57-year-old female with rheumatoid arthritis complains of fatigue. She is jaundiced and has multiple scratch marks on her body. Her autoantibody screen reveals the presence of anti-nuclear antibodies and anti-mitochondrial antibodies.

Which one of the following is the most likely diagnosis in this patient?

A Autoimmune hepatitis type I
B Autoimmune hepatitis type II
C Felty's syndrome
D Primary biliary cirrhosis
E Primary sclerosing cholangitis

4.43 A 55-year-old male presents to the Emergency Department acutely unwell, with sudden-onset abdominal pain. He is confused and uncooperative. On abdominal examination there is caput medusae, rebound tenderness, guarding, shifting dullness and absent bowel sounds. His temperature is 38.3 °C.

Which one of the following is the most likely diagnosis?

A Abdominal aortic aneurysm
B Intra-abdominal abscess
C Mallory–Weiss tear
D Perforated duodenal ulcer
E Spontaneous bacterial peritonitis

4.44 A 57-year-old male with longstanding asthma, hyperuricaemia and essential hypertension presents to his General Practitioner due to recurrent headaches. The patient's average ambulatory blood pressure monitoring reveals an average blood pressure of 151/97 mmHg. The patient is already prescribed the maximum dose of losartan; he is also taking allopurinol and a Symbicort Turbohaler (budesonide and formoterol).

Which one of the following is the most appropriate anti-hypertensive for the General Practitioner to prescribe this patient?

A Bendroflumethiazide
B Bisoprolol
C Doxazocin
D Nifedipine
E Ramipril

4.45 A 43-year-old female is admitted to hospital with a purpuric rash on her legs and a feeling of being constantly tired over the last three months. Initial investigations reveal:

Platelets	$260 \times 10^9/\text{L}$
ESR	53 mm in the first hour
Temperature	38.4 °C

Which one of the following is the most likely diagnosis in this patient?

A Acute myeloid leukaemia
B Cutaneous small-vessel vasculitis
C Disseminated intravascular coagulation
D Meningococcal septicaemia
E Thrombotic thrombocytopaenic purpura

4.46 A 65-year-old male presents to his General Practitioner with weight loss, retrosternal chest pain and dysphagia. His dysphagia was initially to solids but it is now affecting his consumption of liquids.

Which one of the following is the most appropriate investigation in this patient?

A Abdominal ultrasound
B Barium swallow
C CT scan of the chest and abdomen
D Oesophageal manometry
E Upper gastrointestinal endoscopy

4.47 A 49-year-old male with known inflammatory bowel disease develops crampy, intermittent epigastric pain and has vomited dark fluid three times since its onset. On examination the abdomen is slightly distended and there are high-pitched, tinkling bowel sounds. There is no evidence of peritonism and his temperature is 36.9 °C. The abdominal X-ray shows central gas shadows with valvulae conniventes that can be seen to cross the bowel lumen completely.

Which one of the following is the most appropriate initial step in the management of this patient?

A Abdominal ultrasound scan
B Intravenous morphine
C Nasogastric tube and intravenous fluid
D Nil by mouth
E Refer for surgery

4.48 A 41-year-old overweight female on the oral contraceptive pill presents to her General Practitioner with vomiting and gradually increasing pain in both her right upper quadrant and above her clavicle. This pain used to come and go but is now continuous. She has had similar, less severe episodes in the past. The abdominal examination is difficult but pressing on the right upper quadrant is so painful that on palpation it arrests deep inhalation. She is not overtly jaundiced and has a temperature of 37.7 °C.

Which of the following is the most likely diagnosis in this patient?

A Carcinoma of the pancreas
B Cholecystitis
C Cholelithiasis
D Hepatic abscess
E Pyelonephritis

4.49 A 15-year-old male with acute coryzal symptoms is brought to see his General Practitioner by his worried mother who is concerned about him missing school. He has been suffering with a dry cough, sore throat and non-purulent watery nasal discharge for two days.

His vaccinations are all up to date and there is no history of breathing difficulties, nasal congestion, atopy, watering of the eyes, facial pain or hearing impairment. On examination, he appears unwell with a temperature of 38.4 °C; however, the examination of his ears, eyes, tonsils and lymph nodes are all normal.

Which one of the following is the most appropriate management option for this patient?

A Amoxicillin
B Benzylpenicillin
C Intranasal glucocorticoids
D Steam inhalation
E Paracetamol

4.50 A 47-year-old male presents to his General Practitioner after three episodes of collapse. On further questioning it is noted that he has become increasingly short of breath on exercise and also has chest pain during exercise, which is relieved by rest. Auscultation of the precordium reveals an ejection systolic murmur heard loudest over the second right intercostal space that radiates to both carotid arteries.

Which one of the following is the best investigation to perform in order to assess the severity of this patient's condition?

A Chest X-ray
B Coronary angiography
C Doppler echocardiography
D ECG
E Transthoracic echocardiography

4.51 A 45-year-old female presents with increased fatigability, orthopnoea, palpitations and peripheral oedema. She also reports a six-month history of weight loss, dysphagia, odynophagia, retrosternal discomfort and a sensation that neither food nor liquid pass properly down on swallowing. Aside from the presenting complaints, the remainder of the history and examination is unremarkable. A myocardial biopsy is performed and reveals diffuse interstitial fibrosis, widespread lymphocytic infiltration and atrophy of myocardial cells.

Which one of the following organisms is the most likely infectious agent?

A *Borrelia burgdorferi*
B Coxsackievirus
C *Leptospira interrogans*
D *Tropheryma whipplei*
E *Trypanosoma cruzi*

4.52 A mother of two brings her newborn son to the Emergency Department after she noticed yellowing of the whites of his eyes and a lump on his left hand side just below his ribs. On examination there is a mass in the left upper quadrant, which is dull to percussion. Investigations are as follows:

Haemoglobin	11.1 g/dL
Reticulocyte count	7%
Direct antiglobulin test	Negative
Indirect antiglobulin test	Negative

Blood film report: There is evidence of haemolysis with erythrocytes that lack central pallor.

In the laboratory, on immersing the patient's erythrocytes in a hypotonic solution, they are found to have an increased osmotic fragility.

Which one of the following is the most likely abnormality in this child's erythrocytes?

A A defect in a membrane protein which binds the cytoskeleton
B A defect in the gene encoding for the alpha-globulin chain of haemoglobin
C Maternal anti-rhesus-D antibodies are bound to cell surface antigens
D The accumulation of oxidants due to a deficiency in cells' reducing power
E The transposition of valine for glutamate in position 6 of the beta-globulin haemoglobin chain

4.53 A 74-year-old male presents to his General Practitioner with increasing shortness of breath over many months, which gets worse on exertion. A chest X-ray shows diffuse ground glass shadowing, pleural plaques that are geographic in appearance and blunting of the right costophrenic angle.

Which one of the following is the most likely diagnosis?

A Asbestosis
B Idiopathic pulmonary fibrosis
C Sarcoidosis
D Silicosis
E Tuberculosis

4.54 A 73-year-old male is brought into the Emergency Department after experiencing a sudden feeling of tight, squeezing pressure in the middle of his chest whilst sitting and watching television at home. This has now lasted for 40 minutes. The patient reports previous similar episodes that have been shorter and always occur during exertion. Investigations are as follows:

ECG	ST segment depression in the inferior leads
12-hour troponin T	0.01 µg/L

Which of the following is the most likely diagnosis?

A Non-cardiac event
B NSTEMI
C Stable angina
D STEMI
E Unstable angina

4.55 A 67-year-old female presents with a headache and sudden onset of blindness in one eye. She has a temperature of 38 °C and reports having difficulty brushing her hair because of shoulder pain.

Which one of the following is the most appropriate initial treatment?

A Intravenous methylprednisolone
B Oral aspirin

C Oral azathioprine
D Pulsed intravenous cyclophosphamide
E Subcutaneous low-molecular-weight heparin

4.56 A 56-year-old female presents to her GP with a two-day history of dysuria and increased frequency of micturition. She has a past medical history of hypertension and rheumatoid arthritis, for which she is taking ramipril and methotrexate. A urine dipstick yields the following results:

Protein   +
Blood   +
Leukocytes   ++
Nitrites   ++

Which one of the following is the most appropriate treatment option?

A Intravenous amoxicillin-clavulanic acid
B Intravenous piperacillin-tazobactam
C Oral clarithromycin
D Oral nitrofurantoin
E Oral trimethoprim

4.57 A 34-year-old female is about to undergo a total thyroidectomy for papillary thyroid carcinoma.

Which one of the following is the most common short-term complication of a total thyroidectomy?

A Hypercalcaemia
B Hyperthyroidism
C Hypocalcaemia
D Neck haemotoma
E Recurrent laryngeal nerve damage

4.58 A 32-year-old female has a urinalysis, which shows the presence of red cell casts and dysmorphic red blood cells. The patient is subsequently diagnosed with thin glomerular basement membrane disease.

Which one of the following features is most suggestive of thin glomerular basement membrane disease?

A Family history of chronic kidney disease
B Frank haematuria
C Loin pain
D Paternal deafness
E Unremarkable history

4.59 A 23-year-old female presents to her General Practitioner with recurrent episodes of severe central chest pain which occur at rest. She is referred for treadmill stress test, which is unremarkable.

Which one of the following medications is contraindicated in this patient?

A Amiodarone
B Amlodipine
C Digoxin
D Metoprolol
E Verapamil

4.60 A 72-year-old male is brought into the Emergency Department after collapsing whilst out shopping. He has a history of myocardial infarction nine years ago and coronary artery bypass grafting three years ago. An ECG is performed and shows left-axis deviation, right bundle branch block and a PR interval of 0.3 seconds.

Which one of the following is the most appropriate management for this patient?

A 24-hour Holter monitoring
B Coronary angiography
C Echocardiography
D Pacemaker insertion
E Tilt table testing

Paper 4: Answers

4.1

D – *Staphylococcus aureus*

This patient displays clinical signs of infective endocarditis causing tricuspid regurgitation. The two primary events in bacterial endocarditis are endothelial damage (which triggers platelet activation) and a bacteraemia. Platelet activation generates a platelet-fibrin nidus within which bacteria colonise, causing further platelet aggregation and ultimately the formation of valvular 'vegetations'. These cause valvular incompetency. Intravenous drug users are at an increased risk of developing infective endocarditis because they often use dirty needles contaminated with bacteria. Although *Streptococcus viridans* is the most common cause of infective endocarditis, intravenous drug users are more likely to be infected with staphylococcal species found on the skin, of which *Staphylococcus aureus* and *Staphylococcus epidermidis* are most common. Enterococci are a group of bacteria found most commonly in the gut that are also implicated in infective endocarditis. Rarely, the HACEK (*Haemophilus, Actinobacillus, Cardiobacterium, Eikenella* and *Kingella*) group of organisms and *Coxiella burnetii* have also been shown to cause infective endocarditis. Because they grow very poorly in culture mediums these bacteria are causes of culture-negative endocarditis.

Treatment of staphylococcal endocarditis is usually with intravenous flucloxacillin and gentamicin, as opposed to intravenous benzylpenicillin and gentamicin for streptococcal endocarditis. The blood supply to heart valves is so poor that, to ensure complete resolution of the valvular lesion, intravenous antibiotics usually need to be given for four to six weeks.

4.2

D – Idiopathic pulmonary fibrosis

This patient displays clinical features of idiopathic pulmonary fibrosis and has a restrictive lung defect. Idiopathic pulmonary fibrosis (previously called cryptogenic fibrosing alveolitis) classically affects males who are or were smokers, and typically affects the lower zones rather than the upper zones.

Causes of upper lobe fibrosis:

- Berylliosis
- Radiation
- Extrinsic allergic alveolitis
- Ankylosing spondylitis
- Sarcoidosis
- Tuberculosis.

In a restrictive lung defect the FVC is reduced and the FEV_1:FVC ratio is either normal or increased (greater than 0.8).

4.3

D – Post-bronchodilator FEV_1:FVC ratio of 0.58, FEV_1 57% of predicted, haemoglobin 18.5g/dL

This patient's history is highly suggestive of COPD, which is predominantly caused by smoking and is characterised by progressive airflow obstruction that is, in contrast to asthma, not fully reversible with bronchodilator therapy. The diagnosis of COPD should be considered in patients over the age of 35 who have a risk factor (usually smoking) and who present with exertional breathlessness, chronic cough, frequent winter bronchitis, regular sputum production or wheeze. If a patient is considered likely to have COPD, post-bronchodilator spirometry should be performed to confirm the diagnosis. A post-bronchodilator FEV_1:FVC ratio of less than

0.7 confirms the diagnosis of COPD. Percentage of predicted FEV_1 values are used to assess disease severity as shown below:

Percentage of predicted FEV_1	Disease severity
Greater than 80%	Mild
50–79%	Moderate
30–49%	Severe
Less than 30%	Very severe

Note: Option A would be consistent with COPD and asthma.

A chest X-ray should also be performed at this stage to exclude other diagnoses (such as congestive cardiac failure, pleural effusion, malignancy and interstitial lung disease), along with a body mass index calculation and full blood count. This is because patients with COPD develop chronic hypoxia and secondary polycythaemia.

4.4

C – Prednisolone

This patient has allergic bronchopulmonary aspergillosis, a condition characterised by type I and type III hypersensitivity reactions to the fungus *Aspergillus fumigatus*. This usually occurs in patients with a history of asthma. The type I hypersensitivity reaction leads to bronchoconstriction and the type III hypersensitivity reaction, mediated by immune complexes, gives rise to inflammation that damages bronchial walls and causes bronchiectasis. Therefore, the most effective way to treat acute exacerbations is with high-dose oral corticosteroids to reduce the inflammation. Itraconazole, an antifungal agent, has been shown to play a useful role in the management of allergic bronchopulmonary aspergillosis alongside corticosteroids. There is no place for amphotericin B and flucytosine, other antifungal agents, in the treatment of allergic bronchopulmonary aspergillosis. However, these antifungals do play a role in treating invasive aspergillosis, a condition found in immunosuppressed (particularly neutropaenic) patients where *Aspergillus* hyphae invade tissue and cause systemic infection. Inhaled beta agonists such as salbutamol (short acting) and salmeterol (long acting) should be given to patients with allergic bronchopulmonary aspergillosis to help to control their asthma.

4.5

E – Insert a 14-gauge cannula above the third rib

This patient has a left tension pneumothorax and requires immediate treatment with insertion of a normal large-bore cannula (12- or 14-gauge) into the second intercostal space just above the third rib in the midclavicular line. A tension pneumothorax usually occurs as a result of a lung laceration, when air is trapped in the pleural space under positive pressure. This creates a one-way valve effect that allows air to escape into the pleural space but not back again. Progressive build up of pressure in the pleural space results in mediastinal shift, compression of the contralateral lung, reduction of venous return and eventually cardio-respiratory arrest. Tension pneumothorax is an important reversible cause of cardiac arrest. As this patient is haemodynamically unstable and likely to deteriorate further if not treated immediately, he must be treated before undergoing a chest X-ray; waiting for X-ray confirmation of a tension pneumothorax can have devastating consequences. Treatment with a cannula insertion is deemed to be successful if a hiss is heard; this represents trapped air escaping from the pleural space. Once this is performed successfully a chest drain should be inserted on the same side in order to prevent the tension pneumothorax reoccurring. The blood pressure will normalise following release of the left tension pneumothorax.

4.6

E – Mallory body

A Mallory body describes an eosinophilic 'twisted rope' inclusion body found in the hepatocyte cytoplasm. They are most commonly associated with cirrhosis secondary to alcohol but can also be found in the context of cirrhosis secondary to Wilson's disease, primary biliary cirrhosis and hepatocellular carcinoma. A Councilman body is an eosinophilic globule found in the cytoplasm of hepatocytes undergoing apoptosis. Feathery degeneration is a process in which the hepatocyte cytoplasm enlarges in the setting of cholestasis. A ground glass hepatocyte has a uniformly dull, granular cytoplasm and is seen in chronic hepatitis B infection. Kayser–Fleischer rings are found in the irises of patients with Wilson's disease and represent accumulation of copper in Descemet's membrane (the basement membrane that lies between the corneal stroma and the endothelial layer of the cornea).

4.7

C – Acute promyelocytic leukaemia

In acute promyelocytic leukaemia (also known as acute myeloid leukaemia subset M3) the *PML-RARA* fusion gene has formed due to a reciprocal translocation involving the long arms of chromosomes 15 and 17. *RARA* usually codes for a receptor for retinoic acid, a vitamin A derivative that is essential for myeloid lineage maturation. However, in acute promyelocytic leukaemia the *PML-RARA* fusion gene codes for a hybrid protein that inhibits differentiation of the myeloid lineage. Treatment with all-trans-retinoic acid increases production of a functional retinoic acid receptor. This subsequently induces differentiation and maturation of the blast cells of the myeloid lineage that are found in this disease. Sensitivity to retinoic acid is unique to acute promyelocytic leukaemia. Acute leukaemias are due to over-proliferation of immature blood cells and they tend to present acutely in younger patients with the symptoms and complications of bone marrow failure. Chronic leukaemias, on the other hand, occur due to the accumulation of mature blood cells and they tend to present more insidiously (or even on a routine blood test) in older patients.

4.8

A – Patients are at an increased risk of non-Hodgkin's lymphoma

This patient has Sjögren's syndrome and is at an increased risk of developing non-Hodgkin's lymphoma. About 5% of patients with Sjögren's syndrome will eventually develop some form of lymphoid malignancy. Lymphomas are most commonly found in the salivary glands.

Sjögren's syndrome may be primary or secondary (it is associated with other connective tissue diseases). Women are nine times more likely to be affected than men, with the peak age of onset in the fifth decade of life. Rheumatoid factor is positive in 95–100% of patients with Sjögren's syndrome; however, anti-Ro and anti-La antibodies are more sensitive. Anti-mitochondrial antibodies are associated with primary biliary cirrhosis. Patients with Sjögren's syndrome are at an increased risk of other autoimmune diseases, including primary biliary cirrhosis.

4.9

B – Joint replacement

This patient has severe osteoarthritis of her right hip. Although physiotherapy, weight loss, NSAIDs, glucosamine and chondroitin sulphate may all be useful in the conservative management of osteoarthritis of the hip, the most effective treatment is surgery.

4.10

D – Anti-histone

This patient has developed drug-induced lupus erythematosus secondary to treatment with isoniazid. Anti-histone antibodies are found in more than 95% of cases of drug-induced lupus erythematosus. More than 50 drugs are known to cause drug-induced lupus, with isoniazid, hydralazine and D-penicillamine among the most well known. The features of drug-induced lupus erythematosus include arthralgia, myalgia, fatigue, pericarditis and pleuritis. Remission is induced in patients when the drug is stopped. Anti-dsDNA antibodies are almost exclusively found in patients with non-drug-induced systemic lupus erythematosus, although only 60% of patients with systemic lupus erythematosus test positive for these antibodies. Anti-centromere antibodies are most strongly associated with the limited form of scleroderma. Anti-Ro and anti-La antibodies are associated with Sjögren's syndrome and are also found in 20% of patients with systemic lupus erythematosus. Anti-Ro antibodies can cross the placenta and cause congenital heart block in children born to mothers with these diseases.

4.11
C – Hypertensive nephropathy

The normal renal length is 9–12 cm. Most causes of chronic kidney disease cause the kidneys to reduce in size, including hypertension. Of all the options in this question only hypertensive nephropathy gives rise to small kidneys. Hypertension increases glomerular pressure, which causes damage to the glomerulus. Following this, there is a release of cytokines that promote glomerular fibrosis and death of nephrons, leading to glomerulosclerosis. Subsequently, proteinuria may develop. In addition, tubulointerstitial scarring develops as a result of poor perfusion to this region. This combination of fibrosis and scarring leads to a reduction in kidney size.

Autosomal dominant polycystic kidney disease is the most common inherited renal disease and results from mutations either in *PKD-1* (found on chromosome 16) or *PKD-2* (found on chromosome 4). Mutations in *PKD-1* are seven times more common than *PKD-2*. Patients develop multiple cysts in their kidneys that can cause the kidneys to double in length. The liver, spleen and pancreas can also become cystic.

Bilateral hydronephrosis can occur as a result of bladder outlet obstruction, causes of which include an enlarged prostate, a pelvic tumour or bilateral vesico-ureteric reflux (which may result from posterior urethral valves or a neurogenic bladder). Chronic back-flow of urine causes excessive dilatation of the kidneys.

Renal amyloidosis occurs as a result of extracellular deposition of degradation-resistant proteins that form beta-pleated sheets. The two most common types of amyloid are AL (amyloid light chain; due to overproduction of monoclonal light chains by plasma cell dyscrasias) and AA (amyloid serum protein A; due to overproduction of serum amyloid A proteins in the setting of chronic inflammation, e.g. osteomyelitis, rheumatoid arthritis, inflammatory bowel disease). These proteins can be stained with Congo red dye, and display apple-green birefringence when viewed under polarised light. The deposition of amyloid in the mesangium and capillaries can give rise to renal enlargement. Clinically, renal amyloidosis presents with nephrotic syndrome and normal-sized kidneys.

Renal cell carcinoma classically presents with haematuria, pain and a palpable mass. In the vast majority of cases the mass is unilateral, although the primary tumour can occasionally metastasise to the contralateral kidney and cause bilaterally enlarged kidneys.

4.12

B – Bendroflumethiazide

Lithium is a medication used to treat bipolar disorder. Unfortunately, it has a narrow therapeutic index and prescription of certain medications can reduce lithium excretion and potentiate toxicity. This can manifest as:

- Anorexia, diarrhoea and vomiting
- Drowsiness
- Cerebellar signs
- Coarse tremor
- Renal failure
- Hypokalaemia
- Collapse.

Thiazide diuretics, such as bendroflumethiazide, increase serum lithium concentrations. They inhibit the sodium/chloride transporter in the distal convoluted tubule. As a result, there is a compensatory increase in the reabsorption of sodium and lithium in the proximal tubule and a subsequent increase in serum lithium levels. This can give rise to lithium toxicity. Other drugs that potentiate lithium toxicity include ACE inhibitors and NSAIDs. Hyponatraemia is also associated with increased lithium levels, as the kidney reabsorbs lithium in place of sodium. Of the other medications listed in this question, none cause lithium toxicity.

4.13

E – Right middle cerebral artery infarct

This patient has had an infarct affecting the right middle cerebral artery. A cerebral infarction presents with a sudden, focal neurological deficit that results in loss of function. Patients often have vascular risk factors for a cerebral infarction such as increasing age, hypertension, diabetes, hypercholesterolaemia and atrial fibrillation.

The middle cerebral artery is the most common site for cerebral infarction. A middle cerebral artery infarct will have varying presentations depending on the extent of the infarct and the side of the lesion. Common features of a middle cerebral infarct include varying degrees of drowsiness (an intact cerebral cortex is required for consciousness), contralateral hemiparesis, contralateral hemisensory loss (worse in the upper limb and face than the lower limb), contralateral homonymous hemianopia and contralateral neglect and inattention. If the infarct occurs in the dominant hemisphere there may also be aphasia. Depending upon the extent of the infarct this can be a Broca's aphasia, Wernicke's aphasia or global aphasia.

In an anterior cerebral artery infarct the patient is also drowsy and the hemiparesis and hemisensory loss is worse in the lower limb than the upper limb. This is due to somatotopic arrangement of the primary motor and sensory cortices. Gait apraxia, urinary incontinence and emotional lability are also associated with an anterior cerebral artery infarct.

A lacunar stroke is a collective term given when there is occlusion of one of the penetrating arteries that provides blood to the subcortical structures. There are many different types of lacunar infarct depending upon the penetrating arteries affected. The most common lacunar strokes are a pure motor stroke and a pure sensory stroke. A pure motor stroke causes a contralateral hemiparesis and is due to infarction of the striate arteries that supply the posterior limb of the internal capsule through which the corticospinal tract passes. A pure sensory stroke presents with unpleasant sensations on one side of the body and is due to infarction of the arteries that supply the ventral posterolateral nucleus of the thalamus.

The posterior cerebral artery supplies the occipital lobe, the inferomedial temporal lobe, a large portion of the thalamus and the midbrain. Symptoms will vary depending upon the location of the infarct. A proximal infarct will affect all of the areas supplied by the artery whereas more distal infarcts will result in more limited deficits. Common features of a proximal posterior cerebral infarct include a contralateral homonymous hemianopia with macular sparing, cortical blindness, memory difficulties, post-stroke (thalamic) pain, contralateral hemiplegia and oculomotor nerve palsy. The contralateral hemiplegia and oculomotor nerve palsy occur due to occlusion of the paramedian branches, which supply the midbrain. Infarction of the paramedian vessels is known as Weber's syndrome (medial medullary syndrome).

A posterior inferior cerebellar artery stroke (lateral medullary syndrome or Wallenberg syndrome) affects the nuclei of cranial nerves V, VIII, IX and X, the descending sympathetic fibres, cerebellum and the spinothalamic tract (the fibres of which have already decussated). Clinical features include dysarthria, dysphagia, dysphonia, unilateral Horner's syndrome, unilateral cerebellar signs, loss of pain and temperature on the same side of the face and the opposite side of the body (with respect to the side of the lesion).

4.14

E – Stop methotrexate and perform blood cultures

In this patient there is a high index of suspicion of methotrexate pneumonitis, a rare but potentially life-threatening complication of treatment with methotrexate. Most patients present with pneumonitis within the first few months of commencing methotrexate or after a significant increase in dose. Immediate management involves stopping methotrexate and helping to exclude infection by performing blood cultures. Often stopping methotrexate is all that is required. However, there is anecdotal evidence that high-dose corticosteroids accelerate recovery. Folinic acid may also play a role in reversing methotrexate toxicity, but evidence for this is scant. Bronchoalveolar lavage may be needed to rule out *Pneumocystis jirovecii* pneumonia. However, this is not the most appropriate immediate option. If the patient is unable to tolerate methotrexate, they can be commenced on sulphasalazine as an alternative disease-modifying agent. Again, this is not an immediate priority in this scenario.

4.15

E – Warm autoimmune haemolytic anaemia

This patient has developed a warm autoimmune haemolytic anaemia as a result of taking methyldopa. Methyldopa is a centrally acting anti-hypertensive. It does not have the teratogenic profile of other anti-hypertensive medications, most notably ACE inhibitors and angiotensin II receptor blockers, and so is used in the management of hypertension in pregnancy. Twenty percent of patients on methyldopa develop a positive Coombs test; in a small proportion of patients it causes a warm autoimmune haemolytic anaemia.

This patient has a haemolytic anaemia due to the presence of low haemoglobin, increased reticulocyte count and an increase in the levels of serum unconjugated bilirubin. Haemolytic anaemias can be classified according to whether or not the haemolysis is mediated by antibodies directed against a patient's own erythrocytes.

The Coombs test is a useful investigation to distinguish between an autoimmune and non-autoimmune haemolytic anaemia. A positive Coombs test suggests an autoimmune cause of the haemolytic anaemia. There are two types of Coombs test: direct and indirect. In the direct Coombs test, the patient's erythrocytes are mixed with antihuman globulin. If this produces agglutination of erythrocytes it suggests that antibodies are bound to the surface of the erythrocytes. In the indirect test, the patient's serum is mixed with erythrocytes and if agglutination occurs this suggests that the patient's serum contains antibodies that bind to erythrocytes.

There are two broad categories of autoimmune haemolytic anaemia: warm and cold. This depends upon the temperature at which the erythrocytes agglutinate during the Coombs test. The following table highlights the differences between warm and cold autoimmune haemolytic anaemias:

	Warm autoimmune haemolytic anaemia	Cold autoimmune haemolytic anaemia
Site of haemolysis	Extravascular	Intravascular
Type of antibody	IgG	IgM
Temperature at which agglutination of erythrocytes occurs	37 °C	4 °C
Causes	• Idiopathic • Chronic lymphocytic leukaemia • Lymphoma • Systemic lupus erythematosus • Rheumatoid arthritis • Drugs, e.g. methyldopa	• Idiopathic • Chronic lymphocytic leukaemia • Lymphoma • EBV • *Mycoplasma pneumoniae* • HIV • Occasionally systemic lupus erythematosus

Folate deficiency anaemia results in a macrocytic anaemia and a low reticulocyte count. Folate requirements are increased in pregnancy and pregnant women are advised to take supplements when trying for a baby and for the first 12 weeks of pregnancy to aid development of the fetal neural tube. In iron deficiency anaemia there is a microcytic anaemia and low reticulocyte count. Diagnosis is confirmed by a low serum ferritin, low serum iron and raised total iron-binding capacity. Sideroblastic anaemia occurs as a result of failure to incorporate iron into haemoglobin. This results in iron accumulating in the mitochondria. This is identified by the presence of darkly staining ring sideroblasts in bone marrow red cell precursors. In sideroblastic anaemia the mean corpuscular volume can be low, normal or high. This disorder can be primary, as one of the myelodysplastic syndromes, or secondary to malignancy, alcohol, heavy metal poisoning and collagen diseases.

4.16

D – Sarcoidosis

This clinical presentation is typical for acute sarcoidosis. The combination of erythema nodosum and hilar lymphadenopathy is often accompanied by anterior uveitis. Sarcoidosis is a multisystem inflammatory condition of unknown aetiology that commonly presents with non-caseating, granulomatous pulmonary lesions. CT scan of the thorax will often show typical changes of sarcoidosis including bronchovascular beading. Tissue biopsy for sarcoidosis is diagnostic and bronchoscopy with transbronchial biopsy or endobronchial ultrasound-guided lymph node biopsy allows confirmation of the diagnosis. Bronchoalveolar lavage would show an excess of lymphocytes with an increased CD4 to CD8 ratio. Serum ACE levels are raised but not diagnostic as they can be raised in other granulomatous conditions. Five percent of patients will be hypercalcaemic and 40% will have hypercalcuria. Gallium scanning or PET-CT will localise granulomatous tissue.

Causes of erythema nodosum include:

- Infection, e.g. *Streptococcus*, TB
- Sarcoidosis
- Inflammatory bowel disease
- Drugs
- Vasculitis, e.g. polyarteritis nodosa.

4.17

C – Milwaukee shoulder

This patient has a Milwaukee shoulder, a rare arthropathy associated with the deposition of intra-articular or periarticular hydroxyapatite crystals. It leads to a rapid destruction of the glenohumeral joint and rotator cuff muscles. Elderly women are most commonly affected and the diagnosis of Milwaukee shoulder should always be considered in this group of patients who present with a haemarthrosis. Staining of synovial fluid with alizarin red enables identification of hydroxyapatite crystals. Treatment is with NSAIDs, intra-articular steroid injection, physiotherapy and/or joint replacement.

Adhesive capsulitis is also known as frozen shoulder. It is characterised by a deep aching pain and severe limitation of joint movement. There are three phases: a painful phase, a 'frozen' phase and a resolution phase. Gonococcal arthritis presents most commonly as a migratory polyarthritis in young, healthy, sexually active adults. It is associated with rash, skin blisters and tenosynovitis. Gram stain and culture of synovial fluid are often negative; culture of urethral or cervical samples is needed to improve the chances of identifying the organism. Pseudogout is associated with the deposition of intra-articular or periarticular calcium pyrophosphate crystals. Patients often present with an acute painful, swollen large-joint monoarthropathy. Diagnosis is confirmed by the presence of positively birefringent rhomboid crystals on examination of synovial fluid under polarised light. Trauma is unlikely due to the lack of history of injury described by the patient.

4.18

D – Reduce current warfarin dose by 50%

Amiodarone inhibits CYP2C9, a CYP450 isoenzyme responsible for the conversion of warfarin to its major metabolite, 7-hydroxywarfarin. This potentiates the effects of warfarin leading to over-anticoagulation and increased risk of haemorrhagic complications if the current warfarin dose is maintained. Therefore, a pragmatic approach is to reduce the warfarin dose by 50% following amiodarone loading, monitor the international normalised ratio weekly and tailor the dose until the target international normalised ratio is achieved. It is also important to note that this interaction reaches its peak effect six to seven weeks after amiodarone treatment is initiated and persists for a month or more after amiodarone is withdrawn.

As this patient's $CHADS_2$ score is greater than two, stopping warfarin or changing warfarin to aspirin is not appropriate. The $CHADS_2$ score is calculated as follows:

Feature	Score
Congestive heart failure	One point
Hypertension	One point
Age greater than 75	One point
Diabetes mellitus	One point
Previous Stroke or transient ischaemic attack	Two points

Patients with a $CHADS_2$ score of two or more should be commenced on warfarin. This patient has a $CHADS_2$ score of three and therefore warfarin is the most appropriate treatment.

Patients with a $CHADS_2$ score of zero or one should be further risk stratified using the $CHA2DS_2$-VASc scoring system, which includes further modifiable stroke risk factors. The $CHA2DS_2$-VASc scoring system is calculated as follows:

Feature	Score
Congestive heart failure	One point
Hypertension	One point
Age greater than 75 years	Two points
Diabetes mellitus	One point
Previous Stroke or transient ischaemic attack	Two points
Vascular disease (previous myocardial infarction, peripheral vascular disease, mesenteric ischaemia)	One point
Age between 65 and 74 years	One point
Sex (female)	One point

Patients with a CHA2DS$_2$-VASc of one should be treated with either low-dose aspirin or an oral anticoagulant such as warfarin (oral anticoagulant is preferred to aspirin). Patients with a score of zero are very low risk and can therefore be treated with either low-dose aspirin or no antithrombotic therapy (no antithrombotic therapy is preferred).

4.19

B –*Cryptococcus neoformans*

This patient has meningitis due to infection with the fungus *Cryptococcus neoformans*. This infection occurs almost exclusively in immunocompromised patients. In patients who are HIV positive, cryptococcal meningitis is associated with a CD4$^+$ T-lymphocyte cell count of less than 100 cells per ml. Diagnosis is either by India ink staining of cerebrospinal fluid, blood culture or by detection of cryptococcal antigen in the cerebrospinal fluid. Treatment is with amphotericin B and flucytosine.

Toxoplasma gondii is a protozoa associated with HIV-positive patients who have a CD4$^+$ T-lymphocyte cell count of less than 200 cells per ml. Patients present with focal neurological symptoms and signs. Diagnosis is by observing ring-enhancing lesions on CT or MRI scans and by serological investigations. Patients with a CD4$^+$ T-lymphocyte cell count of less than 200 cells per ml are also at an increased risk of developing *Pneumocystis jirovecii* pneumonia. *Mycobacterium tuberculosis* and *Candida albicans* infections are also more commonly found in immunocompromised patients; however, they are unlikely to be found in this scenario.

4.20

D –*Treponema pallidum*

A positive antiphospholipid antibody result can occur either in the setting of positive lupus anticoagulant where there is a prolonged partial thromboplastin time, or in the setting of a positive Venereal Disease Reference Laboratory test. The Venereal Disease Reference Laboratory test is used in the investigation of syphilis, which is caused by the spirochete *Treponema pallidum*. However, it is important to note that this test detects antibodies against negatively charged phospholipid molecules and is not treponema specific. Therefore, positive Venereal Disease Reference Laboratory tests may occur in the setting of systemic lupus erythematosus and other infections, such as *Mycobacterium tuberculosis* and *Mycobacterium leprae*.

4.21

A – Inability to suppress cortisol levels after a high-dose dexamethasone bolus

This patient is likely to have an adrenocorticotropic hormone-secreting lung carcinoma, most likely a small cell carcinoma. In normal subjects, a dexamethasone bolus would act to inhibit the release of corticotropin-releasing hormone and adrenocorticotropic hormone from the hypothalamus and anterior pituitary, respectively. This would subsequently decrease the secretion of cortisol from the zona fasciculata of the adrenal cortex. However, in patients that produce excess adrenocorticotropic hormone, there is an inability to suppress cortisol after a dexamethasone bolus. An inability to suppress cortisol after a high dose of dexamethasone is strongly suggestive that the source of the adrenocorticotropic hormone is exogenous (i.e. not from the anterior pituitary) and is therefore likely to be from an ectopic adrenocorticotropic hormone-secreting tumour.

Pro-opiomelanocortin is the precursor for both adrenocorticotropic hormone and gamma melanocyte-stimulating hormone (which induces skin pigmentation). Ectopic adrenocorticotropic hormone has the ability to increase the activity of gamma melanocyte-stimulating hormone and is responsible for the hyperpigmentation in this patient. Prominent areas for hyperpigmentation are the palmar creases, buccal mucosa and underneath bra-strap lines in females.

The patient in this scenario also has Cushing's syndrome, and the difficulty he experiences rising from a chair is due to the resultant proximal myopathy. However, it is important to note that in Cushing's syndrome caused by a tumour, the malignant cachexia and catabolic state may mask some of the typical features of hyper-cortisolaemia such as central obesity, moon-like facies and striae. Loss of temporal fields bilaterally is suggestive of a pituitary tumour and is not consistent with the respiratory symptoms experienced by this patient. Cortisol has mineralocorticoid activity and acts on the distal tubule of the nephron to reabsorb sodium ions in exchange for excretion of potassium or hydrogen ions. Therefore, patients with excess cortisol will tend towards a hypernatraemic hypokalaemic metabolic alkalosis.

4.22

C – Increase steroid replacement doses

Although the most common cause of Addison's disease in the Western world is autoimmune adrenalitis, tuberculosis is an important and well-recognised cause of adrenal failure worldwide.

This patient has been started on rifampicin, a CYP450 enzyme inducer, as part of her tuberculosis quadruple therapy. Although isoniazid (another anti-mycobacterial medication) is an enzyme inhibitor, it is not powerful enough to fully counteract the effects of rifampicin. Therefore this patient must increase the dose of steroid replacement she is taking for her Addison's disease. Failure to do so will result in increased steroid metabolism and will render the patient Addisonian once again.

The mnemonic 'PC BRAGS' can be used to remember enzyme inducers:

Phenytoin
Carbamazepine

Barbituates
Rifampicin

Alcohol (chronic usage)
Griseofulvin
Sulphonylureas

The mnemonic 'SICKFACES.COM' can be used to remember enzyme inhibitors:

Sodium valproate
Isoniazid
Cimetidine
Ketoconazole
Fluconazole
Alcohol (acute usage)
Chloramphenicol
Erythromycin
Sulphonamides

Ciprofloxacin
Omeprazole
Metronidazole

Midodrine (an alpha-1-adrenoreceptor agonist) is used for symptomatic relief in postural hypotension (a common feature of Addison's disease); however, fludrocortisone is preferred here, as it will correct the mineralocorticoid deficiency. The length of treatment in adrenal and central nervous system tuberculosis is usually 9 to 12 months (not 24 months); this is longer than the standard course of six months for pulmonary tuberculosis. Random serum cortisol has a low sensitivity for adrenal insufficiency and a 9 am serum cortisol should be used instead. Patients with autoimmune Addison's disease should have their thyroid function tested as 40% of patients have autoimmune hypothyroidism.

4.23

A – Digoxin

This patient has developed myocardial AL amyloidosis secondary to her multiple myeloma. Digoxin is usually avoided in patients with myocardial amyloidosis as many studies have documented increased binding of digoxin to amyloid fibrils. This causes increased tissue levels of digoxin in the myocardium and subsequent prolonged exposure to digoxin receptors in the myocardium. As a result, toxicity may occur even with standard therapeutic doses of digoxin.

Myocardial amyloidosis occurs as a result of extracellular deposition of degradation-resistant proteins that form beta-pleated sheets. The two most common types of amyloid are AL (amyloid light chain), which occurs due to overproduction of monoclonal light chains by plasma cell dyscrasias, and AA (amyloid serum protein A), which occurs due to overproduction of serum amyloid A proteins in the setting of chronic inflammation, such as chronic osteomyelitis, rheumatoid arthritis or inflammatory bowel disease. These proteins can be stained with Congo red dye, and display apple-green birefringence when viewed under polarised light.

AL deposition in the myocardium results in the development of a restrictive cardiomyopathy and usually manifests with cardiac failure with a preserved ejection fraction (diastolic dysfunction). This is due to impaired relaxation of the left ventricular myocardium since it has been infiltrated with stiffened amyloid fibrils. Transthoracic echocardiography typically demonstrates non-hypertrophied, non-dilated ventricles with preserved systolic function and dilated atria.

In patients with myocardial amyloidosis, treatment of the associated congestive heart failure is more complicated than in patients who have non-restrictive cardiomyopathies. In AL amyloidosis, possibly because of an associated autonomic neuropathy, angiotensin-converting enzyme inhibitors and angiotensin receptor blockers are rarely tolerated and may provoke profound hypotension even when prescribed in small doses. Beta-adrenoreceptor antagonists have been shown to have no proven benefit and may cause decompensation in severe disease. Calcium channel blockers are also contraindicated since they irreversibly bind amyloid fibrils and can worsen congestive heart failure. Thus, diuretics such as furosemide and spironolactone are virtually the only therapy available to treat heart failure in this condition. However, in patients with cardiac amyloidosis loop diuretics (furosemide) are often prescribed with an alpha-1-adrenoreceptor agonist (midodrine). This is because contrary to standard heart failure management, maintenance of adequate blood pressure with an alpha-1-adrenoreceptor agonist may permit higher doses of loop diuretics, especially in patients with autonomic neuropathy.

Patients with AL amyloidosis are often prothrombotic due to the presence of increased immunoglobulins. As a result, these patients often require long-term anticoagulation to reduce their venous thromboembolic risk. Low-molecular-weight heparin has been demonstrated to reduce the risk of venous thromboembolism in patients with AL amyloidosis.

4.24

C – Sydenham's chorea

Sydenham's chorea is a major manifestation of rheumatic fever, an inflammatory disease that occurs following an infection with *Streptococcus pyogenes*. It is thought to occur as a result of antibody cross-reactivity that can involve the heart, joints, skin and brain. Rheumatic fever is rare in developed countries due to the high availability of antibiotics for streptococcal infections. However, it is still a common cause of morbidity in people from developing countries who have not received appropriate treatment for streptococcal infections.

A diagnosis of acute rheumatic fever can be made according to the modified Jones criteria (see table). Two of the major criteria, or one major criterion plus two minor criteria, along with evidence of streptococcal infection, is diagnostic for rheumatic fever.

Major	Minor
Carditis	Fever
Erythema marginatum	Arthralgia
Painless subcutaneous nodules over bones or tendons	Raised ESR or C-reactive protein
	Leukocytosis
Polyarthritis	ECG showing features of heart block
Sydenham's chorea	Previous episode of rheumatic fever or inactive heart disease

Sydenham's chorea usually develops weeks or months after the primary streptococcal infection and is characterised by:

- Muscle weakness
- Chorea (an involuntary movement disorder)
- Gait disturbances
- Dysarthric speech
- Harlequin tongue (a phenomena in which the tongue pops in and out when the patient tries to hold it out)
- Psychological symptoms (these often precede the onset of the choreiform movements).

Childhood systemic lupus erythematosus generally presents between the ages of 3 and 15, with a four-fold female predominance. Around half of patients develop neuropsychiatric complications that can include chorea. However, this is a rare complication, and therefore, alongside the negative anti-nuclear antibody result, systemic lupus erythematosus is an unlikely diagnosis.

Huntington's disease is a neurodegenerative disease inherited in an autosomal dominant pattern. It occurs because of CAG triplet repeats within a stretch of the Huntington gene. Huntington's disease displays the phenomenon of anticipation in which higher repeat numbers are associated with younger ages of onset. Patients develop neuronal loss in the striatum of the basal ganglia and therefore movement-associated symptoms predominate. Juvenile Huntington's often presents insidiously with stiffness in the legs, choreiform movements of the limbs, behavioural changes and a decline in cognition.

Polycythaemia rubra vera is a myeloproliferative disorder in which the bone marrow makes too many erythrocytes. Polycythaemia rubra vera is known to cause choreiform movements.

Wilson's disease (hepatolenticular degeneration) is an autosomal recessive genetic disorder in which there is a deficiency of caeruloplasmin (which normally binds copper in plasma), and a failure of hepatocytes to excrete free copper. Consequently, in Wilson's disease there is an increase in free copper that can then accumulate in tissues. The excess copper deposits in:

- The basal ganglia, causing chorea or parkinsonian symptoms
- The liver, causing hepatic cirrhosis
- Descemet's membrane (the basement membrane that lies between the corneal stroma and the endothelial layer of the cornea), producing the characteristic Kayser–Fleischer rings.

Wilson's disease is also associated with an autoimmune haemolytic anaemia and a proximal (type II) renal tubular acidosis.

4.25

D – Clarithromycin

Clarithromycin is a macrolide antibiotic known to inhibit the hepatic and intestinal CYP450 3A4 enzyme. Simvastatin is not absorbed in an active form but it is hydroxylated to simvastatin acid. Because this form is more lipid soluble and therefore more readily crosses cell membranes, it has a more active drug profile. As well as being converted to simvastatin acid, simvastatin is also metabolised into a less active metabolite by the CYP450 3A4 enzyme. Inhibition of this enzyme by the macrolide antibiotics reduces metabolism of the drug, allowing it to accumulate and for higher levels of simvastatin acid to be generated. Because of this, the risk of developing side effects is greater with CYP450 3A4 enzyme inhibitors. These include myalgia, myopathy and, in severe cases, rhabdomyolysis. Consequently, patients who require treatment with a macrolide antibiotic (particularly erythromycin) should stop the statin before starting the antibiotic. In patients with non-severe community-acquired pneumonia the antibiotic of choice is amoxicillin unless an atypical organism is suspected or the patient is allergic to penicillin. In these cases, a macrolide is the preferred antibiotic.

4.26

B – Calcium pyrophosphate

This patient has pseudogout, which is one of the crystal arthropathies. Central to the pathogenesis of pseudogout is the accumulation of pyrophosphate and its crystallisation with calcium within the joint space. Most cases of pseudogout are sporadic but acquired causes include:

- Diabetes mellitus
- Haemochromatosis
- Wilson's disease
- All conditions associated with hypercalcaemia (e.g. primary hyperparathyroidism, malignancy).

When viewed microscopically under polarised light, calcium pyrophosphate crystals are small, rhomboid shaped and positively birefringent. There may also be an inflammatory cell infiltrate composed predominantly of macrophages and giant cells. Deposition of calcium pyrophosphate may be asymptomatic but may also cause attacks of an acute mono- or polyarthritis. The knees are the most commonly affected joints.

Deposition of uric acid within the synovium and synovial fluid is characteristic of gout. Unlike calcium pyrophosphate, uric acid crystals are needleshaped and negatively birefringent under polarised light. In 25% of patients the issue is overproduction of uric acid; in 75% of patients there is undersecretion of uric acid.

Haemosiderin deposition is seen in haemochromatosis and can cause an acute arthritis. Although this patient has haemochromatosis, haemosiderin deposition is an unlikely cause of their arthritis as it does not generate crystals that are positively birefringent under polarised light.

AA amyloidosis is a form of amyloidosis associated with serum amyloid A protein which is an acute-phase protein. The formation of serum amyloid A protein occurs in diseases with longstanding cell breakdown due to a chronic inflammatory disease. AA amyloidosis can cause an acute inflammatory arthritis.

Hydroxyapatite is a major component of normal bone matrix and is important for the rigidity of bone. In excess, hydroxyapatite can form crystals that can only be seen under an electron microscope. These crystals may deposit in the joints causing an arthritis, but the most common place for hydroxyapatite deposition is in the rotator cuff tendons causing a frozen shoulder.

4.27

E – Sulphasalazine

This patient has developed oligospermia as a result of taking sulphasalazine for his ulcerative colitis. The oligospermia is reversible on stopping sulphasalazine. Sulphasalazine is a member of the aminosalicylate group of medications that play an important role in the management of inflammatory bowel disease, especially ulcerative colitis. Aminosalicylates pass through the majority of the small bowel, protected by a carrier molecule, before the active salicylate is released in the distal small bowel and large bowel. Here the salicylate has a topical anti-inflammatory action by reducing prostaglandin production.

Ciclosporin is a calcineurin inhibitor that plays a role in rescue therapy to try and avoid colectomy in patients with ulcerative colitis who have poor prognostic signs and a C-reactive protein of greater than 45 mg/L after three days of intravenous hydrocortisone. It can also be used in the management of Crohn's disease that is unresponsive to glucocorticoids or other immunosuppression. Infliximab is an anti-TNF-alpha monoclonal antibody that plays a similar role to ciclosporin in both Crohn's disease and ulcerative colitis. Loperamide is a gastrointestinal-specific mu opioid receptor agonist that, unlike morphine or codeine, does not act on central nervous system mu opioid receptors. It acts to reduce gastrointestinal motility and is therefore used in the symptomatic treatment of diarrhoea. Metronidazole (a nitroimidazole antibiotic) is used to treat anaerobic and protozoal infections. It also plays an important role in the management of perianal fistulae in Crohn's disease.

4.28
E – Type V

This patient's symptoms and thyroid function tests are highly suggestive of Graves' disease, an autoimmune condition caused by autoantibodies against the thyroid-stimulating hormone receptor. This stimulates thyroid hormone synthesis and secretion as well as growth of the thyroid gland.

Hypersensitivity reactions (autoimmune conditions) are classified into five groups according to the underlying immune response. This is known as the Gell and Coombs classification. Type V reactions such as Graves' disease occur when antibodies recognise and bind to cell surface receptors. This can either prevent the intended substrate from binding (e.g. myasthenia gravis) or mimic the substrate's effects (e.g. Graves' disease).

A type I reaction (immediate hypersensitivity) is an allergic reaction provoked by re-exposure to a specific type of antigen. This response is IgE mediated and causes mast cells to degranulate which release histamine. Examples of type I hypersensitivity reactions include anaphylaxis, asthma and atopy.

Type II reactions occur when antibodies (IgG or IgM) bind to cell membranes or tissue antigens. This results in the cells being targeted by the immune response via three main mechanisms. They are opsonin-dependent phagocytosis, complement-dependent antibody lysis and antibody-dependent cell cytotoxicity. Examples of type II (cytotoxic) hypersensitivity reactions are autoimmune haemolytic anaemias and Goodpasture's syndrome.

Type III reactions occurs when antigen-antibody complexes that are not adequately cleared by innate immune cells accumulate, giving rise to an inflammatory response and chemoattraction of leukocytes. These immune complexes can subsequently deposit in small blood vessels, joints and glomeruli. The following are examples of type III hypersensitivity reactions:

- Extrinsic allergic alveolitis
- Henoch–Schönlein purpura
- Post-streptococcal glomerulonephritis
- Systemic lupus erythematosus.

Type IV hypersensitivity reactions are antibody independent and are known as delayed-type hypersensitivity responses since symptoms develop over several days or weeks. This reaction is the result of a cell-mediated immune memory response. Examples of type IV hypersensitivity reactions include chronic transplant rejection, contact dermatitis and the Mantoux test.

4.29

B –Multiple endocrine neoplasia type I

Multiple endocrine neoplasia type I is characterised by parathyroid hyperplasia, pituitary adenomas and pancreatic endocrine tumours. Parathyroid hyperplasia results in hyperparathyroidism and a rise in serum calcium levels due to increased bone turnover and renal calcium reabsorption. Pituitary adenomas in multiple endocrine neoplasia type I are usually prolactinomas, as in this patient. However, they can also be growth hormone- or adrenocorticotropic hormone-secreting tumours, which would result in acromegaly or Cushing's disease, respectively. Endocrine pancreatic tumours can secrete a variety of endocrine hormones, both recognised and unrecognised. Those that we recognise include insulin, glucagon, somatostatin, vasoactive intestinal peptide, pancreatic polypeptide, growth hormone-releasing factor and/or gastrin. This patient has a gastrinoma. The increased secretion of gastric acid causes refractory peptic ulceration, severe oesophagitis and persistent diarrhoea (Zollinger–Ellison syndrome). Seventy-five percent of cases are sporadic and 25% occur as part of multiple endocrine neoplasia type I.

Multiple endocrine neoplasia type II consists of medullary cell carcinoma of the thyroid gland and phaeochromocytoma. It is subdivided into multiple endocrine neoplasia type IIa if there is also hyperparathyroidism, or multiple endocrine neoplasia type IIb if there is Marfanoid habitus and submucosal neurofibromata of the tongue, eyelids and lips.

McCune–Albright syndrome is caused by mutations in the *GNAS1* gene. It is associated with autonomous hypersecretion of multiple endocrine glands, caféaulait spots, hypophosphataemic rickets and precocious puberty. The hallmark symptom of McCune–Albright syndrome is precocious puberty, with it occurring much earlier in girls than boys.

4.30

E – Von Willebrand factor antigen assay

This patient is most likely to have von Willebrand disease, the most common hereditary coagulation abnormality. Von Willebrand disease can also be acquired due to:

- Aortic valve stenosis leading to Heyde's syndrome (perivalvular shear stress causes von Willebrand factor consumption and gastrointestinal bleeding)
- Hypothyroidism
- Presence of autoantibodies
- Thrombocythaemia
- Wilms' tumour.

Von Willebrand disease is due to a deficiency of von Willebrand factor, a protein that is required for platelet adhesion. As a result, patients with von Willebrand disease present with symptoms suggestive of thrombocytopaenia including menorrhagia, spontaneous subcutaneous bruising and epistaxis. However, in von Willebrand disease the platelet count is normal and consequently von Willebrand disease should be considered in patients with a normal platelet count with symptoms of thrombocytopaenia. The best investigation to confirm the diagnosis is to measure the levels of von Willebrand factor using an antigen assay.

Patients with von Willebrand disease can have a mildly prolonged activated partial thromboplastin time which measures the activity of the intrinsic and common pathways of coagulation. Deficiencies of factors in these pathways will result in a prolonged activated partial thromboplastin time. Deficiency of the following results in a prolonged activated partial thromboplastin time:

- Factor VIII
- Factor IX
- Factor XI
- Factor XII.

The activated partial thromboplastin time is mildly prolonged in von Willebrand disease because von Willebrand factor usually binds to and protects factor VIII from rapid breakdown. Factor VIII levels are reduced in von Willebrand disease and should be measured. However, they will not confirm the diagnosis, as there are other causes of reduced factor VIII levels. In patients with hereditary factor VIII deficiency (haemophilia A) or factor IX deficiency (haemophilia B) the activated partial thromboplastin time is likely to be much more prolonged (e.g. greater than 100 seconds) than in von Willebrand disease. Patients with clotting factor deficiencies usually present with internal bleeding such as haemarthrosis and develop recurrent haematomas within subcutaneous tissues and muscles.

Vitamin K is an essential fat-soluble micronutrient required for the maintenance of normal coagulation. The vitamin K-dependent coagulation proteins are synthesised in the liver and are:

Procoagulant	Anticoagulant
Factor II	Protein C
Factor VII	Protein S
Factor IX	
Factor X	

Despite this duality of function, vitamin K deficiency results in an increased bleeding tendency and will cause a prolonged prothrombin time. The prothrombin time measures the activity of the extrinsic clotting cascade. Vitamin K deficiency will therefore reduce the activity of the extrinsic clotting cascade, which manifests as a prolonged prothrombin time. This patient's prothrombin time is normal.

A bone marrow biopsy is usually indicated in patients with a pancytopaenia to determine whether the bone marrow is hypercellular or hypocellular. However, this patient's blood tests are not suggestive of a pancytopaenia as the haemoglobin, total white cell count and platelets are all within normal limits.

4.31

C – Renal biopsy

The presence of microhaematuria and nephrotic-range proteinuria in a patient with known HIV is highly suggestive of HIV nephropathy. The investigation most likely to confirm the diagnosis is a renal biopsy and would typically show a collapsing focal segmental glomerulosclerosis. Patients with HIV nephropathy have persistently enlarged kidneys which helps to differentiate HIV nephropathy from non-collapsing focal segmental glomerulosclerosis. Therefore, imaging can be useful to differentiate HIV nephropathy from other causes of chronic kidney disease, but it is not diagnostic. In patients with HIV nephropathy, the CD4$^+$ T lymphocyte cell count is usually below 200 cells per ml. The CD4$^+$ T lymphocyte cell count is an important marker for prognosis since survival is worse in patients with a low CD4$^+$ T lymphocyte cell count, but again it is not diagnostic of HIV nephropathy. A common feature of HIV nephropathy is a high urea to creatinine ratio; a similarly high ratio occurs in pre-renal acute kidney injury or gastrointestinal haemorrhage.

4.32

A – *Escherichia coli*

This patient has a complicated pyelonephritis as she has a long-term catheter *in situ*. The most likely organism to be implicated in this patient is *Escherichia coli*. This organism accounts for between 20% and 50% of all cases of acute complicated pyelonephritis. All the other organisms listed do occur more commonly in complicated pyelonephritis but are less likely than *Escherichia coli*.

In uncomplicated, community-acquired infections, acute pyelonephritis is usually due to bowel organisms that enter the urinary tract. The most commonly implicated organism in these cases is again *Escherichia coli*, which is responsible for around 80% of infections. *Staphylococcus saprophyticus* (a Gram-positive coagulase-negative staphylococci) and *Enterococcus faecalis* are other, less common organisms implicated in uncomplicated acute pyelonephritis. *Proteus mirabilis* is a Gram-negative, anaerobic, rod-shaped bacterium and a recognised cause of urinary tract infections. It is important to note that *Proteus* organisms produce urease, which can hydrolyse urea to ammonia and therefore alkalinise the urine. This makes *Proteus* species effective in producing an environment in which it can survive. The urine alkalinisation associated with *Proteus* infection can lead to the formation of struvite stones.

Some patients are at an increased risk of developing acute pyelonephritis and certain factors result in patients having a complicated pyelonephritis. These include any structural abnormalities in the urinary tract (e.g. vesicoureteric reflux or kidney stones), recent

urinary tract instrumentation (e.g. catheterisation), metabolic abnormalities (e.g. diabetes mellitus), recent antibiotic use and the isolation of unusual pathogens (e.g. mycobacteria).

4.33

B – Intravenous aciclovir

This patient has meningitis caused by herpes simplex virus and the
treatment of choice is intravenous aciclovir. Fever, nuchal rigidity
(neck stiffness) and photophobia are characteristic features of
meningeal irritation. Herpes simplex virus is associated with erythema multiforme (multiple cutaneous target lesions). The lumbar
puncture profile of this patient is also highly suggestive of viral
meningitis. The table below shows the expected lumbar puncture
results for the different causes of infective meningitis:

Type of meningitis	Cerebro-spinal fluid appea-rance	Cerebro-spinal fluid glucose: serum glucose (mmol/L)	Protein (mg/dl)	Total cell count (mm^3)	Predominant cell type
Acute bacterial	Turbid	<½ serum glucose	>100	100–5000	Polymorphs
Acute viral	Clear to cloudy	Normal but reduced in mumps	Normal but may be slightly elevated	10–300	Mononuclear (lympho-cytes)
Tuberculous	Fibrin web	<½ serum glucose	>100	30–500	Mononuclear and polymorphs
Fungal	Clear to cloudy	<½ serum glucose	50–200	10–200	Mononuclear

If acute bacterial meningitis is suspected, urgent treatment is required as these patients can develop severe complications including

septicaemia and disseminated intravascular coagulation. If a patient is first seen in a primary care setting a single dose of intramuscular benzylpenicillin should be administered before calling for an ambulance. In hospital, patients with suspected bacterial meningitis should be given a third-generation cephalosporin intravenously (e.g. ceftriaxone) before the results of the blood cultures are known. The use of high-dose corticosteroids (e.g. dexamethasone) is also recommended to reduce intracranial oedema.

Amphotericin is an intravenous drug used in severe fungal infections and would be an appropriate treatment in patients with a fungal meningitis (e.g. *Cryptococcus neoformans*). Patients who develop *Cryptococcus* meningitis are usually severely immunocompromised, such as those with poorly controlled HIV infection. Amphotericin is usually only reserved for severe fungal infections as it is highly nephrotoxic.

Tuberculous meningitis is treated with the quadruple therapy of rifampicin, izoniazid, ethambutol and pyrazinamide. The conventional treatment regime lasts 12 months with ethambutol and pyrazinamide being stopped after two months.

4.34

A – Internal carotid artery dissection

This patient's examination findings are highly suggestive of a right-sided Horner's syndrome which is characterised by:

- Ptosis
- Miosis
- Anhydrosis
- Enophthalmos.

Horner's syndrome indicates a problem with the sympathetic nervous system to the affected side of the face and hence all the symptoms are due to a lack of sympathetic innervation. Preganglionic (first-order) sympathetic fibres arise from the hypothalamus and travel through the brainstem and white matter of the spinal cord. They then synapse onto postganglionic (second-order) sympathetic neurons in the paravertebral ganglia (which form the sympathetic chain) from T1 to L2. Second-order neurons from the T1–T4 paravertebral ganglia then coalesce at the superior cervical ganglion, which lies posterior to the internal carotid artery. The postganglionic sympathetic neurons that converge at the superior cervical ganglia supply the sympathetic innervation to the face. To reach the face the postganglionic neurons travel alongside the internal carotid artery.

An interruption of the sympathetic nervous system at any point from the hypothalamus to the face will result in a Horner's syndrome. The most likely cause of a painful Horner's syndrome, as in this patient, is an internal carotid artery dissection. A dissection in the internal carotid artery occurs due to a tear in the tunica intima. This tear allows blood into the middle layer (tunica media), which forces the layers apart, allowing the tear to expand. Dissection of the internal carotid will compress the postganglionic sympathetic fibres travelling alongside the internal carotid artery. Patients may also present with signs of ischaemic brain injury and amaurosis fugax (transient loss of vision). The amaurosis fugax occurs due to impaired blood flow along the ophthalmic artery, which is the first branch of the internal carotid artery. Around 25% of patients with an internal carotid artery dissection may present with a pulsatile tinnitus due to the close proximity of the internal carotid artery to the cochlea and tympanic cavity.

The postganglionic sympathetic fibres that supply the face run close to the apex of the lung, such as a Pancoast tumour. These typically result in a Horner's syndrome that is insidious, painless and associated with other features of a bronchial carcinoma (e.g. haemoptysis, persistent cough and weight loss). In progressive cases, the brachial plexus, which lies close to the apex of the lung, is also affected resulting in wasting of the intrinsic muscles of the hand.

A Horner's syndrome can also occur if there is an interruption of the first-order neuron in the brainstem, which can occur as a result of multiple sclerosis or stroke, or in the spinal cord, which can occur in syringomyelia.

A posterior inferior cerebellar artery stroke (lateral medullary syndrome or Wallenberg syndrome) affects the nuclei of cranial nerves V, VIII, IX and X, the descending sympathetic fibres, cerebellum and the spinothalamic tract (the fibres of which have already decussated). Clinical features include dysarthria, dysphagia, dysphonia, unilateral Horner's syndrome, unilateral cerebellar signs, loss of pain and temperature on the same side of the face and the opposite side of the body (with respect to the side of the lesion).

Posterior communicating artery aneurysms are the most common cause of a surgical oculomotor nerve palsy. This is due to the fact that when the oculomotor nerve emerges from the brain, it passes in close proximity to the posterior communicating artery. Consequently, aneursyms arising here are likely to result in compression of the parasympathetic fibres of the oculomotor nerve resulting in pupil dilation on the affected side. As the aneurysm becomes larger it will compress the motor fibres of the oculomotor nerve, which lie deeper to the parasympathetic fibres. This will result in extraocular and levator palpebrae muscle paralysis. The oculomotor nerve supplies all of the extraocular muscles except the superior oblique (trochlear) and lateral rectus (abducens). Patients with a large posterior communicating artery aneurysm will present with ptosis, a dilated pupil and an eye that faces down and out.

Klumpke's syndrome is due to a traction injury (e.g. motorcycle injury) that results in damage to the brachial plexus (cervical roots C8 and T1). This causes paralysis and affects the intrinsic muscles of the hand and the flexors of the wrist and fingers producing a classical claw hand appearance. If the T1 nerve root is affected, there may also be an accompanying Horner's syndrome due to damage of the sympathetic nerves.

4.35

E – Gentamicin

This patient has myasthenia gravis, an autoimmune neuromuscular disease. It is due to the presence of antibodies that block acetylcholine receptors at the postsynaptic neuromuscular junction, inhibiting the excitatory effects of acetylcholine at neuromuscular junctions. Patients present with muscle weakness and fatigability (particularly the ocular muscles). In patients with myasthenia gravis there are many drugs known to worsen symptoms. Gentamicin (an aminoglycoside antibiotic) is contraindicated in patients with myasthenia gravis as it blocks the presynaptic release of acetylcholine. It can therefore precipitate a myasthenic crisis in which patients can develop reduced function of the respiratory muscles and subsequent respiratory arrest. This neuromuscular transmission defect can be reversed by the administration of calcium and/or neostigmine. All the other antibiotics listed also have the potential to worsen symptoms in myasthenia gravis and should be used with caution.

The major contraindication of amoxicillin is penicillin hypersensitivity. Ceftriaxone (a third-generation cephalosporin) is contraindicated in patients with cephalosporin hypersensitivity or in patients who have previously had an anaphylactic reaction from a previous exposure to a penicillin-containing medication. Ceftriaxone is also contraindicated in neonates less than 41 weeks postmenstrual age and in neonates over 41 weeks postmenstrual age with jaundice, hypoalbuminaemia or acidosis. This is because ceftriaxone is known to cause biliary sludging and obstructive jaundice in neonates. In neonates who require a third-generation cephalosporin, cefotaxime should be used as it is not known to cause this. Ceftriaxone is also contraindicated in neonates over 41 weeks who are receiving intravenous calcium as there is a risk that the calcium can precipitate in the urine and lungs.

Doxycycline (a tetracycline) is contraindicated in pregnant or breastfeeding women and in children less than 12 years of age. This is because tetracyclines deposit in growing bone and teeth (by binding to calcium) which causes staining and occasionally dental hypoplasia. Doxycycline and erythromycin (a macrolide) are contraindicated in patients with acute porphyria as they may precipitate an attack.

4.36

E – Request an HIV test

A ring-enhancing lesion is a radiological finding in which contrast medium accumulates in the periphery of a lesion leaving a central area relatively free of contrast. The major differentials for a ring-enhancing lesion on a contrast CT head include:

- Cerebral abscess
- Cerebral lymphoma
- Cerebral toxoplasmosis
- Intrinsic brain tumour.

Toxoplasmosis and cerebral lymphoma are usually associated with underlying immunosuppression, most commonly due to HIV infection. In this patient, there is a history of recurrent oral candidiasis and therefore a HIV test is the most appropriate next step in this patient's management. If this patient is HIV positive then the most likely diagnosis would be cerebral toxoplasmosis. Toxoplasmosis is caused by the protozoa *Toxoplasma gondii*, which is transmitted to humans mainly via contact with infected cat faeces. The initial infection is often asymptomatic but can present with flu-like symptoms. Following a successful immune response, the parasites remain dormant and encysted in the host tissues (mainly brain, heart and skeletal muscle) for years. They can reactivate if there is immunosuppression. Multiple ring-enhancing lesions are more typical of cerebral toxoplasmosis whereas cerebral lymphoma is more likely to present with a single ring-enhancing lesion. Patients with ring-enhancing lesions without HIV are highly unlikely to have toxoplasmosis. Therefore, the HIV status of a patient should be determined before treating patients for cerebral toxoplasmosis. The treatment for cerebral toxoplasmosis is intravenous sulphadiazine (a sulphonamide antibiotic) and pyrimethamine (a dihydrofolate reductase inhibitor).

If this patient is HIV negative then they should be referred to a neurosurgeon, as the most likely diagnosis would be an intrinsic brain tumour or a cerebral abscess. Both of these conditions would require a neurosurgical evaluation. This patient does not have any signs of meningism and a lumbar puncture is unlikely to aid the diagnosis or management of this patient. Furthermore, this patient has a space-occupying lesion and may have raised intracranial pressure. Performing a lumbar puncture in this patient may therefore precipitate herniation of the brainstem through the foramen magnum. Intravenous aciclovir is usually indicated in patients with suspected herpes simplex encephalitis or meningitis. However, this patient does not have features of meningism (vomiting, nuchal rigidity and photophobia) or encephalitis (fever, headache and altered mental status).

4.37

B – Contact the anaesthetist for intubation

This patient's history of a sudden-onset headache and signs of meningism (stiff neck and photophobia) is highly suggestive of a subarachnoid haemorrhage. Ten to fifteen percent of patients with a subarachnoid haemorrhage die before reaching hospital and approximately 25% of patients die within 24 hours. It is therefore essential that the initial management of patients with a subarachnoid haemorrhage is directed at patient stabilisation. This includes an assessment of the patient's airway, breathing and circulation combined with an evaluation of their consciousness using the Glasgow Coma Scale. The Glasgow Coma Scale is an objective measure of a patient's consciousness, which has a maximum score of 15 (fully awake) and a minimum score of three (deep unconsciousness). This score is comprised of three separate scores for each response tested. The responses tested are eyes with a maximum score of four ('four eyes'), verbal with a maximum score of five ('Jackson Five') and motor with a maximum score of six ('six cylinder engine'). The table below outlines the scoring system for the Glasgow Coma Scale:

	6	5	4	3	2	1
Eyes	N/A	N/A	Opens spontaneously	Opens in response to voice	Opens in response to pain	Does not open eyes
Verbal	N/A	Oriented/ normal conversation	Confused/ disorientated	Inappropriate words	Incomprehensible sounds	No sounds
Motor	Obeys commands	Localises painful stimuli	Flexion/ withdrawal from painful stimuli	Abnormal flexion to painful stimuli	Extension to painful stimuli	No movements

Patients with a Glasgow Coma Scale of less than eight are unable to support their own airway. They therefore require immediate intubation and mechanical ventilation. This patient's Glasgow Coma Scale score is six (eyes two, verbal two, motor two) and the most appropriate initial management is to contact the anaesthetist for intubation. The anaesthetist should also be called to patients with a subarachnoid haemorrhage who have a rapidly decreasing Glasgow Coma Scale score.

Once patients with a suspected subarachnoid haemorrhage have been initially stabilised and appropriate monitoring of vital signs has been established, it is important to confirm the diagnosis with specific investigations. The most appropriate investigation is an urgent non-contrast head CT scan, which, if performed within 48 hours, will identify 95% of subarachnoid haemorrhage cases. In patients with a negative head CT scan where the diagnosis of subarachnoid haemorrhage remains highly likely a lumbar puncture should be performed to detect xanthochromia (partially degraded erythrocytes in the cerebrospinal fluid). A lumbar puncture should never be performed before a head CT scan due to the fact that if there is raised intracranial pressure this may precipitate herniation of the brainstem through the foramen magnum.

Cerebral vasospasm is a complication of a subarachnoid haemorrhage, which can result in an area of secondary ischaemia. It is rare in the first three days after a subarachnoid haemorrhage and its incidence peaks at around 7–10 days. Patients should be commenced on intravenous nimodipine (a calcium channel antagonist) as soon as the diagnosis of subarachnoid haemorrhage is confirmed to reduce the risk of cerebral vasospasm. Intravenous nimodipine is thought to reduce the risk of vasospasm by causing relaxation of the smooth muscles in the cerebral arterial walls.

Patients with a subarachnoid haemorrhage regularly present to a non-neurosurgical unit and often require urgent neurosurgical or neuroradiological intervention. However, it is important to stabilise the patient, confirm the diagnosis and recognise the complications (i.e. commence nimodipine) before they are transferred to a specialist neurosurgical unit.

4.38

A – Co-trimoxazole

This patient has Stevens–Johnson syndrome, a life-threatening dermatological emergency, in which cell death causes the epidermis to separate from the dermis. It is considered part of a spectrum of diseases, which include, in order of increasing severity, erythema multiforme, Stevens–Johnson syndrome and toxic epidermal necrolysis. Both Stevens–Johnson syndrome and toxic epidermal necrolysis have skin and mucous membrane involvement. The major differentiating feature is the percentage of total body skin that is involved; if the area is greater than 30% patients are considered to have toxic epidermal necrolysis.

Stevens–Johnson syndrome usually begins with fever, sore throat and fatigue. Painful ulcers and other lesions then begin to appear in the mucous membranes, almost always in the mouth and lips. These lesions can also occur in the genito-anal regions. Patients can also develop conjunctivitis.

Although most cases of Stevens–Johnson syndrome are idiopathic there are many well-recognised causes. The major causes are medications, infections and rarely neoplasia. Co-trimoxazole is a combination of a sulphonamide and trimethoprim and is prescribed in patients with granulomatosis with polyangiitis as it has been shown to help prevent relapses. Medications containing sulphonamide groups within their structure are well known to cause Stevens–Johnson syndrome. Therefore, trimethoprim on its own is not known to precipitate Stevens–Johnson syndrome.

NSAIDs such as ibuprofen and indomethacin are also recognised to cause Stevens–Johnson syndrome but have no effect on relapse rates in granulomatosis with polyangiitis. Lorazepam is a short-acting benzodiazepine and is the first-line treatment for convulsive status epilepticus. It is not known to cause Stevens–Johnson syndrome. However, many anti-epileptic medications including phenytoin and carbamazepine can cause Stevens–Johnson syndrome.

4.39

D – N-acetylcysteine

Non-immunogenically mediated degranulation of mast cells is termed an anaphylactoid reaction. In an anaphylactoid reaction, a substance binds directly to mast cells, which results in degranulation and subsequent histamine release. Medications known to cause an anaphylactoid reaction are:

- N-acetylcysteine
- Opiates
- Intravenous contrast
- Vancomycin.

Importantly, since anaphylactoid reactions are non-immunologically mediated no prior exposure is required and consequently patients can develop severe signs of anaphylaxis on the first administration of a known precipitant.

Most cases of anaphylaxis are due to an anaphylactic reaction. In an anaphylactic reaction IgE on the surface of mast cells binds to the antigen resulting in degranulation of mast cells and release of histamine. All the medications in the question other than N-acetylcysteine are known to cause an anaphylactic reaction. The most common group of medications known to cause an anaphylactic reaction are the penicillins (e.g co-amoxiclav). Patients who have a true anaphylactic reaction to penicillin should not be prescribed a cephalosporin (e.g. cephalexin) as an alternative antibiotic. This is because penicillins and cephalosporins share a common beta-lactam ring in their structures. Ten percent of patients who have an anaphylactic reaction to penicillin will also develop an allergy to cephalosporins.

Although anaphylactoid and anaphylactic reactions differ in their pathology, they both result in mast cell degranulation and subsequent histamine release. Therefore, both anaphylactic and anaphylactoid reactions can be treated with intramuscular adrenaline in order to stabilise mast cells and reduce vascular permeability.

4.40

D – Progressive supranuclear palsy

The most likely diagnosis for a patient who has negative extrapyramidal symptoms (bradykinesia, rigidity and reduced facial expression) and a gaze palsy is progressive supranuclear palsy. This is a condition of unknown aetiology and develops insidiously in patients over 50 years of age. It is considered one of the Parkinson plus syndromes as the extrapyramidal symptoms can mimic that of idiopathic Parkinson's disease. One of the key features that help to distinguish progressive supranuclear palsy from idiopathic Parkinson's disease is the presence of a gaze palsy. Supranuclear gaze palsies usually first present with impaired downward eye movement followed by a lack of all other eye movements as the disease progresses. A resting tremor is not usually associated with progressive supranuclear palsy whereas it is one of the key features of idiopathic Parkinson's disease. Consequently, patients with progressive supranuclear palsy have rigidity without the presence of cogwheeling (tremor superimposed on rigidity). Patients with progressive supranuclear palsy can also develop cognitive impairment and personality changes. Progressive supranuclear palsy does not respond well to levodopa therapy and death usually occurs within five to seven years of onset.

Multi-system atrophy is a neurodegenerative condition and there are two distinct forms. The first form, which accounts for around two thirds of cases, presents with extrapyramidal symptoms and autonomic failure (usually postural hypotension and bladder symptoms). This is sometimes referred to as Shy–Drager syndrome and can also be considered a Parkinson plus syndrome. The second form is a predominant cerebellar syndrome with upper motor neuron signs. Autonomic failure can also be a feature of this form of multi-system atrophy.

Corticobasal degeneration is a rare neurodegenerative condition and presents with an asymmetrical akinetic-rigid syndrome. It is associated with marked dyspraxia, myoclonus and dementia. Patients may also have an 'alien hand' in which the hand moves purposefully without conscious control.

Wilson's disease (hepatolenticular degeneration) is an autosomal recessive genetic disorder in which there is a deficiency of caeruloplasmin that normally binds copper in plasma and a failure of hepatocytes to excrete free copper. Consequently, in Wilson's disease there is an increase in free copper, which can then accumulate in tissues. The excess copper deposits in:

- The basal ganglia, causing chorea or parkinsonian symptoms
- The liver, causing hepatic cirrhosis
- Descemet's membrane (basement membrane that lies between the corneal stroma and the endothelial layer of the cornea), producing the characteristic Kayser–Fleischer rings.

Wilson's disease is also associated with an autoimmune haemolytic anaemia and a proximal (type II) renal tubular acidosis.

4.41

B – Continue her normal four times daily insulin regimen

This patient is on a basal bolus insulin regimen. The long-acting 'basal' insulin (in the morning and/or night) mimics background pancreatic insulin secretion and the short-acting 'bolus' insulin (usually three times daily) mimics that secreted with meals. A direct effect of infection is hyperglycaemia and therefore insulin requirements typically increase in diabetic patients who have intercurrent infection, rather than decrease. As a result, a patient's insulin regime should never be stopped, as this runs the risk of precipitating hyperglycaemia and diabetic ketoacidosis. However, such patients can also be at an increased risk of hypoglycaemia as they are eating poorly and irregularly, and may also be vomiting. Therefore, the most appropriate option is to admit the patient for intravenous fluids, continue her normal insulin regime and increase the frequency of glucose monitoring. The in-hospital insulin doses may need adjusting accordingly. The following should also be performed in this patient:

- Urine dispstick to check for ketones
- Full blood count, urea and electrolytes, liver function tests and C-reactive protein
- Arterial blood gas
- Stool culture.

4.42

D – Primary biliary cirrhosis

Anti-mitochondrial antibodies are most commonly associated with primary biliary cirrhosis with 95% of patients testing positive for the antibody. Primary biliary cirrhosis is an autoimmune condition that leads to destruction of the intrahepatic bile ducts, cholestasis and back flow of bile, progressing to portal tract inflammation, fibrosis and liver failure. It has strong associations with other auto-immune conditions (e.g. rheumatoid arthritis, systemic lupus erythematosus, Sjögren's syndrome, thyroid autoimmunity and scleroderma), a 9:1 female preponderance and typically presents in middle age. Fatigue and arthralgia are common initial presentations, and there may also be signs of post-hepatic cholestasis (pruritus, jaundice, steatorrhoea, gallstones), portal hypertension (hepatomegaly, splenomegaly, variceal bleeding, ascites), abdominal pain and osteoporosis.

Treatment of primary biliary cirrhosis involves symptomatic relief with the only definitive treatment being liver transplantation. Ursodeoxycholic acid may improve liver function tests and cholestyramine, which binds to bile salts in the gut and prevents their reabsorption, may alleviate pruritus. Rifampicin and naltrexone are alternatives. Patients are deficient in the fat-soluble vitamins A, D, E and K, and appropriate supplements are necessary.

4.43

E – Spontaneous bacterial peritonitis

Abdominal pain and fever in a patient with signs and symptoms of chronic liver disease is strongly suggestive of spontaneous bacterial peritonitis, a well-known complication of liver cirrhosis. The most important initial investigation is a diagnostic paracentesis and peritoneal fluid analysis. Cloudy ascitic fluid with an absolute neutrophil count of greater than 250 cells/mm^3 almost invariably indicates ascitic infection. Aerobic Gram-negative organisms are the most common cause (anaerobes are rare as ascitic fluid is well oxygenated), and are usually of enteric origin (most commonly *Escherichia coli*). Although the exact mechanism by which bacteria appear in the ascitic fluid is still controversial, patients with cirrhosis are at particular risk because of:

- Intestinal bacterial overgrowth (often found in patients with liver cirrhosis)

- Decreased complement levels (impaired hepatic protein synthesis) in the ascitic fluid and serum
- Impaired activity of the reticuloendothelial system.

Until microbiological studies guide management further, antibiotics are given empirically. Cefotaxime or piperacillin-tazobactam are first-line options.

4.44

D – Nifedipine

Nifedipine is a dihydropyridine calcium channel antagonist and is the most appropriate second-line anti-hypertensive agent in this patient. Nifedipine reduces blood pressure through peripheral vasodilation. Bendroflumethiazide is known to increase serum uric acid levels and should be avoided in gout. Bisoprolol is a beta-adrenergic receptor antagonist and can therefore impair the beta-adrenergic relaxation of the airway smooth muscle. It should therefore be avoided in patients with asthma and COPD. Angiotensin-converting enzyme inhibitors such as ramipril are used in preference to an angiotensin II receptor antagonist such as losartan. Patients taking angiotensin II receptor antagonists have likely been switched from angiotensin-converting enzyme inhibitors after developing negative side effects (most commonly dry cough). Doxazocin is an alpha-adrenoreceptor antagonist and a third-line treatment for essential hypertension. It is preferentially used in patients with concurrent prostatism (e.g. benign prostatic hyperplasia) as it causes smooth muscle relaxation in the prostate, the neck of the bladder and the ureters, thus improving urinary symptoms in such patients.

4.45

B – Cutaneous small-vessel vasculitis

The differential diagnosis of this patient's purpuric rash includes all five options; however, a normal platelet count excludes all except cutaneous small-vessel vasculitis. This causes a non-thrombocyto-paenic purpura. Acute myeloid leukaemia tends to present acutely with symptoms of aplastic anaemia; shortness of breath due to aplastic anaemia, signs of infection due to leukopaenia and easy bruising due to thrombocytopaenia. In disseminated intravascular coagulation, there is an overwhelming increase in the activity of circulating thrombin, either by release of procoagulant factors (e.g. malignancy) or by endothelial damage (e.g. in meningococcal sepsis). Laboratory findings reveal a low platelet count, prolonged prothrombin time and activated partial thromboplastin time, grossly prolonged thrombin time and depleted fibrinogen levels. Thrombotic thrombocytopaenic purpura is one of the thrombotic microangiopathies classically characterised by a pentad of:

- Fever
- Microangiopathic haemolytic anaemia, which is character-ised by a low haemoglobin and the presence of fragmen-ted red cells
- Consumptive thrombocytopaenic purpura
- Renal failure
- Neurological symptoms.

4.46

E –Upper gastrointestinal endoscopy

The most important differential diagnosis in this patient is oesopha-geal cancer, for which the investigation of choice is upper gastroin-testinal endoscopy. Gastrointestinal endoscopy can offer diagnostic benefit (visualisation of the oesophagus and biopsy for histological examination) and, if necessary, the option of therapeutic interven-tion (e.g. oesophageal dilation). Dysphagia initially for solids then liquids suggests a luminal obstruction. Barium swallow is used to assess disorders of oesophageal motility (e.g. achalasia). Such patie-nts typically present with difficulty swallowing both solids and liq-uids from the outset. Oesophageal manometry is an evaluation of oesophageal pressures and is an adjunct to the barium swallow; it provides information on peristaltic and lower oesophageal sphincter function. Once the diagnosis of oesophageal cancer is confirmed by endoscopy, CT scanning and endoscopic ultrasound are used to assess tissue invasion and the lesion's operability.

4.47

C – Nasogastric tube and intravenous fluids

This patient has mechanical small bowel obstruction, most likely due to adhesions secondary to inflammatory bowel disease. Adhesive obstructions can settle without the need for surgery and therefore in the initial treatment of small bowel obstruction (particularly ileus and incomplete small bowel obstruction), conservative management is preferable to surgery. Surgery is avoided if possible in order to reduce the chance of developing further adhesions. In contrast, where the cause is a large bowel obstruction, strangulating obstruction or volvulus, surgery is required. The main aim in conservative management of small bowel obstruction is to relieve pressure on the small bowel (which can perforate) and the stomach (which can press on, and splint, the diaphragm), and to rehydrate the patient by administration of intravenous fluids and insertion of a nasogastric tube ('drip and suck'), respectively. Being simply nil by mouth does not relieve the small bowel pressure adequately enough. Analgesia should be considered but is not an initial priority. Blood tests should include:

- Full blood count (a leukocytosis is often common)
- Urea, electrolytes and bone function tests (to check electrolyte balance)
- Inflammatory markers
- Pancreatic enzymes (amylase and lipase).

Failure to improve, or initial clinical concern about the diagnosis should lead to early abdominal CT imaging. The presence of valvulae conniventes, which can be seen to cross the bowel lumen completely, indicate that the small bowel is involved.

4.48

B – Cholecystitis

This patient's history is typical of symptomatic gallstone disease (cholelithiasis) which, in the past, appears to have caused only mild episodes of biliary colic. However, in this acute episode there is likely infection of the gallbladder (calculous cholecystitis) with a resultant inflammatory reaction causing peritonism and fever. Ninety percent of gallstones are asymptomatic. The two main types are due to supersaturation of bile with either cholesterol or pigment, respectively. Risk factors for cholesterol stones include states of high oestrogen and high cholesterol:

- Hormone replacement therapy
- The oral contraceptive pill
- Pregnancy
- A pre-menopausal state
- Obesity
- Hypercholesterolaemia.

Risk factors for pigment stones (which are composed of calcium bilirubinate) are states of high bilirubin (e.g. haemolysis). The absence of haemolysis in this scenario means that this patient is therefore likely to have cholesterol gallstones. The complications of gallstones include:

- Biliary colic
- Choledocholithiasis (stones in the common bile duct)
- Cholangitis (inflammation of the bile ducts)
- Gallstone ileus
- Pancreatitis
- Gallbladder cancer
- Cholecystitis (inflammation of the gallbladder).

Ninety percent of cases of cholecystitis are associated with gall-stones. Cholecystitis occurs because gallstones block the flow of bile, which results in a thickening of the bile and bile stasis. Subsequently increased luminal pressure causes distension of the gallbladder, impaired blood flow and impaired mucosal defences, which, in addition to bile stasis itself, lead to secondary infection with enteric bacteria. A mass may be felt in the right upper quadrant (representing the inflamed gallbladder and the adherent greater omentum and bowel), which, when palpated, arrests deep inspiration. This is known as Murphy's sign. As the patient breathes in and out, the examiner's hand below the right costal cartilage catches the inflamed gallbladder and arrests breathing. The test shows high sensitivity but low specificity for cholecystitis as long as it is negative on the left side.

In this scenario, the patient's right shoulder pain is referred pain that occurs secondary to irritation of the diaphragm on the right (sub-phrenic irritation). Pain is felt in the region of the supraclavicular nerve on the same side. This shares the same cervical nerve root origin as the phrenic nerve. This phenomenon is known as Kehr's sign, and can occur in either shoulder depending on the cause of diaphragmatic irritation. Other causes include intraperitoneal blood/irritants (e.g. ruptured ectopic pregnancy or ruptured spleen) or peridiaphragmatic irritation (pneumonia, pericarditis, cholecystitis, liver abscess, splenic abscess, gastric ulcer).

Finally, Courvoisier's law states that if, in the presence of jaundice, the gallbladder is palpable, then the cause is something other than gallstones. Usually the cause is carcinoma of the pancreas. However, the patient in this scenario was not jaundiced.

4.49

E – Paracetamol

This patient is suffering from an uncomplicated acute coryza (common cold or nasorhinopharyngitis) for which only paracetamol and/or nasal decongestant are of any benefit. The vast majority of upper respiratory tract infections are viral in origin with acute coryza being the most common. However, bacterial infections are the usual causes of otitis media, epiglottitis and acute tonsillitis.

Complications of acute coryza include:

- Bronchitis
- Sinusitis (requiring steam inhalation)
- Pneumonia
- Otitis media (blockage of the Eustachian tubes leads to secondary bacterial infection).

These have all been excluded in this patient and therefore there is no indication to prescribe antibiotics. An analgesic and anti-pyretic such as paracetamol can help to alleviate symptoms and would be a useful prescription in this scenario. Intranasal glucocorticoids are used in the management of allergic rhinoconjunctivitis (hayfever), which is an unlikely diagnosis in this patient. Furthermore, intranasal glucocorticoids are not first-line therapy for allergic rhinoconjunctivitis.

4.50

C – Doppler echocardiography

This patient has aortic valve stenosis. The most common aetiology is different for middle-aged people (bicuspid aortic valve) than for the elderly (degenerative valvular calcification). In this patient, aortic stenosis has presented with the classic triad of syncope (due to impaired cerebral perfusion), ischaemic chest pain (due to the increased oxygen demands of a reactive hypertrophied left ventricle) and heart failure (due to reduced compliance of the hypertrophic left ventricle and pulmonary backflow, resulting in shortness of breath). Another important complication is sudden death, which can occur due to ischaemic changes or a ventricular arrhythmia secondary to myocardial hypertrophy.

This patient's murmur (high-pitched ejection systolic murmur) is classical for aortic stenosis. However, in very severe aortic stenosis the murmur may be inaudible as flow across the aortic valve is so low. Other signs of aortic stenosis include an attenuated carotid pulse with delayed upstroke (an anacrotic, slow-rising pulse) and a paradoxically split-second heart sound (due to the pulmonary valve closing before the aortic valve; the aortic valve usually closes first).

Chest X-ray and ECG are necessary investigations, and a transthoracic echocardiography is useful to diagnose and determine the aetiology of aortic stenosis. However, the best investigation to assess the severity of aortic stenosis is Doppler echocardiography as it can measure the pressure gradients across the aortic valve. For management, symptomatic patients require valve replacement because the survival time from the onset of angina is five years, from the onset of syncope is three years and from the onset of congestive cardiac failure is two years. Coronary angiography may be required to exclude coronary artery disease prior to valve replacement surgery.

4.51

E – *Trypanosoma cruzi*

Trypanosoma cruzi is a flagellate protozoon that causes American trypanosomiasis (Chagas' disease). *Trypanosoma gambiense* and *Trypanosoma rhodesiense* are two other organisms in the same genus as *Trypanosoma cruzi*. *Trypanosoma gambiense* and *Trypanosoma rhodesiense* are the cause of African trypanosomiasis (sleeping sickness).

The vectors for *Trypanosoma cruzi* are insects from the genus *Triatoma*, which are found in houses in Latin America, and transmit *Trypanosoma cruzi* through contact with the wounds, mucous membranes and blood of humans (mainly children). The acute disease often presents with non-specific symptoms including fever, fatigue, myalgia, headache, diarrhoea, vomiting, and lymphadenopathy. Other features of the acute phase include mild hepatosplenomegaly and a local erythematous nodule (chagoma) at the site of infection.

A minority of patients (particularly the young and/or immunocompromised) experience a more severe and potentially fatal acute infection. Features can include:

- Unilateral conjunctivitis
- Periorbital oedema near the wound site (Romana's sign)
- Myocarditis
- Meningoencephalitis.

In the vast majority of patients the acute phase resolves spontaneously after two months. However, even with treatment (nifurtimox or benznidazole), in 30% of patients the infection persists and develops into the life-threatening chronic phase of the disease. Multiorgan invasion induces local inflammation, cell death and fibrosis that primarily affects the following:

- Heart (dilated cardiomyopathy)
- Digestive system (toxic megacolon and megaoesophagus)
- Nervous system (central and peripheral nervous system).

Cardiac involvement is the usual cause of death but the first symptom is often dysphagia due to secondary achalasia and megaoesophagus. The alternative options in this question have different presentations, and most notably, dysphagia is not a feature.

Note: Antitrypanosome therapy does not have a role in the treatment of chronic disease in adults. Nifurtimox and benznidazole are used for acute disease and in children.

4.52

A – A defect in a membrane protein which binds the cytoskeleton

This patient has hereditary spherocytosis, an autosomal dominant disorder that occurs in 1 in 500 live births. It is due to a mutation in one of the several membrane-bound proteins (e.g. spectrin, ankyrin). These proteins are responsible for binding the cytoskeletal matrix to the cell membrane, and are therefore respon-sible for maintaining the normal shape of erythrocytes. The mutations render the erythrocytes less deformable and therefore, as they pass through the splenic microvasculature, some of their membrane is removed. This causes them to appear spheroidal, hyperchromatic and lacking central pallor. The erythrocytes can also be destroyed by the spleen resulting in splenomegaly and haemolytic anaemia. Patients with a haemolytic anaemia are jaundiced (unconjugated hyperbilirubinaemia) and have an increased risk of pigment gallstones. The following investiga-tions should be performed in a patient with suspected hereditary spherocytosis:

- Full blood count to detect anaemia
- Liver function tests to look for a raised serum bilirubin
- Peripheral blood film to look for evidence of haemolysis and spherocytes
- Osmotic fragility (Ham's) test
- Coombs test to rule out an autoimmune cause of the haemolytic anaemia.

The osmotic fragility test involves placing the patient's erythro-cytes in a hypotonic solution. If spherocytes are present, they will rupture more easily because the spherocyte membranes are wea-ker and, unlike biconcave red blood cell membrane, cannot change shape to increase their intracellular volume. The Coombs test is important because spherocytes are also seen in autoimmune haemolytic anaemias, which can present in a similar way.

In this question, glucose-6-phosphate dehydrogenase deficiency results in accumulation of oxidants due to a deficiency in a cell's reducing power, alpha-thalassaemia is a defect in the gene encod-ing for the alpha-globulin chain of haemoglobin, sickle cell disease is due to the transposition of valine for glutamate in position six of the beta-globulin haemoglobin chain and rhesus disease of the newborn is due to maternal anti-rhesus-D antibodies which bind to cell surface antigens. These are all causes of anaemia in the young but will not produce this set of investigation results.

4.53

A – Asbestosis

The most likely diagnosis in this patient is asbestosis and pleural plaques secondary to chronic asbestos exposure, which is associated with certain occupations. These include occupations that produce/ transport asbestos fibres (miners, millers, dockworkers), manufacture insulation products (roofers, floorers, textiles, cements) or work with insulation products (builders, electricians, plumbers, mechanics, firefighters). A detailed occupational history in respiratory patients is vital.

Asbestos is in fibres that are much longer than they are wide. As they're inhaled they align with the airway and can descend down to the small bronchioles. Here they are engulfed by macrophages and coated with ferritin granules, forming inflammatory asbestos bodies. Such exposure is associated with four different pulmonary conditions:

- Pleural plaques: benign patches of calcified pleural thickening that can be seen on X-ray and can cause dyspnoea if large.
- Asbestosis: inflammation and chronic interstitial fibrosis occurring 20–30 years post-exposure; effects range from mild to respiratory failure and death.
- Lung cancer: asbestos increases the risk of both small and non-small cell lung cancer.
- Malignant mesothelioma: a pleural malignancy occurring 40 years post-exposure; mean survival is 8–14 months.

Malignant mesothelioma is a tumour that arises from mesothelial cells, the simple, squamous, epithelial cells which form the lining (serosa/mesothelium) of various body cavities, including the thorax (pleura), abdomen (peritoneum), myocardium (pericardium) and the internal reproductive organs (tunica vaginalis in men; tunica serosa uteri in women). Therefore, although mesothelioma can affect any of these sites, the majority affect the pleura or peritoneum. Over 90% are linked to asbestos exposure (after a roughly 40-year latency period). Pleural malignant mesothelioma are widespread across the pleura, can expand inwards (compressing the lungs and mediastinum) and can cause a pleural effusion. The patient in this question has costophrenic blunting due to pleural thickening, not pleural effusion. Patients with malignant mesothelioma present with chest pain, dyspnoea and/or weight loss. The diagnosis of malignant mesothelioma is an important diagnosis so that patients can claim for compensation. Asbestosis is an interstitial lung disease and is therefore associated with diffuse inspiratory crackles, a reduced PEFR and a chronic dry cough.

4.54

E – Unstable angina

This patient is suffering from pain due to cardiac ischemia which, in this instance, is due to an episode of unstable angina. Unstable angina is a condition that lies on the spectrum of ischaemic heart disease in between stable angina and myocardial infarction. Stable angina lasts less than 20 minutes and occurs on exertion but not at rest. It is due to the presence of a fixed, stable atherosclerotic obstruction of a coronary vessel that occludes the vessel enough to cause cardiac ischaemia but not necrosis. If myocardial necrosis is suspected then such an episode is referred to as the acute coronary syndrome until proven otherwise. Acute coronary syndrome encompasses unstable angina (rest pain without myocardial necrosis) and myocardial infarction. Myocardial infarction causes a rise in cardiac markers and can be further classified into ST elevation myocardial infarction (ST elevation or new left bundle branch block) or non ST elevation myocardial infarction, depending on the ECG changes.

In patients with acute coronary syndrome it is therefore important not only to perform an ECG but also to test cardiac markers to test for necrosis. Patients can then be diagnosed with either unstable angina (negative troponin, no ST elevation), NSTEMI (positive troponin, no ST elevation) or STEMI (positive troponin, ST elevation).

4.55

A – Intravenous methylprednisolone

This patient has temporal arteritis and has lost the vision in one eye. High-dose intravenous methylprednisolone will offer the best chance of preventing loss of sight in the remaining eye. A high ESR and C-reactive protein would support the clinical diagnosis. The diagnosis may be confirmed with a positive temporal artery biopsy but this should not delay treatment with intravenous methylprednisolone. A negative biopsy would not alter the diagnosis because the disease often just affects small segments of the artery (skip lesions) rather than the whole length. After three days of intravenous methylprednisolone high-dose oral prednisolone should be commenced and tapered according to patient response.

The typical patient is female and at least 55 years old. Also known as giant cell arteritis, temporal arteritis causes granulomatous inflammation in the walls of the extracranial branches of the aorta and carotid artery, typically in the temporal and ophthalmic arteries, resulting in turbulent blood flow and downstream ischaemia. Typical symptoms include:

- Fever
- Headache
- Sudden loss of vision
- Diplopia
- Jaw claudication
- Scalp tenderness
- Tinnitus (through hearing the audible, turbulent blood flow).

Half of patients also have polymyalgia rheumatica, which presents with proximal muscle pain and stiffness, but no objective weakness. Cyclophosphamide and azathioprine are both used in the treatment of systemic vasculitis but are not first-line agents for temporal arteritis.

4.56

D – Oral nitrofurantoin

This lady has presented with a urinary tract infection that requires antibiotic treatment. Nitrofurantoin is the most appropriate options of all those listed in this scenario. It has a complex mechanism of action. It is converted to its reduced form by bacterial flavoproteins. This form is highly reactive and damages bacterial DNA, ribosomes and other large molecules. It is also excreted renally, which means that it is at its greatest concentration in the lower urinary tract. It should be noted that nitrofurantoin is not effective at treating urinary tract infections in patients with a creatinine clearance of less than 60 ml/min.

Patients such as the one in this scenario do not require intravenous antibiotics; these are reserved for patients who are systemically compromised or have not improved following a course of oral antibiotics. Clarithromycin is metabolised hepatically and is not excreted via the urinary tract. It is therefore ineffectual at treating urinary tract infections.

Crucially, as this patient is taking methotrexate they must not be given trimethoprim (or, indeed, co-trimoxazole). Methotrexate is primarily an inhibitor of dihydrofolate reductase whereas trimethoprim primarily inhibits bacterial dihydrofolate reductase (although it does have some inhibitory effects on mammalian dihydrofolate reductase). If these two medications are given concomitantly, there is total inhibition of dihydrofolate reductase, which can lead to severe folate deficiency and methotrexate toxicity. The most notable feature of methotrexate toxicity is that of myelosuppression and subsequent pancytopaenia.

4.57

C – Hypocalcaemia

Thyroid carcinoma is the most common indication for thyroidec-tomy, but it is also a suitable treatment option for patients with hyperthyroidism refractory to medical intervention and in patients who have symptoms of mass effect (dysphagia, dyspnoea, hoarse-ness). The most common short-term complication of a total thy-roidectomy is hypocalcaemia secondary to transient primary iatrogenic hypoparathyroidism. This is thought to be as a result of transient intra-operative ischaemia of the parathyroid glands. There are four parathyroid glands within the thyroid gland, and during the thyroidectomy they should be carefully dissected out and left in the thyroid bed. Parathyroid hormone normally acts to increase plasma calcium and decrease plasma phosphate by stimu-lating osteoclastic bone resorption, decreasing renal calcium excre-tion and increasing renal phosphate excretion. Although patients may initially be asymptomatic, worsening hypocalcaemia causes relative depolarisation of the resting membrane potential. Features of hypocalcaemia include:

- Numbness
- Perioral and digital paraesthesia
- Carpopedal spasm
- Chvostek's sign
- Trousseau's sign
- Tetany
- Seizures
- QT prolongation.

Patients undergoing total thyroidectomy are monitored for evi-dence of hypocalcaemia, with provision of calcium and vitamin D supplementation where necessary. Other complications of thyroid-ectomy include:

- Recurrent laryngeal nerve damage (unilateral or bilateral)
- Neck haematoma

- Hyperthyroidism
- Infection (incisional cellulitis or abscess formation).

Bilateral recurrent laryngeal nerve damage paralyses both vocal cords, resulting in aphonia and a high risk of airway obstruction. This situation warrants immediate airway management (e.g. tracheotomy). Patients who develop a neck haematoma (less than 1%) require emergency evacuation (either in theatre or at the bedside) due to the risk of airway compromise. A thyrotoxic storm can be precipitated during thyroid surgery due to thyroid gland manipulation, particularly in patients with pre-existing hyperthyroidism. Therefore one of the contraindications for thyroidectomy is a patient with uncontrolled hyperthyroidism (e.g. Graves' disease). Such patients need cooling, a beta-adrenoreceptor antagonist, propylthiouracil/carbimazole and iodine as necessary. Patients who have a total thyroidectomy require regular long-term follow up to monitor for hypothyroidism.

4.58

E – Unremarkable history

Thin glomerular basement membrane disease, also known as benign familial haematuria, is a common cause of asymptomatic haematuria. The sole abnormality is thinning of the glomerular basement membrane. The important feature of thin glomerular basement membrane disease is that the predominant feature is glomerular haematuria. The diagnosis can only be confirmed by renal biopsy; the prognosis is benign and there are no other features, except that some patients may have mild proteinuria and hypertension. It is a diagnosis of exclusion. During history taking, examination and investigation, other more sinister causes of glomerular haematuria that are associated with a worse prognosis should be actively excluded. These include IgA nephropathy and Alport's syndrome. In Alport's syndrome (a genetic mutation affecting type IV collagen, which is present in the renal, ocular and auditory basement membranes), there is commonly a family history of chronic kidney disease, hearing and ocular impairment and, because the condition is usually X-linked, there is more frequent and severe disease in males. Frank haematuria or loin pain should warrant investigation for other causes such as IgA nephropathy and nephrolithiasis.

4.59

D – Metoprolol

This patient is likely to have variant angina, also known as Prinzmetal's angina. Symptoms typically occur at rest, rather than on exertion (thus attacks usually occur at night). Variant angina should be suspected when the pain occurs at rest or in clusters and in the absence of a positive treadmill stress test. It is associated with ST segment elevation during an acute attack and resolves as the pain subsides. Variant angina is due to vasospasm of the coronary arteries due to dysfunction of the endothelium. Therefore, medications such as beta-blockers (metoprolol) that can induce vasospasm are contraindicated. Calcium channel blockers (both amlodipine and verapamil) and nitrates are used in the management of variant angina as they cause dilation of the coronary arteries. The gold standard investigation for variant angina is coronary angiography with injection of vasospasm-inducing agents into the coronary artery. Rarely, an active spasm can be documented angiographically and if witnessed is diagnostic of variant angina.

4.60

D – Pacemaker insertion

The ECG findings in this scenario are consistent with trifascicular block. The three features of trifascicular block are:

- First-degree atrioventricular block (PR interval of greater than 0.2 seconds)
- Right bundle branch block
- Left bundle hemiblock (this manifests itself as left-axis deviation on an ECG).

Trifascicular block is found in patients with diffuse disease of the conduction system, most commonly as a result of longstanding ischaemic heart disease. The combination of the ECG findings and the episode of syncope mean that this patient requires pacemaker insertion, as without a pacemaker complete (third-degree) heart block is likely to develop.

Twenty-four-hour Holter monitoring is useful in patients who experience paroxysmal arrhythmias, and so is not required in this scenario. Coronary angiography and echocardiography may be indicated in the long term to look for any new atherosclerotic or structural lesions that may be contributing, respectively. Tilt table testing is used to assess patients with suspected vasovagal syncope.

Paper 5

Paper 5: Questions

5.1 A 62-year-old male with a 40-pack year smoking history is being investigated for COPD.

Which one of the following is most likely to suggest an alternative diagnosis to COPD?

A Chronic cough
B Exertional breathlessness
C Frequent winter 'bronchitis'
D Nocturnal wheeze
E Regular sputum production

5.2 A 67-year-old female with a longstanding history of recurrent urinary tract infections develops progressively worsening cough and shortness of breath. Her lung function tests are as follows:

FEV_1	2.4 L
FVC	2.7 L

Which one of the following antibiotics is she most likely to have been taking long term?

A Amoxicillin
B Cefalexin
C Ciprofloxacin
D Nitrofurantoin
E Trimethoprim

5.3 A 26-year-old male presents with haemoptysis and shortness of breath. On examination there are widespread inspiratory crackles bilaterally. Urine dipstick reveals 2+ protein and 3+ blood.

Which one of the following spirometry result profiles is most likely to be found in this patient?

A $FEV_1:FVC$ ratio of 0.72, FEV_1 77% of predicted, kCO 95% of predicted

B $FEV_1:FVC$ ratio of 0.72, FEV_1 77% of predicted, kCO 135% of predicted

C $FEV_1:FVC$ ratio of 0.86, FEV_1 92% of predicted, kCO 65% of predicted

D $FEV_1:FVC$ ratio of 0.88, FEV_1 97% of predicted, kCO 95% of predicted

E $FEV_1:FVC$ ratio of 0.88, FEV_1 75% of predicted, kCO 135% of predicted

5.4 A 44-year-old male presents with a one-year history of excessive daytime sleepiness. His partner mentions that he snores loudly at night and sometimes stops breathing. The patient's body mass index is 34 kg/m^2.

Which one of the following is the most appropriate initial management?

A Assess for mandibular advancement device
B Nasal continuous positive airway pressure
C Refer for bariatric surgery
D Salbutamol inhaler
E Thyroid function tests

5.5 A 23-year-old male presents with a three-month history of cough and shortness of breath. Lateral chest X-ray reveals the presence of a mass in the anterior mediastinum.

Which one of the following is the most likely diagnosis?

A Descending aortic aneurysm
B Neurofibromatosis type I
C Neurofibromatosis type II

D Pericardial cyst
E Teratoma

5.6 A 49-year-old male with haemophilia A presents with jaundice, right upper quadrant pain and weight loss.

Which one of the following is the most likely diagnosis?

A Acute haemolytic transfusion reaction
B Acute viral hepatitis
C Budd–Chiari syndrome
D Hepatocellular carcinoma
E Pancreatic carcinoma

5.7 A 38-year-old male who has recently returned from holiday in Ghana presents shortness of breath, malaise, myalgia and head-ache. He is experiencing alternating fevers and rigors. On examination he is clinically anaemic, icteric and has hepatosplenomegaly. His temperature is 39.1 °C.

Which one of the following is the most appropriate to confirm the diagnosis?

A Blood culture
B Chest X-ray
C Full blood count, urea and electrolytes, liver function tests, blood glucose
D Thick and thin blood films
E Urine dipstick

5.8 A 38-year-old female with systemic lupus erythematosus presents with worsening menorrhagia and easy bruising. On examination there are palatal petechial haemorrhages. Full blood count reveals the following:

Haemoglobin	10.2 g/dL
Mean cell volume	74 fL

| White cell count | $5.2 \times 10^9/L$ |
| Platelet count | $15 \times 10^9/L$ |

A blood film is also performed. An extract from the report is as follows:

'There is a reduction in platelet number. The platelets that are present are larger than normal.'

Which one of the following is the most appropriate initial management for this patient?

A Commence eltrombopag
B Commence intravenous immunoglobulin
C Commence platelet transfusion
D Reassure and repeat blood test in two weeks
E Refer to surgeons for splenectomy

5.9 A 56-year-old male is diagnosed with infective endocarditis and commenced on intravenous antibiotics. Four days later blood tests reveal a markedly raised urea and creatinine.

What is the most likely type of acute kidney injury that has occurred as a result of aminoglycoside prescription?

A Acute interstitial nephritis
B Acute tubular necrosis
C Mesangiocapillary glomerulonephritis
D Post-infectious immune complex glomerulonephritis
E Pre-renal acute kidney injury

5.10 A 39-year-old male with chronic kidney disease is seen in the nephrology outpatients clinic. His estimated glomerular filtration rate is found to be 18 ml/minute/1.73 m^2. He has a history of Crohn's disease, has had several abdominal operations, and has ongoing problems with adhesions. He is currently on no regular medication.

What is the next most appropriate step in management of this patient?

A Haemodialysis
B Peritoneal dialysis

C Referral for arteriovenous fistula construction
D Referral to palliative care
E Renal transplantation

5.11 A 73-year-old female with type II diabetes is started on enalapril after a routine check up identifies proteinuria. Soon after commencing enalapril, she becomes dyspnoeic. Chest X-ray reveals interstitial shadowing.

What is the most likely cause of this scenario?

A Acute respiratory distress syndrome
B Anaphylaxis
C Atheromatous renal artery stenosis
D Fibromuscular dysplasia
E Hereditary angioedema

5.12 A 43-year-old female receiving treatment for highly active relapsing-remitting multiple sclerosis presents with a five-week history of progressively worsening weakness of the left arm and leg, aphasia and memory loss. MRI of the brain revealed multiple new areas of hyperintensity on T2-weighted and fluid attenuation inversion recovery images and hypointensity on a T1-weighted image. Polymerase chain reaction detection of JC virus in the cerebrospinal fluid was positive.

Which one of the following medications is this patient most likely to have been taking?

A Efalizumab
B Glatiramer
C Methylprednisolone
D Natalizumab
E Rituximab

5.13 A 28-year-old male allergic to NSAIDs presents with back pain radiating to the buttocks and early morning stiffness that improves throughout the day. X-ray of his sacroiliac joints reveals bilateral sacroiliitis.

Which one of the following is the most appropriate treatment option in this patient?

A Bisphosphonates
B Indomethacin
C Physiotherapy
D Rest
E Spinal steroid injection

5.14 A 38-year-old female presents with joint pain. Examination reveals the presence of nail pitting and itchy, scaly pink plaques on the elbows and knees bilaterally.

Which one of the following statements regarding her condition is true?

A Arthritis mutilans is the most common pattern of joint involvement
B Nail pitting occurs more commonly in those with arthritis
C Rheumatoid factor is positive in the majority of patients
D The arthritis always predates the skin changes
E Women are more likely to be affected than men

5.15 A 53-year-old female with longstanding rheumatoid arthritis is found to have a nodular lesion on the superior aspect of the sclera. There is exposure of the underlying dark uveal tissue. Abnormal blood vessels are found running over this area.

Which one of the following is the most likely diagnosis?

A Episcleritis
B Keratoconjunctivitis sicca
C Pinguecula
D Pterygium
E Scleromalacia perforans

5.16 A 51-year-old female presents with chest tightness, shortness of breath, wheeze and cough. She was diagnosed with asthma ten years ago and now requires daily oral steroids to control her symptoms. On examination there is a purpuric rash present on both legs, decreased sensation over the lateral three and a half digits of the left hand and weakness of abductor pollicis brevis of the left hand. Blood tests reveal an eosinophil count of $3.4 \times 10^9/L$.

Which one of the following is the most likely diagnosis?

A Acute eosinophilic pneumonia
B Allergic bronchopulmonary aspergillosis
C Eosinophilic granulomatosis with polyangiitis
D Loeffler's syndrome
E Sarcoidosis

5.17 A 77-year-old female presents with muscle weakness and generalised bony pain. On examination the patient displays a 'waddling' gait. Investigations are as follows:

Serum calcium	2 mmol/L
Serum phosphate	0.6 mmol/L
Serum alkaline phosphatase	400 IU/L
Serum vitamin D	15 nmol/L
Serum parathyroid hormone	6 pmol/L

An X-ray of the left femur shows an abnormality at the femoral neck.

Which one of the following is the most likely abnormality to be found on the X-ray of this patient?

A Loss of joint space
B Periarticular osteopaenia
C Pseudofracture
D Subchondral cysts
E Subchondral sclerosis

5.18 A 47-year-old HIV-positive male presents with a two-week history of worsening vision and the presence of floaters in his visual field. Fundoscopy reveals a 'mozzarella and tomato' appearance of the retina.

Which one of the following is the most appropriate first-line treatment of this patient?

A Aciclovir
B Ganciclovir

C Ribavirin
D Tenofovir
E Zidovudine

5.19 A 46-year-old male presents with a three-day history of fever, cough, headache and severe muscle pains. On examination there is bilateral conjunctival haemorrhage, lymphadenopathy, splenomegaly and a purpuric rash over the lower limbs. The patient has photophobia but there is no nuchal rigidity. Urine dipstick reveals the presence of 2+ protein and 3+ blood.

What is the most likely infectious agent to have caused this presentation?

A *Borrelia burgdorferi*
B *Brucella melitensis*
C *Legionella pneumophila*
D *Leptospira interrogans*
E *Streptococcus pyogenes*

5.20 A 57-year-old female receiving chemotherapy for non-Hodgkin's lymphoma develops malaise, lethargy and a fever of 39.1 °C. The patient states that they developed shortness of breath and an itchy, erythematous rash when they were given penicillin in the past.

Which one of the following is the most appropriate treatment option for this patient?

A Intravenous benzylpenicillin and gentamicin
B Intravenous ceftriaxone and gentamicin
C Intravenous ciprofloxacin, teicoplanin and gentamicin
D Intravenous co-amoxiclav and gentamicin
E Intravenous tazocin and gentamicin

5.21 An eight-year-old male presents with his mother to his General Practitioner with a two-day history of a purpuric rash on his buttocks, thighs and legs. In addition, his mother mentions that he also complains of arthralgia in his right ankle and diffuse abdominal pain.

Which one of the following investigations is most appropriate to perform?

A Abdominal ultrasound
B Blood cultures
C Joint aspiration
D Lumbar puncture
E Urine dipstick

5.22 A 62-year-old male presents to his General Practitioner with a three-month history of progressive weakness. Neurological examination reveals the presence of fasciculations with upper and lower motor neuron signs.

Which one of the following conditions causes both upper and lower motor neuron degeneration?

A Amyotrophic lateral sclerosis
B Primary lateral sclerosis
C Progressive bulbar palsy
D Progressive muscular atrophy
E Pseudobulbar palsy

5.23 A 65-year-old male who had a prosthetic valve insertion 12 months previously presents to his General Practitioner with increasing shortness of breath, fever and night sweats. On auscultation a new murmur is heard.

Which one of the following organisms is the most likely causative agent?

A *Candida albicans*
B *Mycobacterium tuberculosis*
C *Staphylococcus epidermidis*
D *Streptococcus bovis*
E *Streptococcus viridans*

5.24 A 36-year-old male who has just arrived back from a holiday in Spain presents with myalgia, a non-productive cough, headache and fever of 38.2 °C. On examination of the chest there is dullness to percussion with crackles on auscultation over the right lung base. Chest X-ray shows consolidation in the right lower zone with a blurred right heart border. Further investigations reveal the presence of *Legionella* antigen in the urine.

Which one of the following antibiotic regimens would be the most appropriate in this patient?

A Amoxicillin and rifampicin
B Benzylpenicillin and clarithromycin
C Cefuroxime and clarithromycin
D Clarithromycin and rifampicin
E Co-amoxiclav and clarithromycin

5.25 A 32-year-old female presents with a two-day history of increasing shortness of breath accompanied by pleuritic chest pain. Her observations are as follows:

Heart rate	112 beats per minute
Blood pressure	100/60 mmHg
Respiratory rate	20 breaths per minute
Oxygen saturations	92% on room air
Temperature	36.8 °C

Further questioning revealed that she had suffered three miscarriages over the last three years and has also suffered from a posterior cerebral artery infarct.

Which one of the following is the most likely underlying diagnosis in this patient?

A Anti-phospholipid syndrome
B Factor V Leiden deficiency
C Nephrotic syndrome
D Protein C deficiency
E Protein S deficiency

5.26 A 29-year-old male is found to have a blood pressure of 190/110 mmHg. Blood tests are requested and the subsequent results make the physician consider Conn's syndrome as the diagnosis.

Which one of the following metabolic profiles is most likely to occur in a patient with Conn's syndrome?

A Hyperkalaemic, hyponatraemic metabolic acidosis
B Hyperkalaemic, hypernatraemic metabolic acidosis
C Hypokalaemic, hypernatraemic metabolic acidosis
D Hypokalaemic, hypernatraemic metabolic alkalosis
E Hypokalaemic, hypochloraemic metabolic alkalosis

5.27 A 65-year-old female was recently started on a new medication by her General Practitioner. A subsequent routine blood test reveals a serum potassium of 3.2 mmol/L.

Which one of the following medications is most likely to have caused hypokalaemia in this patient?

A Amiloride
B Bendroflumethiazide
C Benzamil
D Furosemide
E Spironolactone

5.28 A 29-year-old pregnant female attends her booking appointment at nine weeks. A routine urine culture reveals the presence of *Escherichia coli*. The patient has no urine frequency or dysuria.

Which one of the following management options is most appropriate in this patient?

A Admit to hospital for intravenous co-amoxiclav
B Prescribe oral amoxicillin
C Prescribe oral ciprofloxacin
D Prescribe oral trimethoprim
E Reassure and send home

5.29 A 68-year-old female receiving chemotherapy for breast cancer attends the outpatient clinic. She explains that her grandson has become unwell and developed a rash consistent with chickenpox yesterday. The patient had been present at his birthday party two days ago. The patient has no history of chickenpox and currently feels well.

Which one of the following is the most appropriate initial management option?

A Intravenous aciclovir
B No action required
C Oral aciclovir
D Serum VZV antibody titres
E VZV immunoglobulin

5.30 A five-year-old male has been referred to a neurologist due to several episodes of abrupt onset of staring blankly, which last for 20 seconds. During each episode he is unresponsive and there is a brief upward rotation of the eyes. The child's mother states that these episodes usually occur after the child has been hyperventilating. A sleep-deprived electroencephalogram reveals the presence of 3 hertz generalised spike-wave discharges that correlate to an episode of staring blankly.

Which one of the following medications is most likely to worsen this child's condition?

A Carbamazepine
B Ethosuximide
C Lamotrigine
D Topiramate
E Valproate

5.31 A 60-year-old female undergoes a surgical resection of the colon for presumed colorectal cancer. Histological analysis reveals the presence of a moderately differentiated adenocarcinoma that penetrates the muscularis propria but not the subserosal fat. There is no evidence of lymph node involvement.

According to the adapted Dukes' classification which one of the following is the stage of this patient's adenocarcinoma?

A Stage A
B Stage B1
C Stage B2
D Stage C1
E Stage C2

5.32 A 36-year-old female with a history of anorexia nervosa presents with increasing shortness of breath on exertion. On examination she is noted to have a resting heart rate of 102 beats per minute, swollen ankles and bibasal inspiratory crackles on auscultation of the lung fields. An echocardiogram reveals an ejection fraction of 70%.

Which one of the following is the most likely diagnosis?

A Aortic stenosis
B Dilated cardiomyopathy
C Ischaemic heart disease
D Iron deficiency anaemia
E Left ventricular hypertrophy

5.33 A 45-year-old male has the following thyroid function tests:

Thyroid-stimulating hormone   Undetectable
Free thyroxine   55 nmol/L

He is commenced on treatment but two weeks later is admitted to hospital with a sore throat and fever. An urgent blood test reveals a neutrophil count of 0.7×10^9/L.

Which one of the following medications is most likely to have caused this complication?

A Clozapine
B Levothyroxine
C Propranolol
D Propylthiouracil
E Radioiodine

5.34 A 67-year-old female attends the Emergency Department complaining of severe right-sided periorbital pain that started three hours ago. She also states that she can see haloes around most objects and that the pain is made worse when she is sitting in a dimly lit room. On examination of the right eye, there is an erythematous sclera and an oval-shaped, semi-dilated pupil.

Which one of the following is the most appropriate initial management option in this patient?

A Intravenous acetazolamide, topical timolol and topical prednisolone
B Intravenous mannitol, oral prednisolone and topical pilocarpine
C Intravenous mannitol, oral prednisolone and topical timolol
D Oral acetazolamide, oral prednisolone and topical timolol
E Topical pilocarpine, topical prednisolone and intravenous acetazolamide

5.35 A 54-year-old HIV-positive male with Kaposi's sarcoma presents with fever, night sweats and weight loss. On examination, there is axillary and inguinal lymphadenopathy. A summary of his blood tests is as follows:

Haemoglobin	10.2 g/dL
White cell count	3.5×10^9/L
Interleukin-6	Elevated

Which one of the following is the most likely diagnosis?

A Castleman's disease
B Kikuchi's disease
C Multiple myeloma
D *Mycobacterium avium* infection
E *Pneumocystis jirovecii* pneumonia

5.36 A 65-year-old female is referred to a neurologist due to increasing bilateral incoordination that was initially unilateral. She has also noticed that her speech has become increasingly slurred over the previous two months. On examination there is severe truncal and neck ataxia, accompanied by an ataxic gait. There is also a mild horizontal nystagmus. The neurologist requested a contrast-enhanced MRI of the brain which was unremarkable. Examination of the cerebrospinal fluid showed a raised protein and white cell count; all other investigations were normal.

Which one of the following is the most likely diagnosis in this patient?

A Alcoholic cerebellar degeneration
B Cerebellar haemangioblastoma
C Late-onset multiple sclerosis
D Paraneoplastic cerebellar degeneration
E Systemic lupus erythematosus

5.37 A 55-year-old male presents with a two-month history of arthralgia, weight loss and diarrhoea. On further questioning it is also noted that he has become increasingly confused and has recently been diagnosed as having epilepsy. Selected blood tests are as follows:

Serum calcium   1.95 mmol/L
Albumin   35 g/L

Endoscopy and duodenal biopsy is performed. Peroidic acid-Schiff staining is performed on the tissue and when examined under the microscope shows magenta-coloured macrophages in the lamina propria.

Which one of the following is the most likely diagnosis in this patient?

A Coeliac disease
B *Entamoeba histolytica* infection
C *Giardia lamblia* infection
D Ulcerative colitis
E Whipple's disease

5.38 A 56-year-old male presents with a right-sided foot drop. Examination reveals weakness of ankle dorsiflexion. Ankle jerk is intact.

Which one of the following additional features on examination is most likely to confirm the diagnosis of common peroneal nerve palsy?

A   Ability to evert the ankle
B   Ability to invert the ankle
C   Inability to plantarflex the ankle
D   Loss of sensation over the big toe
E   Wasting of the gastrocnemius

5.39 An 80-year-old female with Alzheimer's disease presents to the Emergency Department. Her daughter reveals that she had a fall two weeks previously and since then has become increasingly confused. On examination the patient has a Glasgow Coma Score of 12. A CT scan reveals the presence of a left-sided hypodense bi-concave lesion, which crosses several suture lines.

Which one of the following is most likely to explain this patient's symptoms?

A   Damage to the bridging veins
B   Damage to the middle meningeal artery
C   Damage to the posterior cerebral artery
D   Damage to the posterior inferior cerebellar artery
E   Damage to the striate arteries

5.40 A 40-year-old male is found to have the following blood results:

Fasting cholesterol	7.7 mmol/L
Low-density lipoprotein	5 mmol/L

His father had a myocardial infarction aged 47 and a diagnosis of familial hypercholesterolaemia is under consideration. He has not had his serum cholesterol previously tested.

Which one of the following is the most appropriate first step in management?

A   Give appropriate dietary and lifestyle advice
B   Initiate bezafibrate
C   Initiate ezetimibe

D Initiate high-dose simvastatin
E Send off further blood samples for glucose, urea and electrolytes, fasting lipids, thyroid function tests and liver function tests

5.41 A 62-year-old male with longstanding, well-controlled type II diabetes mellitus is called to his General Practitioner for his six-monthly check up.

Which one of the following is the most appropriate investigation to screen for microalbuminuria?

A 24-hour urine collection
B Renal ultrasound and biopsy
C Routine urine dipstick
D Spot urine test for albumin:creatinine ratio
E Urea and electrolytes

5.42 An 18-year-old male presents with vomiting, drowsiness and extreme thirst. The doctor notices he has fruity-smelling breath.

Which one of the following is the most appropriate initial investigation?

A Arterial blood gas
B Blood cultures
C Chest X-ray
D ECG
E Urine dipstick

5.43 A 17-year-old female with known sickle cell disease presents to the Emergency Department with acute severe pain in her right thigh, which has not improved with naproxen. On examination she is well hydrated, and aside from a mild tachycardia and tachypnoea, her basic observations (urine output, oxygen saturations, temperature and blood pressure) are within the normal range.

After initial resuscitation, the administration of which one of the following medications is the most appropriate next step in management?

A Antibiotics
B Intravenous 0.9% sodium chloride

C NSAIDs
D Opiate analgesia
E Oxygen supplementation

5.44 A 68-year-old male with known alcoholic liver cirrhosis who regularly attends the Emergency Department is admitted and started on a full alcohol detoxification regimen. After two days of improvement he develops constipation, confusion, disorientation and sleep disturbance. On examination there is asterixis and constructional apraxia but no signs of psychosis, seizure or focal neurology.

Which one of the following is the most appropriate first step in the management of this patient?

A CT head
B Lactulose
C Neomycin
D Thiamine
E Zopiclone

5.45 A 28-year-old male has been undergoing investigation for increasing exertional dyspnoea and fatigue. After a chest X-ray demonstrated a cardiothoracic ratio of 0.8 he is referred for echocardiogram, which demonstrates four enlarged, globular chambers with thin, hypokinetic walls, impaired systolic and diastolic function and no septal hypertrophy. Further tests are subsequently requested in an attempt to elucidate a unifying diagnosis.

Which one of the following is most associated with a normal echocardiogram and can therefore be ruled out as a differential in this patient?

A Alcohol abuse
B Chagas' disease
C Haemochromatosis
D Thyrotoxicosis
E Vitamin B_{12} deficiency

5.46 A 73-year-old female undergoes a routine blood test and is found to have the following results:

Haemoglobin	17.3 g/dL
Mean corpuscular volume	80 fL
Haematocrit	0.55
Red cell mass	126% of predicted
White cell count	$13.0 \times 10^9/L$
Platelets	$490 \times 10^9/L$

Subsequent investigation reveals:

Serum erythropoietin	2.7 U/L

Which one of the following is the most likely diagnosis?

A Chronic kidney disease
B COPD
C Polycythaemia rubra vera
D Relative polycythaemia
E Von Hippel–Lindau disease

5.47 A 41-year-old female presented to her General Practitioner six months ago with a scaly, pruritic, well-demarcated annular rash with a central clearing in her left axilla. There was an inflammed, raised, erythematous edge that was about 5 cm in diameter at the time. Eczema was diagnosed and she has since been prescribed several courses of topical steroid creams. Many months later, she returns, requesting yet another prescription. This is because, although the creams make the rash less red and irritating, since stopping the cream the itching has got worse. The itching has never been as bad as it is on this occasion. On examination of the lesion, although the margin now appears less raised and scaly, the rash itself is less well demarcated, pustular and has expanded to over 15 cm in diameter. In addition, there is some skin thinning and telangiectasia around the site of the lesion, which was not present initially.

Which one of the following is the most likely diagnosis in this patient?

A Cutaneous candidiasis
B Erythrasma
C Flexural psoriasis
D Tinea corporis
E Tinea incognito

5.48 A 76-year-old female presents to the Emergency Department following a fall at home. She was found on the floor by her neighbour and states that she had been lying on her floor for approximately 24 hours. On examination she is dehydrated and has a large bruise over her left buttock. She has passed a small quantity of dark brown urine whilst in the Emergency Department. She has no previous history of renal impairment and her past medical history is notable only for hypercholesterolaemia, for which she is taking simvastatin. She is currently receiving 1 L of 0.9% sodium chloride over 4 hours. Selected investigations reveal the following:

Serum sodium	152 mmol/L
Serum potassium	6.3 mmol/L
Serum urea	9 mmol/L
Serum creatinine	493 μmol/L

Urine dipstick:

Protein	+
Blood	+++
Leukocytes	−
Nitrites	−
Urine microscopy	'No red cells, no casts'

ECG showed 90 beats per minute, normal sinus rhythm and no T wave changes

Which one of the following is most in keeping with an alternative clinical diagnosis?

A Low calcium
B Raised alkaline phosphatase
C Raised aspartate transaminase

D Raised phosphate
E Raised uric acid

5.49 A 48-year-old male has undergone routine endoscopic surveillance in order to monitor his longstanding Barrett's oesophagus. He is once again reassured that no pre-cancerous or cancerous changes have been detected.

Which one of the following histological findings is most likely to be found on his biopsy report?

A Columnar metaplasia
B High-grade dysplasia
C Low-grade dysplasia
D Malignant neoplasia
E Squamous metaplasia

5.50 A 45-year-old male is admitted with a creatinine of 325 μmol/l, associated with an eosinophilia and eosinophiluria. The patient had been taking regular naproxen for a painful neck for the last six weeks. His baseline urea and electrolytes were normal prior to starting the naproxen.

Which one of the following is the most likely cause of his acute kidney injury?

A Acute interstitial nephritis
B Ischaemic acute tubular necrosis
C Mesangial IgA disease
D Mesangiocapillary glomerulonephritis
E Renal vein thrombosis

5.51 A 66-year-old male has presented to his General Practitioner with shortness of breath and a persistent cough. His dyspnoea has been getting progressively worse and more laboured over the last few months and is now present even at rest. His cough is non-productive and has also been worsening. There is no significant past medical history, drug history or family history, he is a non-smoker and the systems review is also unremarkable. He is clubbed, his pulse is 90 beats per minute and regular, jugular venous pressure is not elevated, heart sounds are normal, and on respiratory examination he is tachypnoeic and has bibasal end inspiratory crackles. Spirometry referral reveals a restrictive lung defect.

Which one of the following is the most likely diagnosis?

A Caplan's syndrome
B Idiopathic pulmonary fibrosis
C Pulmonary oedema
D Sarcoidosis
E Tuberculosis

5.52 A 39-year-old female who has been complaining to her General Practitioner of painful mouth ulcers for many months has begun to develop multiple flaccid blisters on her trunk that are easily friable. Most of them have ruptured, leaving behind widespread areas of painful, haemorrhagic and exudative ulceration, which has now become dry and crusted. They are non-purulent and Nikolsky's sign is positive.

Which one of the following is the most likely diagnosis?

A Behcet's disease
B Bullous pemphigoid
C Insect bites
D Pemphigus vulgaris
E Scalded skin syndrome

5.53 A 45-year-old male presents with a six-week history of loose stools. The remainder of the history and examination is unremarkable. Investigations reveal the following:

Haemoglobin	11.1 g/dL
Mean corpuscular volume	73 fL
Serum iron	9 µmol/L
Serum ferritin	8 µg/L
Total iron-binding capacity	89 µmol/L

Which one of the following is the most appropriate next step in the management of this patient?

A Commence the patient on ferrous sulphate
B Reassure and prescribe Fybogel
C Referral to a haematologist
D Referral for routine colonoscopy
E Referral for urgent colonoscopy

5.54 A 35-year-old male who returned from Bangladesh ten days ago presents with an intermittent fever and headache. He has also had several episodes of diarrhoea, which he describes as yellow-green in colour. On examination he has several clusters of red macules and mild splenomegaly. He has a positive Widal test and no parasites are seen on thick and thin blood cultures.

Which one of the following antibiotics should this patient be commenced on?

A Ceftriaxone
B Clarithromycin
C Co-amoxiclav
D Doxycycline
E Metronidazole

5.55 A 66-year-old male with metastatic lung cancer presents with increasing pain. He was initially controlled on 60 mg MST modified release every 12 hours. He is now requiring three additional doses of 20mg Oromorph® to control the pain.

Which one of the following is the most appropriate decision option regarding MST modified release prescription?

A 40 mg MST modified release every 6 hours
B 60 mg MST modified release every 8 hours
C 80 mg MST modified release every 12 hours
D 90 mg MST modified release every 12 hours
E 120 mg MST modified release every 12 hours

5.56 A 58-year-old female with metastatic breast cancer presents with a two-month history of progressively worsening shortness of breath that is worse on lying flat. Auscultation of the lung fields reveals bilateral coarse inspiratory crackles. There is bilateral pitting oedema up to the knees.

Which one of the following medications is the most likely cause of this patient's symptoms?

A Carboplatin

B Docetaxel

C Gemcitabine

D Tamoxifen

E Trastuzumab

5.57 A 73-year-old female presents to the Emergency Department with confusion. On examination she is found to have periorbital oedema, alopecia and slow-relaxing reflexes. Her observations are as follows:

Heart rate	48 bpm
Blood pressure	120/60 mmHg
Respiratory rate	10 bpm
Oxygen saturations (room air)	91%
Temperature	35.1 °C

Selected blood tests are as follows:

Serum thyroid-stimulating hormone	12 mU/L
Serum free thyroxine (T_4)	1.6 nmol/L
Serum cortisol (9 am)	80 nmol/L

Which one of the following initial treatment options is most appropriate in this patient?

A Adrenaline

B Fludrocortisone

C Hydrocortisone

D Thyroxine

E Triiodothyronine

5.58 A 73-year-old male who is currently on warfarin for a previous deep vein thrombosis is commenced on clarithromycin. Three days later he develops left-sided weakness. His international normalised ratio is 6.9. An urgent CT head scan reveals the presence of an intracerebral haemorrhage.

Which one of the following treatment options is most appropriate in this patient?

A Omit warfarin and commence fresh frozen plasma with intravenous vitamin K

B Omit warfarin and commence oral vitamin K

C Omit warfarin and commence prothrombin complex with intravenous vitamin K

D Omit warfarin and commence prothrombin complex with oral vitamin K

E Omit warfarin until international normalised ratio is within therapeutic range

5.59 A 17-year-old male is brought to his General Practitioner by his mother. He has been suffering frequent falls. On examination he has a high-arched palate, an ejection systolic murmur and a marked kyphoscoliosis. The following signs are elicited on neurological examination of the lower limbs:

Inspection	Distal wasting. Pes cavus. No asymmetry or fasciculations
Tone	Normal
Power	Generalised weakness, distal > proximal, extensors > flexors
Reflexes	Absent ankle and knee reflexes. Upgoing plantar reflexes
Co-ordination	Impaired heel-shin test. Positive Romberg's test. Intention tremor
Gait	Broad-based
Sensation	Impaired vibration and proprioception in the feet

Which one of the following is the most likely diagnosis?

A Amyotrophic lateral sclerosis
B Charcot–Marie–Tooth disease
C Conus medullaris lesion
D Friedreich's ataxia
E Marfan's syndrome

5.60 A 60-year-old male is admitted to hospital for observation following a head injury. There is no focal neurology, and CT head and initial blood tests performed in the Emergency Department are normal. On the following day, the patient becomes confused. Examination is normal and the patient is clinically euvolaemic. Subsequent investigations are as follows:

Serum sodium	123 mmol/L
Serum potassium	3.8 mmol/L
Serum urea	7 mmol/L
Serum creatinine	95 µmol/L
Serum urate	98 µmol/L
Plasma osmolality	255 mmol/kg
Urine osmolality	558 mmol/kg

Which one of the following is the most appropriate treatment option for this patient?

A Amiloride
B Demeclocycline
C Desmopressin
D Hydrocortisone
E Thyroxine

Paper 5: Answers

5.1

D – Nocturnal wheeze

COPD is predominantly caused by smoking and is characterised by progressive airflow obstruction that is not fully reversible. Diagnosis of COPD should be considered in patients over the age of 35 who have a risk factor (usually smoking) and who present with exertional breathlessness, chronic cough, frequent winter 'bronchitis', regular sputum production or wheeze. Nocturnal wheeze specifically is not seen in COPD as it implies that airway reversibility is present. Nocturnal wheeze is commonly seen in asthma and if it is found in a patient with presumed COPD, an alternative diagnosis should be sought.

5.2

D – Nitrofurantoin

This patient has a restrictive lung defect. In a restrictive lung defect the FVC is reduced and the FEV_1:FVCratio is either normal or increased (greater than 0.8). All of the antibiotics listed in the question can be used in the treatment or prevention of urinary tract infections; however, nitrofurantoin, an antibiotic that acts by damaging bacterial DNA, has an association with pulmonary fibrosis. Patients on long-term nitrofurantoin should be monitored for lung function changes and nitrofurantoin should be discontinued if there are any signs of lung damage. Amoxicillin (a penicillin) and cephalexin (a cephalosporin) are members of the beta-lactam group of antibiotics. Beta-lactams inhibit penicillin-binding proteins, a group of proteins that are involved in the final stage of cell wall trans-peptidation. Ciprofloxacin is a member of the quinolone family of antibiotics. Quinolones act by inhibiting bacterial DNA gyrase and are associated with tendon rupture. Trimethoprim inhibits the enzyme dihydrofolate reductase, which prevents DNA replication.

5.3

E – FEV_1:FVC ratio of 0.88, FEV_1 75% of predicted, kCO 135% of predicted

This patient has anti-glomerular basement membrane disease, an autoimmune condition characterised by the presence of autoanti-bodies against type IV collagen that damage alveoli and the glomerular basement membrane. The clinical features are haemoptysis, cough and shortness of breath. Lung function tests reveal a restrictive defect and an increased kCO if alveolar haemorrhage is present. In a restrictive lung defect the FVC is reduced and the FEV_1:FVC ratio is either normal or increased (greater than 0.8). The kCO is increased in cases of alveolar haemorrhage (granulomatosis with polyangiitis and systemic lupus erythematosus are other causes) because the erythrocytes that line the alveoli take up CO readily and 'falsely' increase the measurement. (In contrast the kCO is reduced when alveoli are destroyed, such as in emphysema, or thickened, such as in pulmonary fibrosis.) Renal involvement in anti-glomerular basement membrane disease is characterised by haematuria, proteinuria and renal failure. Renal biopsy reveals a crescentic glomerulonephritis that is rapidly progressive and there is linear basement membrane deposition of IgG detectable by immunofluorescence. Management is with high-dose steroids and cyclophosphamide. Dialysis may be necessary.

5.4

E – Thyroid function tests

Obstructive sleep apnoea is defined as upper airway narrowing, provoked by sleep, that results in sufficient sleep fragmentation to cause significant daytime symptoms, which is usually excessive sleepiness. Initially, it is important to exclude treatable causes of obstructive sleep apnoea such as hypothyroidism and also offer simple advice on weight loss, evening alcohol consumption and sleeping position. Other initial investigations include body mass index, and arterial blood gas measurement if respiratory failure is suspected. Patients with suspected obstructive sleep apnoea will then undergo a sleep study assessment, which usually only involves pulse oximetry at night. If a sleep study reveals mild obstructive sleep apnoea then a mandibular advancement device can be offered to the patient. Mandibular advancement devices are also important in reducing snoring. If significant obstructive sleep apnoea is detected then nasal continuous positive airway pressure and bariatric surgery can be offered. Salbutamol inhalers play no role in the management of this condition.

5.5

E – Teratoma

Teratomas arise from immature germ cells and tend to present in the anterior mediastinum as a well-defined mass with spicules of calcification. They represent 80% of germ cell tumours and most commonly present in young adults. The anterior mediastinum consists of the area behind the sternum and in front of the pericardium. The differential diagnosis for anterior mediastinal masses can be remembered by the 'five Ts': thymus, teratoma (and other germ cell tumours), thyroid, thoracic (ascending) aortic aneurysm and 'terrible' lymph nodes (lymphoma). The descending aorta is found in the posterior mediastinum and aneurysms of this vessel are usually asymptomatic. If an aortic aneurysm is suspected the best imaging modality is with a CT or MRI scan. Neurofibromatosis types I and II are peripheral nerve sheath tumours and arise mainly in the posterior mediastinum. They are often asymptomatic. However, enlargement significant enough to cause spinal cord compression can occur. The posterior mediastinum is defined as the area in front of the vertebrae and behind the pericardium. It contains the spinal nerve roots, the descending aorta, the oesophagus, the azygous and hemiazygous veins, the thoracic duct, and the vagus and splanchnic nerves. Pericardial cysts occupy the middle mediastinum; this is the area containing the heart and pericardium, the ascending aorta, the lower half of the superior vena cava, part of the azygous vein, the pulmonary vessels, the tracheal bifurcation, the phrenic nerves and the inferior vena cava.

5.6

D – Hepatocellular carcinoma

This patient has developed hepatocellular carcinoma as a result of receiving pooled factor VIII derived from blood products contaminated with hepatitis C, a single-stranded RNA virus. Prior to the 1990s, pooled blood was used for the treatment of haemophiliacs, before the advent of recombinant factor VIII. Pooled blood was not screened for infections such as hepatitis C, and, given this patient's age, it is likely that he has become chronically infected with this virus. Eighty percent of patients exposed to hepatitis C become chronically infected, with 10–30% progressing to liver cirrhosis. Cirrhosis is a prerequisite for hepatocellular carcinoma, and 1–3% of patients with cirrhosis go on to develop hepatocellular carcinoma every year. Patients with hepatocellular carcinoma classically present with jaundice, a right upper quadrant mass that can cause pain and weight loss.

An acute haemolytic transfusion reaction occurs rapidly, usually within minutes of transfusion, as a result of ABO blood group incompatibility. Natural, preformed antibodies against the A or B antigens mediate erythrocyte destruction. Patients present with fever and rigors, and can also develop jaundice and haemoglobinuria if there is massive erythrocyte destruction. Acute viral hepatitis is most commonly associated with hepatitis A, which is also a single-stranded RNA virus. It can cause jaundice but right upper quadrant pain and weight loss are unlikely, because these patients do not have cirrhosis. Pancreatic carcinoma is classically associated with jaundice and a palpable, non-tender gallbladder. This is known as Courvoisier's law. It implies that the gallbladder has been enlarged due to an obstruction of the common bile duct by a pancreatic carcinoma that has prevented the drainage of bile into the duodenum via the ampulla of Vater. Budd–Chiari syndrome occurs as a result of hepatic vein thrombosis. It presents with abdominal pain, ascites, hepatomegaly and jaundice. The presence of weight loss in this patient makes this diagnosis unlikely.

5.7
D – Thick and thin blood films

It is highly likely that this patient has malaria. While all of the options in this question are important in the management of patients with suspected malaria, thick and thin blood films are required to confirm the diagnosis. Thick films are used to assess if parasites are present or not; thin films are used to assess the burden of parasitaemia and to identify the *Plasmodium* species (*falciparum, ovale, vivax* or *malariae*). Blood samples should be repeated over several hours if the patient is unwell and the initial blood films are negative for malaria. An experienced individual should examine at least three sets of thick and thin films. In addition to blood films, malaria rapid antigen testing can also be performed to help confirm the diagnosis. Blood cultures need to be performed to exclude typhoid or a Gram-negative septicaemia (that may be present alongside malaria infection). A chest X-ray is required to exclude community-acquired pneumonia and to assess if there is any pulmonary oedema or signs of acute respiratory distress syndrome. Full blood count is useful as anaemia, leukopaenia and thrombocytopaenia suggest *Plasmodium falciparum* infection. Acute kidney injury and haemoglobinuria occur in severe *Plasmodium falciparum* infection; therefore urea and electrolytes and urine dipstick is warranted. Liver function tests are important as elevated (unconjugated) bilirubin reflects haemolysis. Hypoglycaemia can occur as a complication of *Plasmodium falciparum* infection and therefore blood glucose needs to be measured.

5.8

B – Commence intravenous immunoglobulin

This patient has an autoimmune thrombocytopaenic purpura secondary to systemic lupus erythematosus. Features include easy bruising, petechial haemorrhages and menorrhagia in women. Autoimmune thrombocytopaenia occurs as IgG anti-platelet autoantibodies directed against the glycoprotein IIb–IIIa or Ib complex result in premature removal of platelets from the circulation by macrophages of the reticuloendothelial system, especially in the spleen. Patients only require treatment once the platelet count drops below 50×10^9/L, as it is at this stage that the risk of bleeding increases significantly. Treatment is with immunosuppressive agents such as steroids and intravenous immunoglobulin. Intravenous immunoglobulin binds to Fc receptors on the surface of macrophages, therefore inhibiting their ability to bind to and remove platelet-antibody complexes from the circulation. Concomitant immunosuppressant administration with steroids acts to reduce autoantibody production.

Eltrombopag is a thrombopoietin-receptor agonist that acts to stimulate thrombopoiesis and had been indicated to treat patients with disease refractory to steroids and intravenous immunoglobulin. However, recent guidance recommends that it should not be used to treat patients with autoimmune thrombocytopaenic purpura, as it does not provide enough benefit to justify its high cost. Platelet transfusions are futile, as the benefit will only last for a few hours before the platelets are removed from the circulation by the autoantibodies. However, they may be utilised in patients with acute life-threatening bleeding to provide short-term benefit. Patients with a platelet count greater than 50×10^9/L can be monitored every two weeks to assess their bleeding risk. Splenectomy is indicated in symptomatic patients that have a platelet count less than 30×10^9/L after three months of steroid or intravenous immunoglobulin therapy.

5.9

B – Acute tubular necrosis

Acute tubular necrosis is the most common cause of intrinsic acute kidney injury and occurs either directly as a result of administration of a nephrotoxic agent such as contrast dye or aminoglycoside antibiotics, or secondary to renal ischaemia. Aminoglycosides, such as gentamicin, are antibiotics that inhibit bacterial protein synthesis and play an important role in the treatment of infective endocarditis because of their high level of bioavailability when administered intravenously. However, aminoglycosides, along with being nephrotoxic, also have a narrow therapeutic index and are renally excreted. These factors ensure that peak and trough serum aminoglycoside levels need to be taken regularly, and that urea and electrolytes must also be frequently monitored.

Acute interstitial nephritis occurs in response to drugs. Allopurinol, the beta-lactam antibiotics (penicillins, cephalosporins and carbapenems), NSAIDs, rifampicin and sulphonamides are the most common medications implicated. Acute interstitial nephritis is thought to be associated with an immune-mediated hypersensitivity reaction towards the offending drug.

Mesangiocapillary glomerulonephritis, also known as membranoproliferative glomerulonephritis, is associated with the glomerular deposition of cryoglobulins in the setting of chronic hepatitis C infection. Post-infectious immune complex glomerulonephritis is a sequela of streptococcal infection and occurs approximately three weeks following the initial infection. Pre-renal acute kidney injury may occur in infective endocarditis secondary to hypovolaemia, sepsis or cardiac failure as a result of a defective valve. The ensuing ischaemia can also easily lead to acute tubular necrosis. This is due to the fact that the renal tubules have a relatively poor blood supply (from the vasa recta), in order to maintain a high concentration gradient between the medulla and tubules. However, the specific question being asked in this scenario excludes these options.

5.10

C – Referral for arteriovenous fistula construction

Chronic kidney disease is staged according to estimated glomerular filtration rate. The table below summarises the stages of chronic kidney disease:

Stage	Estimated glomerular filtration rate (ml/minute/1.73m^2)
I	90 or more
II	60–89
III	30–59
IV	16–29
V	15 or less

This patient has stage IV chronic kidney disease and should be prepared for renal replacement therapy before he develops end-stage renal failure. Options for renal replacement therapy include haemodialysis, haemofiltration, peritoneal dialysis or transplantation. His history of Crohn's disease and ongoing problems with adhesions rule out peritoneal dialysis.

Preparation for haemodialysis involves either insertion of a central venous catheter or construction of an arteriovenous fistula. An arteriovenous fistula needs to be constructed at least six weeks before haemodialysis is to be commenced in order to allow the fistula to mature, so planning is crucial in this respect. It is also important to remember that patients with end-stage renal failure may not be suitable for renal replacement therapy due to pre-existing co-morbidities or may not wish to undergo renal replacement therapy. In these patients, it is appropriate to refer them to palliative care.

5.11

C – Atheromatous renal artery stenosis

The most likely cause in a patient of this age is atheromatous renal artery stenosis. Patients with renal artery stenosis who are commenced on an ACE inhibitor, such as enalapril, can develop pulmonary oedema due to acute renal failure. In the setting of renal artery stenosis perfusion pressure in the efferent end of the arteriole is reduced. An increased afferent arterial tone maintains the glomerular pressure — this relies on angiotensin II. ACE inhibitors inhibit angiotensin II and consequently reduce afferent arteriole tone and glomerular filtration pressure.

Acute respiratory distress syndrome and anaphylaxis are not associated with this scenario. Patients with fibromuscular dysplasia who start taking ACE inhibitors can also develop similar problems. However, the patient's age in this scenario makes fibromuscular dysplasia a less likely cause; usually younger women are affected. Hereditary angioedema is due to C1 esterase inhibitor deficiency. In the absence of C1 esterase inhibitor, activation of the complement cascade leads to increased levels of vasoactive peptides that increase capillary permeability, most notably bradykinin. Bradykinin is usually inactivated by ACE; however, in patients taking ACE inhibitors, such as enalapril, this level can rise such that it causes facial and laryngeal oedema with subsequent airway obstruction. In this situation the chest X-ray changes consistent with pulmonary oedema wouldn't be present.

5.12

D – Natalizumab

This patient has developed progressive multifocal leukoencephalopathy secondary to taking natalizumab. Natalizumab is a humanised monoclonal antibody against the cell adhesion molecule α4-integrin, which prevents the egress of leukocytes from the blood into the central nervous system. It is used to treat highly active relapsing-remitting multiple sclerosis. Progressive multifocal leukoencephalopathy is a rare but often fatal neurological disorder caused by reactivation of the polyomavirus JC virus that leads to lytic infection of glial cells. The features of progressive multifocal leukoencephalopathy are of progressive neurological and/or intellectual impairment. Progressive multifocal leukoencephalopathy occurs in severely immunosuppressed patients that either have HIV, have undergone chemotherapy or treatment with the monoclonal antibodies natalizumab, efalizumab or rituximab. There is no specific antiviral drug that improves survival in progressive multifocal leukoencephalopathy, and so treatment centres on restoring the adaptive immune response to JC virus by withdrawal of any of the aforementioned immunosuppressant medications that the patient may be taking, or by placing the patient on combination antiretroviral therapy if they are HIVpositive. (Such patients should also be treated with steroids to prevent a subsequent immune reconstitution inflammatory syndrome.)

Efalizumab is a formerly available monoclonal antibody against CD11a that was used to treat moderate to severe chronic plaque psoriasis that hadn't responded to other medication. It was withdrawn from the market after it was decided that the risks of developing progressive multifocal leukoencephalopathy outweighed the benefits of treating the psoriasis. Efalizumab was never shown to be effective in treating multiple sclerosis and so is not an appropriate answer to this question.

Glatiramer is an immunomodulatory agent that, through an unknown mechanism, has been shown to decelerate disease progression in patients with relapsing-remitting multiple sclerosis. Methylprednisolone is a corticosteroid used to treat acute relapses of multiple sclerosis. It does not alter long-term outcomes in multiple sclerosis. Both glatiramer and methylprednisolone are not associated with progressive multifocal leukoencephalopathy.

Rituximab is an anti-CD20 monoclonal antibody that acts to reduce B-cell proliferation and plays an important role in the treatment of lymphomas and autoimmune diseases.

5.13

C – Physiotherapy

This patient has ankylosing spondylitis, a chronic inflammatory disorder that affects the spine and sacroiliac joints. Patients should undergo intense physiotherapy and continue to exercise in order to prevent loss of flexibility and formation of the classic 'question mark' posture found in ankylosing spondylitis. NSAIDs, such as indomethacin, also play a role in relieving symptoms; however, they would not be used in this patient due to his allergy. Spinal steroid injections can also be used in order to temporarily reduce pain and stiffness; however, they would not form part of the initial treatment of this patient. Bisphosphonates don't form part of the initial treatment of ankylosing spondylitis; however, they can be used to prevent osteoporotic fractures in this group of patients.

5.14

B – Nail pitting occurs more commonly in those with arthritis

This patient has psoriatic arthritis, which affects upwards of 50% of patients with psoriasis. It is important to note that nail pitting is more than twice as common in patients with psoriatic arthritis (90%) than in those with psoriasis alone (40%). The arthritis may predate the skin lesions. There are five different patterns of joint involvement in psoriatic arthritis:

- I: Oligoarthritis
- II: Symmetrical polyarthritis resembling rheumatoid arthritis
- III: A pattern resembling osteoarthritis with Heberden's and Bouchard's nodes
- IV: Sacroiliitis (usually unilateral) resembling ankylosing spondylitis
- V: A destructive pattern termed arthritis mutilans.

Arthritis mutilans is a rare, destructive form of psoriatic arthritis and affects about 5% of patients. Periarticular osteolysis leads to collapse of the soft tissue in the digits, leading to a 'telescoping' appearance in the fingers.

Psoriatic arthritis is one of the seronegative spondyloarthropathies. Nevertheless, up to 10% of patients are positive for rheumatoid factor. Women and men are equally affected in psoriatic arthritis.

5.15

E – Scleromalacia perforans

This patient has scleromalacia perforans, a rare ocular complication of rheumatoid arthritis. It occurs when rheumatoid nodules erode through the sclera and expose the underlying uveal tissue. If left untreated, the uveal tissue can herniate through the damaged sclera and cause perforation of the globe. Treatment is with high-dose corticosteroids. Scleromalacia perforans is often painless, as opposed to scleritis, which is usually intensely painful.

Episcleritis can also occur as an ocular manifestation of rheumatoid arthritis. The eye is erythematous, painless and the episcleritis is benign and resolves by itself. Keratoconjunctivitis sicca is the most common ocular complication of rheumatoid arthritis and is characterised by dry, painful, gritty eyes. It results from a reduction in tear production and is treated with artificial tears. A pinguecula is a benign yellow conjunctival nodule that occurs at the limbus (the border between the cornea and conjunctiva), and needs no treatment. This is in contrast to a pterygium, another type of benign yellow conjunctival growth that occurs at the palpebral fissure (the junction between the upper and lower eyelids). A pterygium can grow onto the cornea, and therefore will need to be removed to maintain normal vision.

5.16

C – Eosinophilic granulomatosis with polyangiitis

Eosinophilic granulomatosis with polyangiitis (Churg–Strauss syndrome) is a small- to medium-vessel vasculitis that affects predominantly the lungs and the skin. Asthma and eosinophilia in the setting of vasculitis are associated with eosinophilic granulomatosis with polyangiitis. Patients can often develop a mononeuritis multiplex. Eosinophilic granulomatosis with polyangiitis is most associated with p-ANCAs, which are antibodies against the perinuclear antigen myeloperoxidase. Remisssion is induced with corticosteroids, given in conjunction with another immunosuppressant agent such as cyclophosphamide or azathioprine.

Acute eosinophilic pneumonia presents with shortness of breath, cough, fever and myalgia in the absence of fungal, parasitic or other infection and responds promptly to corticosteroids. There is no blood eosinophilia despite the fact that bronchoalveolar lavage yields a significant amount of eosinophils.

Allergic bronchopulmonary aspergillosis is a condition character-ised by type I and type III hypersensitivity reactions to the fungus *Aspergillus fumigatus* in patients with asthma. The type I hypersensitivity reaction leads to bronchoconstriction and the type III hypersensitivity reaction, mediated by immune complexes, gives rise to inflammation that damages bronchial walls and causes bronchiectasis. Patients have a blood eosinophilia, a positive skin prick test to *Aspergillus* and IgG precipitins to *Aspergillus fumigatus*. Serum IgE levels are also raised.

Loeffler's syndrome is found in patients returning from overseas and presents with shortness of breath, cough, fever, anorexia and night sweats. It is caused by parasitic infections, namely *Ascaris lumbricoides*, *Strongyloides stercoralis* and *Ankylostoma* species. Treatment is with anti-helminthic agents such as mebendazole or ivermectin, and corticosteroids.

Sarcoidosis is a multisystem inflammatory condition of unknown cause that commonly presents with non-caseating, granulomatous pulmonary lesions. It is not usually associated with a markedly raised blood eosinophil count.

5.17

C – Pseudofracture

Osteomalacia is characterised by defective bone and cartilage mineralisation with accumulation of unmineralised bone matrix. The classical radiological findings of osteomalacia are pseudofractures, which are also termed Looser's zones. They appear as wide, transverse hypolucent areas that commonly occur at right angles to the affected cortex. Pseudofractures are most commonly found on the ribs, clavicles, outer borders of the scapulae, femoral necks, pubic rami and metatarsals. Patients with osteomalacia present with muscle weakness, bony pain and often display a 'waddling' gait, which occurs as a result of bone deformity and proximal muscle weakness. Reduced serum calcium and phosphate with a raised serum alkaline phosphatase is associated with osteomalacia.

Loss of joint space, subchondral cysts and subchondral sclerosis are associated with osteoarthritis. Periarticular osteopaenia is found radiologically in rheumatoid arthritis, along with soft tissue swelling, loss of joint space, erosions and deformity.

5.18

B – Ganciclovir

This patient has CMV retinitis. This usually occurs in immunocompromised patients, such as those who are HIV positive. CMV is also known as HHV-5. Usually after the acute infection it becomes latent; however, in immunocompromised patients it can re-activate and cause disease. In patients with HIV, CMV has a predilection for infecting the retina, causing visual problems and the characteristic 'mozzarella and tomato' appearance on fundoscopy. Treatment for CMV retinitis is with intravenous ganciclovir, a guanine analogue that is phosphorylated and incorporated into viral DNA, which then results in termination of DNA elongation. Aciclovir also acts in identical fashion; however, ganciclovir has better ocular bioavailability and so is used for CMV retinitis. Ribavirin is an antiviral agent used in hepatitis C infection, and zidovudine and tenofovir are nucleoside analogue reverse transcriptase inhibitors that are used in highly active anti-retroviral therapy for HIV infection.

5.19

D – *Leptospira interrogans*

The most likely infectious agent to have caused this presentation is *Leptospira interrogans*, a spirochetal organism that is carried by rodents and is passed onto humans via contact with water that has been contaminated with their urine. Clinical features include fever, cough, headache, photophobia, bilateral conjunctival haemorrhage, lymphadenopathy, splenomegaly, jaundice and features of disseminated intravascular coagulation. Renal involvement is also common. Treatment is with doxycycline, a tetracycline antibiotic. Dialysis may be required if there is severe renal failure.

Borrelia burgdorferi is another spirochetal organism that is spread to humans by infected *Ixodes* ticks; it is the causative agent of Lyme disease. In Lyme disease, there is a characteristic rash at the site at which the tick bites called erythema chronicum migrans. The rash of erythema chronicum migrans is often described as looking like a bull's-eye on a dartboard. Other features include myalgia, arthralgia, carditis and neurological involvement.

Brucella melitensis is a Gram-negative coccobacillus that is most commonly transmitted to humans from unpasteurised milk and cheese. Symptoms include episodic fevers, sweating, myalgia and migratory arthralgia.

Legionella pneumophila is a Gram-negative bacterium associated with contaminated water used in air-conditioning and swimming pools. It causes a pneumonia associated with myalgia, fever and a dry cough. Abdominal pain and haematuria are also common in *Legionella pneumophila* infection.

Streptococcus pyogenes is a group A beta haemolytic streptococcus and is the most common bacterial cause of acute pharyngitis. Immunological sequelae of untreated infection include rheumatic fever and acute glomerulonephritis.

5.20

C – Intravenous ciprofloxacin, teicoplanin and gentamicin

This patient must be presumed to have neutropaenic sepsis until another diagnosis is established and must be treated accordingly for this with intravenous antibiotics that provide cover against both Gram-positive and Gram-negative organisms. The situation is complicated in this patient as she describes an anaphylactic reaction to penicillin. The only combination of antibiotics that doesn't contain a penicillin derivative or beta-lactam (which can also cause anaphylactic reactions in patients with penicillin allergy) is that of ciprofloxacin, teicoplanin and gentamicin.

Ciprofloxacin is a member of the quinolone family of antibiotics. Quinolones act by inhibiting bacterial DNA gyrase. Teicoplanin is a glycopeptide antibiotic that inhibits polymerisation of the peptides N-acetylmuramic acid and N-acetylglucosamine. These peptides are important in forming the backbone strands of the bacterial cell wall. Gentamicin is an aminoglycoside antibiotic that inhibits bacterial protein synthesis. It plays an important role in providing cover against Gram-negative organisms.

All of the other options in this question have a high chance of inducing an anaphylactic reaction in this patient. Co-amoxiclav is also known as augmentin, and is a combination of amoxicillin (a penicillin) and clavulanic acid. Ceftriaxone is a member of the cephalosporin family of antibiotics. A significant proportion of patients with a penicillin allergy also have an anaphylactic response to this family of antibiotics. Benzylpenicillin is a penicillin derivative. Tazocin is a combination of piperacillin (a penicillin) and tazobactam (a beta-lactamase inhibitor). In patients who do not have a penicillin allergy, intravenous tazocin and gentamicin is the antibiotic combination of choice for neutropaenic sepsis.

5.21

E – Urine dipstick

This boy's symptoms are typical of Henoch–Schönlein purpura, a systemic vasculitis of unknown aetiology that primarily affects children of ages two to ten years old. It is characterised by IgA immune complex deposition in the small vessels, including those of the glomerulus (IgA nephropathy). Renal involvement may involve haematuria, and therefore performing a urine dipstick to exclude nephropathy is the most appropriate investigation to perform in this child. In the acute setting 40–50% of patients will develop some degree of renal impairment, and 1–2% of children will develop chronic kidney disease.

Abdominal ultrasound can be used if gastrointestinal symptoms are present but it is rarely of diagnostic or prognostic value. In this situation, the clinical history is characteristic of Henoch–Schönlein purpura and an abdominal ultrasound is unlikely to yield any further benefit in the management of the child. If the diagnosis were uncertain, an abdominal ultrasound would be appropriate to rule out other causes of diffuse abdominal pain. Arthritis is a common presenting feature of Henoch–Schönlein purpura and typically involves the large, lower joints; it is self-limiting and benign. Joint aspiration is not usually performed since it is of little diagnostic benefit but in an atypical presentation where there is diagnostic uncertainty a joint aspirate may be required to rule out other more serious pathology, such as septic arthritis.

Classically, patients with Henoch–Schönlein purpura have a purpuric rash that is present on the lower extremities and buttocks, but it can be widespread. A widespread purpuric rash in a child with a fever should be managed as a *Neisseria meningitidis* (meningococcal) septicaemia until proven otherwise.

5.22

A – Amyotrophic lateral sclerosis

Amyotrophic lateral sclerosis, also known as Lou Gehrig's disease, is a form of motor neuron disease caused by the degeneration of both upper and lower motor neurons. Motor commands generated in the primary motor cortex reach their target muscle by travelling along two types of motor neurons (upper and lower motor neurons). Upper motor neurons are first-order neurons originating in the primary motor cortex. Upper motor neurons travel entirely within the central nervous system and synapse with the cell bodies of lower motor neurons that lie within the central nervous system. Lower motor neurons are second-order neurons and the axons of these neurons leave the central nervous system to form synapses with muscles of the body. All peripheral and spinal neurons with motor control are lower motor neurons.

The upper motor neurons which supply the cranial motor nerves run within a different tract to those that supply the spinal motor neurons, namely the corticobulbar tract. Degeneration of the upper motor neurons within the corticobulbar tract leads to a pseudobulbar palsy whereas degeneration of the lower motor neurons, which form the cranial nerves, leads to a bulbar palsy.

In contrast to the corticobulbar tract, the corticospinal tract is composed of upper motor neurons that terminate on spinal motor neurons. Degeneration of the upper motor neurons within the corticospinal tract is called primary lateral sclerosis (named due to the lateral position of the corticospinal tract within the white matter of spinal cord). Degeneration of lower motor neurons within the peripheral spinal nerves is termed progressive muscular atrophy.

In amyotrophic lateral sclerosis there is usually degeneration of the peripheral spinal lower motor neurons and corticospinal tracts simultaneously. The degeneration can also spread to involve the corticobulbar tract and lower motor neurons within the cranial nerves.

5.23

E – *Streptococcus viridans*

When considering the pathogen involved in infective endocarditis it is important to distinguish between native and prosthetic valve. The organism implicated in patients with prosthetic valves differs depending upon the length of time that the infection occurs after surgery. If the infection occurs within six months of surgery the most likely causative agents are *Staphylococcus aureus* and coagulase-negative *Staphylococcus* (*Staphylococcus epidermidis*). However, if the infection occurs more than six months after surgery the organisms are the same as for a native valve. Therefore, the most likely organism in this patient is *Streptococcus viridans*.

Streptococcus bovis is a rare cause of infective endocarditis and is associated with dysplasia in the lining of the colon. As a result, all patients who have *Streptococcus bovis* positive endocarditis should undergo colonoscopy.

Candida albicans is a fungal cause of infective endocarditis and only accounts for around 4% of all cases.

Tuberculosis would be a differential diagnosis in a patient with night sweats, fever and breathlessness. However, there is no other history to support a diagnosis of tuberculosis and infective endocarditis is more likely given the recent history of prosthetic valve implantation and the presence of a murmur.

5.24

D – Clarithromycin and rifampicin

This patient has an atypical pneumonia caused by *Legionella pneumophila*, a Gram-negative organism. The most appropriate treatment regimen is clarithromycin (a macrolide antibiotic) and rifampicin. *Legionella pneumophila* is spread by contaminated water (classically hotel water cooling systems). Symptoms include high fever, confusion, myalgia, non-productive cough and headache. On examination, patients often have few chest signs but can have signs of a lobar pneumonia (e.g. focal consolidation). This patient has characteristic examination and chest X-ray findings suggestive of a lobar pneumonia affecting the right lower lobe.

In patients with a mild to moderate community-acquired pneumonia, oral amoxicillin (a penicillin derivative) alone is usually prescribed. This is because the most common causative organisms for community-acquired pneumonia, such as *Streptococcus pneumoniae*, are sensitive to amoxicillin. Oral clarithromycin (a macrolide) can be prescribed if an atypical organism is suspected or the patient is allergic to penicillin.

Severe community-acquired pneumonia requires hospital admission and can be treated initially with a number of different broad-spectrum antibiotics. Commonly, patients are treated with intravenous co-amox-iclav and oral clarithromycin.

In patients with *Legionella pneumophilia*, the combination of clarithromycin and rifampicin has been shown to be the most effective antibiotic regime. In the setting of community-acquired pneumonia, rifampicin is generally only prescribed when the causative organism is *Legionella pneumophilia*.

5.25

A – Anti-phospholipid syndrome

This patient's symptoms and initial observations are highly suggestive of a pulmonary embolism. In young patients developing a pulmonary embolism, it is important to think about an underlying pathological process that may be leading to a hypercoagulable state. In this patient, who has a history of previous miscarriages and thrombotic events, the diagnosis of anti-phospholipid syndrome should be considered.

Anti-phospholipid syndrome is an autoimmune, hypercoagulable state caused by antibodies against cell-membrane phospholipids that provokes arterial and venous thrombosis. In patients with anti-phospholipid syndrome, thrombosis can occur in any vessels but the most common venous event is deep vein thrombosis of the lower extremities. This can lead to the development of a pulmonary embolus. The most common arterial event in patients with anti-phospholipid syndrome is cerebral thrombosis. Anti-phospholipid syndrome also causes pregnancy-related complications including miscarriage, stillbirth, preterm delivery or severe pre-eclampsia. If a clinical diagnosis of anti-phospholipid syndrome is suspected, then the following tests should be ordered:

- Antibodies against beta$_2$-glycoprotein
- Anticardiolipin IgM and IgG antibodies
- Lupus anticoagulant.

Anti-phospholipid syndrome can occur in the absence of any other related disease (primary) or be associated with other autoimmune diseases, particularly systemic lupus erythematosus (secondary).

The most common inherited thrombophilia is factor V Leiden, an autosomal dominant disorder that occurs in up to 5% of Caucasians. Factor V Leiden is a result of a specific gene mutation in factor V that increases its resistance to degradation by activated protein C and leads to a hypercoagulable state. It should not be confused with the rare disorder factor V deficiency, which is associated with haemorrhagic complications of varying severity. In the normal person, factor V functions as a cofactor to allow factor Xa to activate thrombin. Thrombin in turn cleaves fibrinogen to form fibrin, which polymerises to form the dense meshwork that makes up the majority of a clot. Factor V Leiden, in comparison to anti-phospholipid syndrome, is almost entirely associated with venous thrombosis and is unlikely in this patient due to the previous history of cerebral artery infarction.

Inherited deficiencies in protein C and S are rare causes of thrombophilia. Both protein C and S are vitamin K-dependent physiological anticoagulants and deficiencies of these proteins result in decreased degradation of factor Va and factor VIIIa. This results in an increased propensity to form venous thrombosis but deficiencies in protein C or S do not increase the risk of arterial thrombosis.

Nephrotic syndrome results in a prothrombotic state due to the loss of antithrombin III via the glomerulus. Patients with reduced antithrombin III are at increased risk of venous thrombosis, particularly in atypical locations, e.g. the hepatic vein (Budd–Chiari syndrome) or the renal vein. This patient does not display any of the features associated with nephrotic syndrome, making this diagnosis unlikely.

5.26

D – Hypokalaemic, hypernatraemic metabolic alkalosis

Conn's syndrome is an aldosterone-producing adenoma and a cause of primary hyperaldosteronism. In the collecting ducts of the kidneys, aldosterone acts to enhance exchange of sodium for potassium or hydrogen ions. When too much aldosterone is present, as in Conn's syndrome, there is excess sodium reabsorption and increased loss of potassium and hydrogen. Consequently, patients develop a hypokalaemic, hypernatraemic metabolic alkalosis. The hypernatraemia associated with Conn's syndrome results in increased water reabsorption in the kidneys and thus patients with Conn's syndrome will develop secondary hypertension.

In Addison's disease, there is decreased production of aldosterone and consequently too much sodium will be lost from the collecting ducts in exchange for potassium and hydrogen. These patients will therefore develop a hyperkalaemic, hyponatraemic metabolic acidosis. The hyponatraemia associated with Addison's disease results in increased water loss due to a direct osmotic effect in the kidneys. This increased water loss leads to the development of postural hypotension in these patients. Aldosterone receptor antagonists such as spironolactone can also produce the same metabolic profile as Addison's disease.

Patients in the latter stages of a salicylic acid (aspirin) overdose may develop a hypokalaemic, hypernatraemic metabolic acidosis. Salicylic acid inhibits aerobic respiration and as a result there is increased ketone production, which accounts for the metabolic acidosis. Additionally, there is increased loss of potassium and fluid via the kidneys. Increased fluid loss results in dehydration and thus an apparent hypernatraemia.

Patients admitted with diabetic ketoacidosis have a metabolic acidosis due to high levels of ketones. They also lose high quantities of potassium via the kidneys but because they are initially severely dehydrated, have an apparent hyperkalaemia and hypernatraemia. Regular electrolyte monitoring is required when rehydrating patients with diabetes as they may become hypokalaemic due to total body potassium being low.

Patients with pyloric stenosis have an obstruction of the gastric outlet. As a result, they vomit up gastric contents, which contain high quantities of potassium and hydrochloric acid. Therefore, patients with pyloric stenosis develop a hypokalaemic, hypochloraemic metabolic alkalosis.

5.27

B – Bendroflumethiazide

Thiazide diuretics (bendroflumethiazide) and loop diuretics (furosemide) can both cause hypokalaemia. However, thiazide diuretics are more likely to cause hypokalaemia. Unlike loop diuretics, thiazides do not affect potassium transport directly but instead stimulate potassium secretion indirectly.

Thiazide diuretics inhibit the sodium/chloride co-transporter in the distal collecting tubule, which leads to increased sodium delivery to the collecting ducts. As the sodium concentration in the distal convoluted tubules and collecting ducts increases, so does aldosterone activity. Aldosterone acts to reabsorb sodium in exchange for potassium or hydrogen to maintain electrical neutrality in the cells of the collecting ducts.

Furosemide acts to inhibit the sodium/potassium/chloride co-transporter in the thick ascending limb of the loop of Henle. A compensatory response for the increased sodium concentration in the renal tubules occurs in the distal convoluted tubule. In the distal convoluted tubule the increased sodium is reabsorbed in conjunction with chloride, which maintains electroneutrality. Therefore, unlike with thiazide use, potassium is not secreted into the tubules in exchange for sodium.

Thiazides also lower the luminal calcium concentration in the distal convoluted tubule. This activates aldosterone-controlled epithelial sodium channels (which are inhibited by calcium) and further favours potassium secretion. Loop diuretics increase calcium delivery to the distal convoluted tubules and consequently reduce activity of the aldosterone-driven sodium/potassium exchanger.

Spironolactone, amiloride and benzamil are all potassium-sparing diuretics and can increase the risk of developing hyperkalaemia. Amiloride and benzamil both inhibit the epithelial sodium channel whose activity is modulated by aldosterone. Blocking the epithelial sodium channel inhibits sodium reabsorption in exchange for potassium excretion in the distal convoluted tubule. Spironolactone inhibits the effect of aldosterone by competing for intracellular aldosterone receptors in the cortical collecting duct. This decreases the activity of the epithelial sodium channel and consequently reduces the reabsorption of sodium, while decreasing the secretion of potassium.

5.28

B – Prescribe oral amoxicillin

This patient has asymptomatic bacteriuria that should be treated during pregnancy. Asymptomatic bacteriuria occurs in around 2–7% of all pregnancies and the most likely causative organism is *Escherichia coli*. It has been shown that asymptomatic bacteriuria increases the risk for developing acute pyelonephritis, which is a risk factor for preterm labour. Asymptomatic bacteriuria itself has been demonstrated to be an independent risk factor for preterm birth but the mechanism for this is not fully known. In pyelonephritis it has been established that production of phospholipase A2 by microorganisms can initiate labour through the activation of prostaglandins.

As a result of the link between pyelonephritis and preterm labour, patients are screened for asymptomatic bacteriuria at their booking visit. If there is the presence of more than 10^5 colony-forming units per ml of microorganisms in a urine sample, then the patient is treated with a course of antibiotics. Oral amoxicillin is a good first-line treatment option, as it is not known to pose any major risks to the developing foetus.

Intravenous co-amoxiclav is not required to treat asymptomatic bacteriuria but would be appropriate if the patient developed acute pyelonephritis. Trimethoprim inhibits dihydrofolate reductase and should be avoided during the first trimester. This is because it interferes with folate metabolism which increases the risk of neural tube defects in the developing foetus. It can be used in the second and third trimesters. Ciprofloxacin can be used to treat urinary tract infections but should be avoided in pregnancy because animal studies have demonstrated that it can reduce the length of the epiphyseal growth plate.

Nitrofurantoin may be used in the first and second trimesters but is to be avoided in the third due to the risk of neonatal haemolysis if the neonate has glucose-6-phosphate dehydrogenase deficiency. Cephalexin may be safely used in pregnancy.

5.29

D – Serum VZV antibody titres

This immunocompromised patient with no history of chickenpox has been exposed to VZV. Before giving this patient VZV immunoglobulin it is necessary to check her serum VZV antibody titres; VZV immunoglobulin would only be given if VZV antibody titres were negative. As this patient currently feels well there is no clinical indication for aciclovir. People with VZV are infectious from three to four days before the rash appears until all the blisters have crusted over (usually five days later). Patients who are at special risk of VZV infection include:

- Pregnant women
- Newborn babies
- Immunocompromised patients.

Patients who are vulnerable to chickenpox complications can be offered the chickenpox vaccine in order to prevent scenarios such as the one in this question occurring.

5.30

A – Carbamazepine

This child is likely to have absence seizures, which present with episodes of staring blankly or daydreaming during which the child is unresponsive. Absence seizures are a form of generalised seizure because there is loss of consciousness during the episode. In contrast, in a partial seizure consciousness remains intact.

Typical childhood absence epilepsy usually begins before the age of ten years and has a peak at five to six years of age. Absences are frequent (tens or hundreds each day) and respond well to treatment with remission within two to five years from onset.

The pathophysiology of absence seizures is thought to involve an abnormal thalamo-cortical circuit that activates abnormal oscillatory rhythms. This generates the generalised 3 hertz spike and wave discharges on an electroencephalogram. Gamma-aminobutyric acid signalling within the reticular nucleus and the ventrobasal complex of the thalamus is critical to the neurophysiology of absence seizures. It has been demonstrated that potentiation of gamma-aminobutyric acid signalling worsens absence seizures whilst antagonising gamma-aminobutyric acid receptors suppress absences. One of the mechanisms of action of carbamazepine is to potentiate gamma-aminobutyric acid receptors and it is therefore contraindicated in patients with absence seizures. Carbamazepine has also been demonstrated to aggravate other types of generalised seizures including juvenile myoclonic epilepsy. The major use of carbamazepine is in the treatment of partial seizures, trigeminal neuralgia and as a second-line treatment for bipolar disorder.

Valproate is a weak antagonist of sodium ion channels and is also a weak inhibitor of enzymes that deactivate gamma-aminobutyric acid such as gamma-aminobutyric acid transaminase. Because of its many mechanisms of action, sodium valproate has efficacy in all partial and generalised seizures including absence seizures. Both ethosuximide and sodium valproate can be used as a first-line treatment in the management of absence seizures. They are of equal efficacy and control around 75% of seizures. Unlike sodium valproate, ethosuximide is usually only used in the treatment of absence seizures.

Lamotrigine can be used in children with absence seizures who are not controlled with a combination of ethosuximide and valproate or if these medications are contraindicated. Lamotrigine, like carbamazepine, is also used as a first-line treatment in patients with focal seizures. In patients with tonic-clonic seizures, lamotrigine is used when sodium valproate is either ineffective or not tolerated. If a patient has myoclonic seizures or is suspected of having juvenile myoclonic epilepsy, it is important to be aware that lamotrigine may exacerbate myoclonic seizures.

Topiramate is generally reserved as an adjunct for the treatment of epilepsy disorders that have not responded to either first- or second-line treatments. Topiramate is known to inhibit carbonic anhydrase and should be used with caution in patients already on a carbonic anhydrase inhibitor (e.g. acetazolamide) as it increases the risk of developing kidney stones. It is also an inducer of the CYP450 3A4 enzyme and has been known to reduce the efficacy of digoxin and the oral contraceptive pill.

5.31

B – Stage B1

Colorectal cancer is staged according to the level of penetration of the bowel wall, lymph node involvement and metastatic spread. There are two widely used classifications: TNM (Tumour, Node, Metastases) and the Dukes' classification (not to be confused with the modified Duke criteria for infective endocarditis). The Dukes' classification is widely adopted and when it was first introduced had four stages A–D. This has since been adapted with stages B and C being divided into 1 and 2. The following outlines the criteria for each stage:

Stage	Level of spread
A	Limited to mucosa
B1	Extending into muscularis propria but not penetrating through it; nodes not involved
B2	Penetrating through muscularis propria; nodes not involved
C1	Extending into muscularis propria but not penetrating through it;nodes involved
C2	Penetrating through muscularis propria; nodes involved
D	Distant metastatic spread

The patient in this question has a tumour that is Dukes' stage B1. The tumour extends into the muscularis propria but does not penetrate through it, as it has not reached the subserosal fat (the layer beneath the muscularis propria). There is also no lymph node involvement or evidence of metastatic spread.

The Dukes' classification gives valuable information on the prognosis and management of patients with colorectal cancer. Post-surgical five-year survival rates are approximately 90% for stage A and 50% for stage C. The main treatment of colorectal cancer is surgery and adjuvant (post-surgical) chemotherapy for patients who are at Dukes' stage B2 and C.

5.32

D – Iron deficiency anaemia

Heart failure is defined as the inability of the heart to supply sufficient blood flow to meet the needs of the body. The most frequent cause of heart failure is due to conditions that affect the myocardium itself, causing the cardiac output to decrease (low-output heart failure). However, heart failure can also occur when the body's requirements for oxygen and nutrients are increased and the heart is unable to keep up with this demand. This form of heart failure is termed high-output since the myocardium is still able to maintain a cardiac output within normal limits.

The underlying problem in high-output heart failure is a reduction in systemic vascular resistance. This causes a reduction in systemic blood pressure, which also occurs in low-output heart failure. A decreased blood pressure leads to sympathetic activation, which causes a compensatory rise in cardiac output, and neurohormonal activation (activation of the renin-angiotensin-aldosterone system). This results in increased salt and water retention and subsequent heart failure. Thus, salt and water retention occur both in low- and high-output heart failure due to neurohormonal activation in response to hypotension.

The reduction in systemic vascular resistance that occurs in high-output heart failure can be due to either systemic arteriovenous shunting or peripheral vasodilatation. The major causes of high-output heart failure include:

- Severe chronic anaemia
- Septicaemia
- Beriberi (vitamin B_1/thiamine deficiency)
- Thyrotoxicosis
- Arteriovenous fistulae and arteriovenous malformations
- Paget's disease.

In severe anaemia there is a physiological adjustment to maintain tissue perfusion and oxygenation. This includes peripheral vasodilation and a subsequent reduction in systemic resistance. This peripheral dilatation is in part due to increased vascular nitric oxide synthase activity and a low blood viscosity.

All of the other options in this question are causes of low-output cardiac failure since they affect the myocardium itself. Ischaemic heart disease and dilated cardiomyopathy are causes of systolic dysfunction, which can simply be described as failure of the pump function of the heart. It is characterised by a decreased ejection fraction (the fraction of blood pumped out of the ventricle with each heart beat). In contrast left ventricular hypertrophy, a consequence of a chronically elevated systemic resistance (e.g. due to aortic stenosis), causes diastolic dysfunction. Diastolic dysfunction occurs when the ventricles fail to adequately relax and is usually due to a 'stiffened' left ventricle. This results in reduced ventricular filling and therefore a decreased stroke volume. An inadequate stroke volume results in a low cardiac output (as cardiac output = stroke volume × heart rate). Although the cardiac output is reduced in diastolic dysfunction the ejection fraction is preserved. This is because the ejection fraction is highly dependent upon the contractility of the myocardium and in diastolic dysfunction the contractility of the heart is still intact.

5.33

D – Propylthiouracil

The most likely medication to have been prescribed in this scenario is propylthiouracil. The two most commonly used medications to treat hyperthyroidism are carbimazole and propylthiouracil, both of which are thioamides. The thioamides inhibit the actions of thyroid peroxidase, the enzyme that iodinates tyrosine residues on thyroglobulin. Thioamides thus decrease the production of thyroxine and triiodothyronine. The most important side effect of the thioamides is agranulocytosis, where there is a failure to make granulocytes (neutrophils, eosinophils and basophils). Patients with a neutrophil count below $1 \times 10^9/L$ are highly immunocompromised and at risk of serious infections, which may be fatal. Consequently, all patients on a thioamide should be warned to seek medical attention for an urgent full blood count if they develop a sore throat or feel slightly unwell.

Clozapine (an atypical antipsychotic) is also known to cause agranulocytosis. Its primary role is in the management of treatment-resistant schizophrenia and plays no role in the treatment of hyperthyroidism.

Propranolol (a beta-blocker) can be used for rapid symptom control such as tremor in patients with hyperthyroidism. Radioiodine is used as a definitive treatment for hyperthyroidism by ablating the thyroid gland. Neither of these medications is known to cause agranulocytosis.

Levothyroxine is a synthetic form of thyroxine and is primarily used to treat hypothyroidism. It is also used, alongside a thioamide, as part of the 'block and replace' strategy for hyperthyroidism. Levothyroxine is not known to cause agranulocytosis but can cause symptoms of hyperthyroidism if overprescibed.

5.34

A – Intravenous acetazolamide, topical timolol and topical prednisolone

This patient's history is highly suggestive of acute closed-angle glaucoma. This is a condition in which the iris is pushed anteriorly and blocks the trabecular meshwork at the angle of the anterior chamber of the eye, between the cornea and iris. When the trabecular meshwork is blocked, the outflow of aqueous humour from the eye via the canal of Schlemm is interrupted, which causes a rise in intraocular pressure. If closure of the angle occurs suddenly, as in this patient, symptoms are severe and require urgent treatment. Patients with acute closed-angle glaucoma should be admitted to hospital for treatment to reduce the intraocular pressure and preserve the patients' sight by preventing optic nerve damage. The initial treatment includes intravenous acetazolamide (a carbonic anhydrase inhibitor), topical timolol (a beta-blocker) and topical prednisolone (a corticosteroid).

Both beta-blockers and acetazolamide are thought to decrease aqueous humour production and enhance opening of the angle between the cornea and iris, allowing for increased drainage of aqueous humour. In addition to raised intraocular pressure, inflammation is an important part of the pathophysiology. Therefore, topical steroids are important in the initial treatment as they decrease the inflammatory reaction and reduce optic nerve damage.

After the initial intervention, the patient should be reassessed, which includes evaluating intraocular pressure and considering the need for further medical or surgical intervention. Topical pilocarpine (a muscarinic agonist) should be administered approximately one hour after commencing the initial treatment. Pilocarpine is a miotic agent (causes the pupil to constrict) and therefore causes opening of the angle. In the initial phase of acute glaucoma, there is ischaemic paralysis of the iris due to the increased intraocular pressure. Therefore, pilocarpine is ineffective in the initial management. However, after one hour the primary treatment should have lowered the intraocular pressure sufficiently to reduce the ischaemic paralysis and thus pilocarpine becomes beneficial.

An osmotic agent must be considered if the intraocular pressure is not reduced 30 minutes after a second dose of pilocarpine. Osmotic agents cause a total body fluid reduction and thus reduce vitreous volume, which, in turn, decreases intraocular pressure. The decreased intraocular pressure also improves the responsiveness to other medications such as pilocarpine by reducing the iris ischaemia. Oral osmotic agents such as glycerol are usually prescribed unless the patient is diabetic in which case oral isosorbide is preferred. Intravenous mannitol is usually reserved for patients who are unable to tolerate oral intake or in whom the intraocular pressure does not decrease despite treatment with oral osmotic agents.

The definitive treatment for acute open-angle glaucoma is laser peripheral iridotomy, which is performed 24–48 hours after the intraocular pressure is controlled.

5.35

A – Castleman's disease

This patient's generalised lymphadenopathy combined with a history of Kaposi's sarcoma makes Castleman's disease the most likely diagnosis. This is a benign lymphoproliferative disorder that is also referred to as angiofollicular hyperplasia. Using clinical and radiological findings Castleman's disease can be classified as unicentric or multicentric. This patient has multicentric Castleman's disease, which presents with generalised lymphadenopathy and 'B' symptoms including severe fatigue, night sweats, fever and weight loss. These 'B' symptoms are typically driven by overproduction of interleukin 6. Overproduction of interleukin 6 results in an acute-phase reaction with elevated ESR, C-reactive protein, fibrinogen, a thrombocytosis and hypergammaglobulinaemia. Patients with multicentric Castleman's disease may also suffer from a non-iron-deficient microcytic anaemia and there may be hepatosplenomegaly. About 50% of multicentric Castleman's disease is caused by HHV-8, a gammaherpesvirus trophic to B-lymphocytes. HHV-8 is also the cause of Kaposi's sarcoma. The presence of Kaposi's sarcoma provides further evidence to support a diagnosis of Castleman's disease in this patient. Multicentric Castleman's disease in patients who are HIV positive usually has a poorer prognosis as patients more frequently progress to develop non-Hodgkin's lymphoma.

Unicentric Castleman's disease involves lymphadenopathy in one location (most commonly mediastinal) and presents with no symptoms other than those directly associated with the physical enlargement of the lymph node. Acute-phase proteins are not elevated in unicentric Castleman's disease and this may account for the lack of 'B' symptoms seen in this form of the disease.

Patients with HIV are at risk of developing a variety of opportunistic infections including *Mycobacterium avium* and *Pneumocystis jirovecii*. *Mycobacterium avium* is an atypical *Mycobacterium*. Infection with *Mycobacterium avium* can present with weight loss, night sweats, fever malaise and lymphadenopathy. However, most patients also have a history of diarrhoea and as a result *Mycobacterium avium* infection should always be considered in a person with HIV infection presenting with diarrhoea. The risk of *Mycobacterium avium* infection is inversely related to the patient's CD4 cell count, and increases significantly when the CD4 cell count decreases below 50 cells/mm³.

Pneumocystis jirovecii is a yeast-like fungus that causes pneumocystis pneumonia, which usually presents with dry cough, shortness of breath and rapid oxygen desaturation on exercise. Patients with a CD4 cell count of less than 200 cells/mm³ are at an increased risk of developing pneumocystis pneumonia.

Kikuchi's disease, also termed histiocytic necrotising lymphadenitis, is classically a self-limiting cause of lymphadenitis. The most common clinical manifestation of Kikuchi's disease is cervical lymphadenopathy with a fever that resolves after several weeks or months. Although the cause is currently unknown, many studies suggest a link between Kikuchi's syndrome and systemic lupus erythematosus.

Multiple myeloma is a condition in which there is malignant prolif-eration of plasma B-cells. This produces diffuse bone marrow infil-tration causing bone destruction, bony pain, hypercalcaemia and bone marrow failure. There is also overproduction of a monoclonal antibody by the malignant plasma cells. Immunoglobulin light chains are detectable in the urine as Bence Jones proteins. Patients can also present with immunodeficiency and renal failure.

5.36

D – Paraneoplastic cerebellar degeneration

This patient has developed cerebellar symptoms (incoordination, slurred speech, ataxia and nystagmus) most likely secondary to a paraneoplastic phenomenon. It occurs as a result of anti-neuronal antibodies produced by the primary malignancy that are specific for antigens expressed on Purkinje cells and possibly other cerebel-lar cells. These antibodies mediate damage of these cells, thus pro-ducing the cerebellar symptoms. It is important to note that clinical manifestations of paraneoplastic cerebellar degeneration can pre-cede those of an underlying malignancy by months or years.

Paraneoplastic cerebellar degeneration is most associated with ovar-ian carcinoma but has also been described secondary to breast and small cell lung cancer and Hodgkin's lymphoma. Further investiga-tions involve screening for anti-neuronal antibodies (anti-Yo, anti-Ri, anti-Hu, anti-CV2, anti-mGluR1 and anti-Tr) and appropriate imag-ing to try and identify the primary malignancy. Anti-Hu and anti-CV2 are most associated with small cell lung cancer; anti-Yo with ovarian and breast cancer; anti-Ri with breast and small cell lung cancer; and anti-mGluR1 and anti-Tr with Hodgkin's lymphoma. Treatment of this paraneoplastic syndrome is by surgical removal of the source of the antibodies (i.e. the primary malignancy).

Alcoholic cerebellar degeneration is associated with shrinkage of the cerebellum on MRI scanning and normal protein and white cell count on cerebrospinal fluid analysis. In addition, there is no sig-nificant alcohol history mentioned in the stem of this question.

Cerebellar haemangioblastomas are benign neoplasms associated with von Hippel–Lindau disease; these neoplasms are likely to be identified on an MRI. Haemangioblastomas produce ectopic erythropoietin and so patients can also develop polycythaemia. Multiple sclerosis can also produce cerebellar signs. However, there are no white matter lesions identified on MRI, which makes this diagnosis less likely. Systemic lupus erythematosus is a disease characterised by autoimmune-mediated, systemic inflammation that can affect multiple organs. Again, if there were neurological involvement secondary to systemic lupus erythematosus, it would be likely that lesions would be identified on an MRI.

5.37

E – Whipple's disease

Whipple's disease is a rare cause of malabsorption due to infection with the bacteria *Tropheryma whipplei*. The majority of patients are white, middle-aged males who present with arthralgia, diarrhoea, weight loss and abdominal pain. Central nervous system features include a reversible dementia and oculomasticatory myorhythmia, which describes pendular vergence oscillations of the eyes with concomitant contractions of the muscles of mastication. It is pathognomonic of Whipple's disease. Hyperpigmentation, clubbing and seizures are also well described. Diagnosis is usually made however by small bowel biopsy that reveals the presence of magenta-coloured periodic acid-Schiff-positive macrophages and the presence of trilaminar-walled *Tropheryma whipplei* bacteria within macrophages on electron microscopy. Treatment for Whipple's disease involves intravenous ceftriaxone for two weeks then oral co-trimoxazole for one year.

Coeliac disease is characterised by gluten-induced inflammation of the upper small bowel that results in indigestion, bloating and diarrhoea or steatorrhoea. Mouth ulcers, infertility, polyneuropathy and neuropsychiatric symptoms including epilepsy can also occur. If the disease is left untreated, osteoporosis and gross malnutrition may result. Patients with coeliac disease may also develop dermatitis herpetiformis, an itchy, blistering rash most commonly found on the elbows. Duodenal biopsy reveals subtotal villus atrophy and crypt hyperplasia.

Entamoeba histolytica is a unicellular parasite that causes a diarrhoeal illness which, when severe, results in dysentery. Diagnosis is by stool microscopy (which reveals *Entamoeba histolytica* trophozoites, blood and inflammatory cells) and faecal antigen testing. Treatment is with oral metronidazole. *Giardia lamblia* is another unicellular parasite; it causes malabsorptive symptoms. Treatment is again with metronidazole. Ulcerative colitis does not affect the small bowel and so would not present with features of malabsorption.

5.38

B – Ability to invert the ankle

The common peroneal nerve acts to dorsiflex and evert the ankle, therefore patients with common peroneal nerve palsy are unable to do these actions. It is important to assess ankle inversion in this patient (who has impaired ankle dorsiflexion and an intact ankle jerk) in order to distinguish between a common peroneal nerve palsy and an L4 root lesion. Ability to invert the ankle tells the examiner that L4 nerve root is intact, and so the lesion is along the common peroneal nerve instead. The common peroneal nerve is most commonly injured by compression against the head of the fibula, usually secondary to prolonged leg crossing, pressure from a plaster cast or by repetitive kicking.

Inability to plantarflex the ankle occurs as a result of Achilles tendon rupture. Loss of sensation over the big toe occurs in an L5 nerve root lesion. The gastrocnemius is supplied by S1 and S2 nerve root; therefore wasting of the gastrocnemius occurs if there is a lesion in these nerve roots. The S1 and S2 nerve roots also supply the ankle jerk reflex.

5.39

A – Damage to the bridging veins

This patient's history of increasing confusion after a fall combined with the findings on the CT scan are highly suggestive of a chronic subdural haematoma. Subdural haematomas occur when there is a bleed between the dura mater (the outermost layer of dura) and the arachnoid mater (the second layer of dura), which usually results from tears in the bridging veins that cross the subdural space. Since the dura is attached to the underlying cerebral hemispheres, an atrophied brain will stretch the dura and bridging vessels that run within it. Stretched bridging veins are more prone to rupture and consequently subdural haematomas are more common in patients who have atrophied cerebral hemispheres, such as in patients with Alzheimer's disease or alcoholics.

Extradural haematomas occur outside of the dura in the space between the cranium and the dura mater. The majority of extradural haematomas are as a result of a traumatic blow to the side of the head. The region where the parietal bone, the temporal bone, the greater wing of the sphenoid bone and the frontal bone join (called the pterion) is the weakest part of the cranium. The middle meningeal artery, which runs in the extradural space, lies just below the pterion and is particularly prone to rupture from traumatic blows to the head in this region. Since the cause of the majority of extradural haematomas is due to rupture of an artery, blood accumulates at a much higher rate than in subdural haematomas. Patients initially present with a lucid interval after the injury but will then decline rapidly as the increased intracranial pressure rises above the threshold for which the brain can compensate. The consequence of a rapid rise in intracranial pressure is brainstem herniation and in order to reduce the risk of this, emergency evacuation of the haematoma is required. On CT imaging, extradural haematomas usually appear convex in shape because their expansion stops at the skull's sutures, where the dura mater is tightly attached to the skull. They are often referred to as being lens shaped and are hyperdense on CT due to accumulation of fresh blood.

The posterior inferior cerebellar artery is a branch of the vertebral artery and is one of three arteries to supply the cerebellum. The posterior inferior cerebellar artery also supplies the lateral medulla of the same side. Infarction of the territory supplied by the posterior inferior cerebellar artery results in a characteristic syndrome termed lateral medullary syndrome. The cerebellar features include dysarthria (slurred speech), ipsilateral limb ataxia, vertigo and nystagmus (due to vestibulo-floccular connections). The brainstem signs include an ipsilateral Horner's syndrome (due to ischaemia of the preganglionic sympathetic fibres which run in the lateral medulla), ipsilateral pain and temperature loss to the face (due to ischaemia of the spinal trigeminal nucleus and tract), contralateral loss of pain and temperature of the limbs and trunk (due to ischaemia of the lateral spinothalamic tract), and ipsilateral pharyngeal and laryngeal paralysis (due to ischaemia of the nucleus ambiguus which gives rise to the efferent motor fibres for cranial nerves IX and X). Pharyngeal and laryngeal paralysis gives rise to:

- Dysarthria
- Dysphonia
- Dysphagia.

The posterior cerebral arteries are two in number; there is one for each cerebral hemisphere and they arise from the basilar artery. The major structures that are supplied by the posterior cerebral arteries include parts of the midbrain, the subthalamic nucleus, the thalamus, the occipital cortex and parts of the inferior temporal lobe. The major cause of pathology associated with the posterior cerebral artery is an infarction of the territory supplied by it. This usually presents with a homonymous hemianopia with macular sparing and unilateral sensory loss. An unenhanced CT scan will not reveal any meningeal pathology but there may be an area of hypodensity in the region supplied by the posterior cerebral artery.

The striate arteries supply the internal capsule through which the corticospinal tract runs. Infarction of the territory supplied by the striate arteries leads to the development of a pure motor loss on the contralateral side. This is known as a lacunar syndrome. These patients will initially have a flaccid paralysis followed by the development of upper motor neuron signs.

5.40

E – Send off further blood samples for glucose, urea and electrolytes, fasting lipids and thyroid and liver function tests

It is important to first rule out secondary causes of hypercholesterolaemia when assessing a patient for familial hypercholesterolaemia. Elevated blood lipid levels can be due to thyroid, liver and kidney disease, as well as type II diabetes mellitus, Cushing's syndrome and drugs (e.g. thiazides, steroids, ciclosporin and beta-blockers). After excluding secondary hyperlipidaemias, dietary and lifestyle advice would be the first line of management. Patients should be advised to eat foods containing low levels of saturated fats and cholesterol and high levels of polyunsaturated and mono-unsaturated fats, as well as exercising more. Patients with familial hypercholesterolaemia (autosomal dominant, tendon xanthomas are characteristic) should also be started on a statin. Statins inhibit HMG CoA-reductase, the rate-limiting step in hepatic cholesterol synthesis.

Ezetimibe and bezafibrate are second-line therapy in familial hypercholesterolaemia. Ezetimibe localises in the gut wall to inhibit cholesterol absorption in the small intestine; it can be used alone, or in combination with a statin. Bezafibrate is a type of fibrate medication, which is useful in patients with mixed hyperlipidaemia.

5.41

D – Spot urine test for albumin:creatinine ratio

Microalbuminuria is an albuminuria of 30–300 mg/day and the most appropriate test is a spot urine test for the albumin:creatinine ratio (ideally in the morning because albumin excretion varies throughout the day; heavy exercise should be avoided in the previous 24 hours). In microalbuminuria, the urine levels of albumin are too low to be detectable on routine urine dipstick but could be detected with special albumin-specific urine dipsticks. Imaging is not necessary as part of routine diabetes mellitus surveillance. Renal biopsy is not routinely indicated for diabetic nephropathy and only plays a role if nephrotic syndrome or de novo renal failure develops rapidly.

The albumin:creatinine ratio compensates for variations in urine concentration. Microalbuminuria is defined as an albumin:creatinine ratio of greater than or equal to 2.5 mg/mmol in a male and 3.5 mg/mmol in a female. A positive test should be repeated three months after the first to confirm the first result.

5.42

E – Urine dipstick

Confusion, drowsiness and vomiting, especially in conjunction with polyuria and polydipsia in a young patient, is diabetic ketoacidosis until proven otherwise. This is the initial presentation for 25% of patients with type I diabetes mellitus. A urine dipstick test for ketones and glucose is the most appropriate initial investigation. Diabetic ketoacidosis is due to insulin deficiency, which results in an inability to utilise blood glucose. The resultant hyperglycaemia results in glycosuria and an osmotic diuresis. Also, in the absence of insulin the switch to a catabolic state results in lipolysis and generation of free fatty acids, some of which are converted to ketones in the liver resulting in a high anion gap metabolic acidosis and associated vomiting. In addition to the glycosuric osmotic diuresis, vomiting also contributes to the patient's state of dehydration, which if severe can progress to hypotension, pre-renal acute kidney injury and shock. Shock triggers a stress response (release of catecholamines, cortisol, growth hormone and antidiuretic hormone), which further opposes insulin and worsens the acidosis, hyperglycaemia and state of dehydration.

The most common precipitating factor is infection (found in 50% of cases) and therefore subsequent investigations could include blood cultures, midstream urine, chest X-ray, sputum samples and swabs of any wound sites. Other precipitating factors include myocardial infarction, trauma and stroke (which all increase catecholamine release and therefore the physiological insulin requirement), as well as cessation or omission of insulin therapy. In 10–15% of cases no identifiable cause is found. After urine dipstick, the laboratory investigations that should follow are plasma glucose, urea and electrolytes and an arterial blood gas. Unless an underlying cardiac cause is suspected, an ECG is not routinely recommended.

5.43

D – Opiate analgesia

In sickle cell anaemia, factors including acute stress, infection, inflammation, dehydration, hypoxia, excessive exercise and the cold encourage sickling of red blood cells, predisposing patients to painful vaso-occlusive crises. Patients are therefore advised to avoid such precipitating factors as much as possible. Such crises can occur in many different organs of the body with different frequency and severity. When they do occur, patients need prompt resuscitation and treatment both to correct the precipitant and to reduce the pain (which is often severe and intractable). In this scenario, initial resuscitation has been done and it is clear from her examination and basic observations that such precipitating factors are absent and/or corrected. Therefore, the most appropriate next step in management is to control her pain, which has not been eased by naproxen (an NSAID). Therefore opiates should be administered.

Importantly, patients with recurrent admission for painful crises may require hydroxyurea, a drug that increases production of the non-sickling haemoglobin F in place of haemoglobin S, thereby reducing ischaemic crises.

5.44

B – Lactulose

This patient has developed hepatic encephalopathy secondary to constipation, and therefore the most appropriate management is lactulose. He is already having thiamine as part of his alcohol detoxification regimen. Hepatic encephalopathy is a neuropsychiatric condition that occurs in chronic liver disease. Toxic nitrogenous waste products (particularly ammonia) of protein metabolism undergo hepatic bypass due to portosystemic shunting, and pass into the brain. Here, astrocytic clearance involves the conversion of glutamate to glutamine, which accumulates, resulting in an osmotic imbalance and a shift of fluid into the cells (cerebral oedema). Symptoms range from sleep disturbance, poor concentration, drowsiness and poor intellect to marked confusion, disorientation and coma, and can be graded clinically from grades I to IV. Signs include constructional apraxia (inability to draw simple configurations such as stars, clocks and intersecting pentagons), asterixis (the reverse of myoclonus; brief interruptions of forearm extensor tone leads to a wrist and finger weakness; 'flapping tremor') and dyscalculia (poor mental arithmetic). If there are focal neurological signs then other causes should be sought. The differential diagnosis of hepatic encephalopathy includes intracranial bleed (if suspected, a CT scan should be performed), drug/alcohol intoxication, alcohol withdrawal, delirium tremens, Wernicke's encephalopathy, primary psychiatric disorders, hypoglycaemia, Wilson's disease and post-ictal states. Common precipitating factors of hepatic encephalopathy include alcohol, dehydration (e.g. diuretics, paracentesis), drugs (e.g. sedatives, antidepressants), increased protein load (e.g. oesophageal variceal haemorrhage), hypokalaemia and infection (e.g. spontaneous bacterial peritonitis).

The diagnosis is clinical, and management involves treating the cause and reducing the concentration of toxic nitrogenous waste products produced by gut bacteria. In this scenario, lactulose addresses both of these steps as it first produces an osmotic laxative effect, and second reduces absorption of ammonia by reducing the pH in the colon (through bacterial conversion of lipids to short-chain fatty acids). This favours the formation of the non-absorbable ammonium ion from ammonia. Other aspects of management to consider are further reducing the nitrogenous load (by performing regular enemas and reducing protein intake) and reducing cerebral oedema (by tilting the head up combined with another osmotic diuretic such as mannitol). Although neomycin and metronidazole were previously used to reduce the number of toxin-producing bacteria, their side effects (ototoxicity and peripheral neuropathy, respectively) now contraindicate their use. Sedatives such as zopiclone should be avoided as they may mask the symptoms of encephalopathy.

5.45

E – Vitamin B_{12} deficiency

This patient has a dilated cardiomyopathy. All of the options listed are associated with cardiomyopathy except for vitamin B_{12} deficiency. Cardiomyopathy is the pathological deterioration of myocardial function and can be classified, based on the functional abnormality, into dilated, hypertrophic and restrictive cardiomyopathies (the three most common types). Each of these functional classifications of cardiomyopathy has extrinsic and intrinsic causes depending on whether or not an identifiable extrinsic cause can be identified. Although the term cardio- ('heart') myo- ('muscle') -pathy ('disease') technically applies to a disease that affects the heart, practically speaking it is reserved for severe myocardial disease that leads to congestive cardiac failure. In addition, there are causes of myocardial disease (for example, ischaemic injury or valvular heart disease) that cause the same cardiac dysfunction as (and therefore can mimic) these cardiomyopathies. However, these are not true cardiomyopathies. Dilated and hypertrophic cardiomyopathy are the most common cardiomyopathies, each with a prevalence of 0.2%.

In dilated cardiomyopathy the ventricular walls become stretched, weakened and hypertrophied (dilatation masks ventricular hypertrophy) so that the lumens of all four chambers dilate (the heart becomes 'globular' in shape). Forty percent of cases are X-linked congenital (e.g. a muscular dystrophy). Non-genetic extrinsic causes include:

- Toxins (alcohol and anthracyclin chemotherapies like doxorubicin)
- Hypertension
- Haemochromatosis
- Infections (viral, e.g. post-myocarditis, and parasitic, e.g. Chagas' disease)
- Nutritional deficiencies (vitamin B_1)
- Peri- or post-partum
- Thyrotoxicosis.

Most patients with dilated cardiomyopathy have a normal quality of life, and progression can be halted with medication combined with avoidance of secondary risk factors (hypertension, alcohol, etc.). However, the disease can still slowly progress into fulminant congestive cardiac failure. Stretching of the valve bases (annuli) can lead to mitral and tricuspid incompetence. Patients also have an increased risk of arrhythmias and arterial emboli.

5.46
C – Polycythaemia rubra vera

The most likely diagnosis in this scenario is polycythaemia rubra vera, a type of myeloproliferative disorder in which there is primarily an increase in erythrocyte production; thrombocytosis and a leukocytosis can also occur. The myeloid proliferative disorders are a spectrum of disorders in the myeloid lineage of the bone marrow (the precursors to all mature non-lymphocytic blood cells). They can be divided into those which are Philadelphia chromosome positive or Philadelphia chromosome negative, whereby chronic myeloid leukaemia comprises the former group and polycythaemia rubra vera, essential thrombocytosis and myelofibrosis comprise the latter. The Philadelphia chromosome is a reciprocal transloca- tion in which the long arms of chromosome 9 and 22 are exchanged, which forms the *BCR-ABL* fusion gene on chromosome 22. The Philadelphia chromosome negative myeloproliferative disorders are associated with the JAK2 kinase mutation, particularly poly- cythaemia rubra vera, of which 80% are JAK2 kinase positive.

Polycythaemia is defined as an increase in haemoglobin concentra- tion above the normal range for the patient's age and sex. It can be divided into two subsets:

- Absolute polycythaemia, where the haematocrit (the vol- ume percentage of red cells in the blood) and the red cell mass are greater than expected
- Relative polycythaemia, where the red cell mass is normal but the plasma volume is reduced (often as a result of dehydration).

Once absolute polycythaemia has been confirmed, it can be further subdivided into:

- Primary polycythaemia, where there is a mutation in an erythroid progenitor cell and low erythropoietin levels (e.g. polycythaemia rubra vera)
- Secondary polycythaemia, where the increased haemoglo- bin concentration is driven by raised erythropoietin levels (e.g. high altitiude, chronic lung disease and erythropoie- tin-producing tumours such as renal cell carcinoma).

In this scenario, the raised red cell mass rules out relative poly- cythaemia. The low serum erythropoietin levels rule out secondary causes such as COPD and von Hippel–Lindau disease.

Chronic kidney disease is associated with anaemia, not polycythae- mia, so the best answer in this scenario is polycythaemia rubra vera.

5.47

E – Tinea incognito

Fungal pathology affecting the skin is common, usually as a result of either dermatophyte (multicellular filaments that multiply asexually via spore formation) or yeast (unicellular forms that replicate by budding) infections. It is usually confined to the superficial stratum corneum (horny layer) of the epidermis. Tinea refers to a variety of fungal skin infections, usually as a result of dermatophyte infection.

Dermatophytes obtain their nutrients from keratin and do not invade more deeply owing to the presence of the host's defence mechanisms. Dermatophyte infections of the skin or nails induce inflammation as they spread centrifugally across the skin. Therefore the typical lesion slowly enlarges to produce an inflamed, ringed appearance (hence 'ring worm') with a centralised clearing that can also be described as 'annular', 'discoid' or 'serpiginous' (snake-like). Lesions are also often scaly, crusty, plaque-like, papular and/ or vesicular (especially at the advancing border).

Typical examples of annular lesions include:

- Tinea
- Pityriasis rosea
- Granuloma annulare
- Sarcoidosis
- Leprosy
- Urticaria
- Subacute cutaneous lupus erythematosus
- Erythema annulare centrifugum.

Although flexural psoriasis, cutaneous candidiasis and erythrasma typically cause lesions in flexural areas, they do not tend to cause annular lesions with a central clearing as seen initially in this patient. The name, symptoms and differential diagnosis of tinea infections depend on their location. For example, they can affect the trunk and limbs (tinea corporis), groin (tinea cruris or 'jock itch'), hand (tinea manuum), scalp (tinea capitis), nail bed (tinea unguium or onychomycosis), foot (tinea pedis or 'athlete's foot') and face (tinea faciei).

Common differential diagnoses of a tinea corporis includes atopic dermatitis (eczema), cutaneous candidiasis, erythema multiforme, erythema annulare centrifugum, erythrasma, granuloma annulare, impetigo, leprosy, subacute cutaneous lupus erythematosus, annular, plaque or flexural psoriasis, pityriasis rosea, sarcoidosis, seborrheic dermatitis, tinea versicolour (caused by the commensal yeast *Malassezia*) and urticaria.

This patient presented with classical tinea corporis, which was misdiagnosed as eczema and treated with immunosuppressive topical steroids. During the time that topical immunosuppression is applied to tinea infections, the inflammation, erythema, itching and scaliness improve. However, the margin becomes less well demarcated, and can become pustular. The infection itself spreads, unimpeded by the host-response, such that upon removal of the immunosuppressive cream, the inflammation becomes much worse than it was before. The symptoms then improve upon restarting the topical cream, and therefore a cycle of steroid cream prescriptions can ensue which increasingly allows a florid tinea infection to emerge. The subsequent rash that develops is known as tinea incognito, and may be accompanied by signs of long-term topical steroid use, such as skin atrophy, telangiectasia and striae. The topical steroid should be discontinued, and anti-pruritic emollient lotions and antifungal treatment should be initiated (e.g. ketoconazole, itraconazole, terbinafine, griseofulvin).

5.48

B – Raised alkaline phosphatase

This patient has developed rhabdomyolysis as a result of a prolonged time lying on the floor following a fall. This is a relatively common clinical presentation in such patients and occurs because damaged skeletal muscle is broken down rapidly. Other causes of rhabdomyolysis include sepsis, status epilepticus, prolonged exertion, burns, electrocution and drugs (e.g. statins, fibrates). The intracellular contents of damaged myocytes, which are released into the circulation, include:

- Creatinine: this leads to a disproportionately raised creatinine compared to urea
- Creatine kinase: this is usually greater than five times the upper limit of normal in rhabdomyolysis; it can be 100 times the normal
- Aspartate transaminase: another muscle enzyme released from damaged myocytes
- Potassium: leading to hyperkalaemia and subsequent arrhythmias
- Phosphate: leading to hyperphosphataemia
- Myoglobin: this saturates haptoglobin (responsible for binding haem-containing substances) and is freely filtered in the glomerulus, causing myoglobinuria
- Uric acid: the breakdown product of DNA purines. It forms obstructive casts and creates an acidic urinary environment that permits the binding of myoglobin to Tamm–Horsfall protein (the most abundant urinary protein) resulting in further tubulopathic cast formation.

The release of the above intracellular contents result in the following abnormalities:

- Hypocalcaemia: calcium binds damaged muscle and circulating phosphate
- Myoglobinuria: dark brown 'coca cola' urine that is dipstick positive for blood but is absent for red cells or casts on microscopy is highly suggestive of myoglobinuria. This is because myoglobinuria gives a false positive result for blood on a urine dipstick
- Acute kidney injury: myoglobinuria, uricosuria and dehydration all lead to cast nephropathy and acute tubular necrosis, worsening the electrolyte imbalance

- Disseminated intravascular coagulation: due to mass activation of the coagulation system by damaged myocytes.

Hypernatraemia in this scenario is due to dehydration. Management is supportive. Rehydration dilutes the urine and reduces tubular cast formation. Alkalinisation of the urine reduces precipitation of myoglobin with Tamm–Horsfall protein.

The indications for renal replacement therapy (such as haemodialysis or haemofiltration) in acute kidney injury are as follows:

- Uraemic symptoms (encephalopathy, pericarditis)
- Persistent hyperkalaemia (potassium greater than 7 mmol/L)
- Refractory pulmonary oedema
- Refractory acidosis (arterial pH less than 7.1, bicarbonate less than 12 mmol/L).

5.49

A – Columnar metaplasia

At the normal gastroesophageal junction the epithelial cell type changes from distal oesophageal non-keratinised stratified squamous epithelia to gastric simple columnar epithelia. However, in Barrett's oesophagus, due to prolonged reflux of gastric contents (notably acid), there is metaplasia (the replacement of one differentiated cell type into another differentiated cell type) of oesophageal squamous epithelia to gastric columnar epithelia, known as columnar metaplasia. Squamous metaplasia is the reverse process, which can occur at the cervical os (metaplasia of the endocervical simple columnar epithelium to ectocervical squamous epithelium) if there is prolonged exposure to the acidic environment of the vagina.

Dysplasia refers to the presence of abnormally or incompletely differentiated cell types, and is deemed to be a pre-malignant change likely to progress to neoplasia (the abnormal proliferation of cells). In patients with Barrett's oesophagus, the classification of dysplasia is divided into either low-grade or high-grade dysplasia. Barrett's

oesophagus is associated with increased risk of developing oesophageal adenocarcinoma and therefore is surveyed regularly by endo-
scopical biopsy.

5.50

A – Acute interstitial nephritis

NSAIDs such as naproxen can cause two separate forms of acute
kidney injury: acute interstitial nephritis or pre-renal acute kidney
injury as a result of renal haemodynamic compromise.

Acute interstitial nephritis is associated with an eosinophilia and
eosinophiluria, and evidence of renal failure may also be present.
Patients can present with malaise, fever, rash and arthralgia. Acute
interstitial nephritis is an acute inflammation of the renal interstitium, which surrounds the tubules of the nephron, and is most commonly caused by an allergic reaction to medication. Renal biopsy
in acute interstitial nephritis reveals a dense infiltration of the
interstitium with lymphocytes, monocytes and eosinophils. The
most common medications implicated are:

- Allopurinol
- Beta-lactam antibiotics (penicillins, cephalosporins and
  carbapenems)
- NSAIDs
- Rifampicin
- Sulphonamides.

The second form of NSAID-induced acute kidney injury is pre-
renal acute kidney injury, which occurs as a result of reduced prostaglandin production secondary to cyclo-oxygenase inhibition.
Prostaglandins are normally responsible for dilation of the afferent
arteriole, and therefore NSAID administration can cause unop-
posed constriction of the afferent arteriole, resulting in an increased
risk of ischaemia to the nephron. Prolonged renal ischaemia particularly affects the tubules, which are more susceptible due to their

high metabolism and relatively poor perfusion. Therefore acute tubular necrosis can arise secondary to pre-renal acute kidney injury. However, these haemodynamic causes of acute kidney injury are not associated with eosinophiluria or eosinophilia.

5.51

B – Idiopathic pulmonary fibrosis

Idiopathic pulmonary fibrosis is a progressive fibrotic condition with a median survival of up to four years. Lung function tests reveal a restrictive pattern. Males are affected more commonly than females; patients are typically non-smokers and are usually clubbed. The diagnosis is usually confirmed with a high-resolution CT scan of the lungs with the patient prone. Bilateral predominantly basal and subpleural reticulation with traction bronchiectasis and basal honeycombing with minimal ground glass shadowing is typical. The pathogenesis is complex – an aberrant wound-healing response following lung injury in a genetically susceptible person is the current theory. Immunosuppression is not effective and the current treatment regimen is oral *N*-acetylcysteine.

Caplan's syndrome is the association between rheumatoid arthritis and pneumoconiosis. Sarcoidosis is a recognised cause of pulmonary fibrosis but the fibrosis typically affects the upper zones, basal crackles would be unusual and the patients are not usually clubbed. Tuberculosis causes predominantly upper zone fibrosis. The patient is not in heart failure.

Chronic restrictive lung diseases are either intrinsic to the lung parenchyma or extrinsic to it (e.g. neuromuscular diseases, disorders of the chest wall and pleural thickening, obesity).

Intrinsic restrictive lung diseases (or 'interstitial lung diseases') are characterised by diffuse lung injury with inflammation and fibrosis which results in reduced FEV_1 and FVC, a normal or high FEV_1:FVC ratio and impaired gas exchange (a restrictive pattern of lung disease).

Causes of intrinsic restrictive lung disease include:

- Idiopathic pulmonary fibrosis
- Infections, e.g. tuberculosis
- Drugs (e.g. amiodarone, bleomycin, methotrexate, sulpha-salazine, nitrofurantoin)
- Occupation-related (e.g. asbestosis, berylliosis, silicosis, coal worker's pneumoconiosis, Caplan's syndrome, hypersensitivity pneumonitis)
- Connective tissue diseases (e.g. rheumatoid arthritis, systemic lupus erythematosus, scleroderma, polymyositis)
- Sarcoidosis
- Radiotherapy (radiation fibrosis).

5.52

D – Pemphigus vulgaris

A blister (bulla) is a collection of fluid that forms within the skin. It is an important medical presentation and differentiating different types of blisters can aid diagnosis.

The skin is made up of three layers, the epidermis, the dermis and the subcutis (the innermost layer of fat and connective tissue). The dermis is a tough interwoven collagen matrix that supports the epidermis, a stratified squamous epithelium made up of keratinocytes that mature as they migrate outwards. The epidermis is divided into four layers (each representing the increasing maturation of keratinocytes), the outermost of which (the corneal layer) is comprised of sheets of dead, anucleated keratinocytes whose cytoplasm is almost entirely keratin. The keratinocytes are bound together by intercellular desmosomes.

Blisters can be either subepidermal, intraepidermal or subcorneal. Subepidermal blisters are tense and sturdy, and occur in conditions such as bullous pemphigoid, dermatitis herpetiformis, linear IgA disease, insect bites and thermal injury (burns). On the other hand, intraepidermal and subcorneal blisters are flaccid and easily ruptured, and occur in conditions such as pemphigus vulgaris, pustular psoriasis, bullous impetigo, acute eczema and herpes virus infection. As they rupture early, these conditions can instead present with a non-purulent exudative, crusty surface, which, because the skin barrier is broken down, can easily develop secondary bacterial infection.

Pemphigus vulgaris and bullous pemphigoid, although rare, are the two most important primary bullous disorders to be aware of. Although they are both autoimmune blistering disorders, they present with different types of blisters because the target of the IgG autoantibodies that are formed is different; in pemphigus vulgaris the antibodies are against the desmosomes (cell to cell adhesion), whereas in bullous pemphigoid the antibodies are against the basement membrane of epidermis. Therefore, in pemphigus vulgaris, slight rubbing of the skin causes exfoliation of the outermost layer of skin (positive Nikolsky's sign), which can cause bleeding. This can also occur in scalded skin syndrome. However, early mouth ulceration is a specific feature of pemphigus vulgaris. Behcet's disease causes the triad of aphthous mouth ulcers, genital ulcers and uveitis, but does not cause skin blistering.

5.53

E – Referral for urgent colonoscopy

Microcytic anaemia is most commonly due to iron deficiency (as in this case). Other causes to consider are thalassaemia and sideroblastic anaemia (particularly if iron supplementation is unsuccessful). However, thalassaemia and sideroblastic anaemia both cause an accumulation of iron (which will be reflected by raised iron and ferritin with a low total iron-binding capacity) and are therefore unlikely in this scenario.

Iron deficiency is not a diagnosis, and a cause must always be sought. This patient has a recent change in bowel habit and a search for a convincing reason for his iron deficiency (e.g. overt haemorrhage, malabsorption, vegetarianism) other than from the colon was unsuccessful. Therefore an urgent colonoscopy in two weeks or less is required to exclude a colonic tumour. Medical management of this patient's loose stools (e.g. loperamide) or iron deficiency (e.g. ferrous sulphate) would not be helpful, and Fybogel (a high-fibre supplement) would actually worsen his loose stools. Finally, a haematology opinion may be required but not before an occult gastrointestinal malignancy is excluded.

5.54

A – Ceftriaxone

This patient's history and examination findings are highly suggestive of typhoid and he should be treated with ceftriaxone. Typhoid is caused by subspecies of the Gram-negative organism *Salmonella enterica* of which there are two main serotypes: *Salmonella typhi* and *Salmonella paratyphi*. Typhoid is mainly spread via food substances contaminated with faecal matter and is endemic in most developing countries in Asia and Africa. Consequently, typhoid should be considered in all patients who present with fever and diarrhoea and have travelled to an endemic area within the last month. The incubation time for typhoid is around 10–20 days but may be as short as three days. Initially it may present with intermittent diarrhoea, fever, headaches and non-productive cough. As the illness progresses patients become increasingly unwell. Examination findings in patients with typhoid may reveal a slightly distended abdomen and splenomegaly. Patients may also develop Rose spots, which are caused by bacterial emboli and are crops of macules 2–4 millimeters in diameter that blanch on pressure. Blood cultures or the Widal test, which measures agglutinating antibodies against the flagellar and somatic antigens of *Salmonella typhi*, can confirm the diagnosis of typhoid.

In patients who are systemically unwell and have a toxic appearance, intravenous antibiotics are usually required. If the patient is likely to have contracted the illness in Asia, empirical treatment with an intravenous third-generation cephalosporin such as ceftriaxone is required. This patient is systemically unwell and has

travelled to Asia. Therefore, they require treatment with intravenous ceftriaxone.In all other patients with typhoid who are systemically unwell intravenous quinolones such as oxofloxacin can
be used as an empirical treatment. In patients who do not appear
systemically unwell, oral antibiotics can be used. The empirical
treatment for these patients is an oral quinolone such as oxofloxacin. However, if the patient has travelled to Asia oral azithromycin
is the preferred antibiotic.

Metronidazole (a nitroimidazole antibiotic), co-amoxiclav (amoxicillin and clavulanic acid), doxycycline (a tetracycline) and quinine
have no role in the management of typhoid. Doxycycline and quinine are used in the treatment of malaria. However, this patient
does not have malaria as the thick and thin blood films, which
detect the presence of malaria parasites, are negative.

5.55

D – 90 mg MST modified release every 12 hours

When calculating opiate requirements for patients with pain, the
first thing to assess is the total amount of morphine received in
24 hours. This patient is requiring two doses of 60 mg MST modified release and three doses of 20 mg Oromorph®. This equates to
180 mg of MST.

Modified release preparations (e.g. Morphgesic®, MST Continus®)
can be given every 12 hours and have maximum effect after 4 hours.
Therefore the correct answer is 90 mg MST modified release every
12 hours. This should be prescribed on the regular side of the drug
chart.

Immediate release preparations of morphine (e.g. Sevredol® tablets, Oramorph® oral solution) should be prescribed on the *pro re
nata* (as required) side of the drug chart for breakthrough pain.
These preparations have maximum effect after 20 minutes and can
be given every 4 hours. The maximum amount of morphine that
can be taken on the 'as required' side of the drug chart should equal

the amount of modified release morphine. Therefore in this patient a maximum of 180 mg can be given to the patient on the 'as required' side (i.e. 30 mg 4-hourly).

It is customary to calculate the strength of opiates in comparison to morphine. Below are some useful rules of thumb for converting oral morphine doses to other opiate medications:

0.1: codeine phosphate
0.1: tramadol
1: oral morphine
1.5: oral diamorphine
2: parenteral morphine
2: oral oxycodone
3: parenteral diamorphine
4: parenteral oxycodone

The strength of parenteral preparations (intravenous, intramuscular or subcutaneous) tends to be twice that of oral.

To convert an oral morphine dose to a fentanyl patch dose, the following approximation can be used: 60 mg of oral morphine per 24 hours equates to a 25 microgram/hour fentanyl patch.

For all patients taking strong opioids it is best practice to co-prescribe regular simple analgesia (paracetamol and an NSAID), a regular stimulant laxative (e.g. senna), an as required antiemetic (e.g. metoclopramide) and an as required naloxone (in case of overdose). Finally, whenever a patient's opiate dose is increased it is vital to monitor for signs of opioid toxicity:

- Drowsiness/confusion
- Slurred speech
- Myoclonus
- Hallucinations
- Pupil constriction.

5.56

E – Trastuzumab

Trastuzumab, which is also known by its brand name as Herceptin, is a monoclonal antibody against the HER2 receptor. It is recommended as an option to treat advanced breast cancer that strongly expresses HER2. The major side effect of trastuzumab is cardiotoxicity and it is associated with the development of congestive cardiac failure, as has occurred in this patient. Other chemotherapeutic agents associated with cardiotoxicity are the anthracyclines, such as daunorubicin and doxorubicin.

Carboplatin is a chemotherapeutic agent that crosslinks DNA and is used to treat a wide variety of malignancies but is not routinely used in breast cancer. It has many side effects including vestibulocochlear nerve palsy, neurotoxicity and nephrotoxicity. It is also highly emetogenic and so should be given in combination with an antiemetic agent. Docetaxel is an anti-mitotic agent that can be given first-line for HER2-negative advanced breast cancer. Gemcitabine is also a first-line agent used to treat HER2-negative advanced breast cancer. Both of these agents are cytotoxic and so are associated with many side effects, including bone marrow suppression. Tamoxifen is an oestrogen receptor antagonist that plays an important role in treating oestrogen receptor–positive breast cancer. Long-term tamoxifen treatment is associated with an increased risk of endometrial cancer.

5.57

C – Hydrocortisone

This patient has presented with features of severe hypothyroidism and also has co-existent Addison's disease. The underlying diagnosis in this case, given that the serum thyroid-stimulating hormone is raised, is most likely autoimmune polyendocrine syndrome type II rather than panhypopituitarism.

It is essential that this patient is given intravenous hydrocortisone before replacement of thyroid hormones. This is because administration of thyroid hormones alone will initially increase the basal metabolic rate and therefore may precipitate an Addisonian crisis. Thyroid hormone replacement can then be initiated once hydrocortisone has been commenced. It is preferable to use triiodothyronine initially because it has a shorter half-life and duration of effect than thyroxine. Thyroxine maintenance can then be introduced after a few days of treatment with triiodothyronine.

In the long term, this patient will require fludrocortisone, which has a greater mineralocorticoid effect than hydrocortisone. This should only be started once the patient has been converted to oral hydrocortisone.

Adrenaline plays no role in the management of myxoedema coma. Aside from hormone replacement, the focus of management should be on:

- Mechanical ventilation if there are signs of respiratory compromise
- Careful fluid balance assessment
- Initiation of broad-spectrum antibiotics (infection is a common precipitant)
- Treatment of hypothermia using warming blankets.

5.58

C – Omit warfarin and commence prothrombin complex with intravenous vitamin K

Clarithromycin inhibits CYP3A4, a CYP450 isoenzyme that metabolises warfarin. Consequently, this patient has developed warfarin toxicity. The management of excessive warfarin anticoagulation depends upon the international normalised ratio, the indication for anticoagulation and whether there is major bleeding as a consequence of the over-anticoagulation. Major bleeds (e.g. intracerebral haemorrhage) should be urgently treated with prothrombin complex concentrate and intravenous vitamin K. The table below highlights the management of excessive warfarin anticoagulation:

International normalised ratio	Management
4.5–6	Reduce warfarin dose or omit. Restart when international normalised ratio is less than 5
6–8	Stop warfarin. Restart when international normalised ratio is less than 5
Greater than 8 with no bleeding or minor bleeding (e.g. epistaxis)	Stop warfarin. Give oral vitamin K if risk factors for bleeding
Any value with major bleeding including intracerebral haemorrhage	Prothrombin complex concentrate and intravenous vitamin K

Prothrombin complex concentrate contains all the vitamin K–dependent clotting factors and is preferred to fresh frozen plasma as it provides a more complete and rapid reversal of warfarin. Additionally, large volumes of fresh frozen plasma may often be required which may result in the patient becoming fluid overloaded.

Vitamin K may take several hours to work and can cause prolonged resistance when restarting warfarin. Therefore, in patients with metallic heart valves, who have a high risk of valve thrombosis, intravenous vitamin K should be avoided.

5.59

D – Friedreich's ataxia

This young male has features of a cerebellar syndrome, mixed upper and lower motor neuron signs, dorsal column dysfunction, pyramidal weakness, ejection systolic murmur and high plantar and palate arches. The most likely diagnosis is Friedrich's ataxia, an autosomal recessive condition in which the mutation is a trinucleotide repeat gene expansion. Other repeat expansion diseases include:

- Huntingdon's disease
- Spinocerebellar ataxia
- Fragile X syndrome
- Myotonic dystrophy
- Juvenile myoclonic epilepsy.

Friedreich's ataxia is primarily a neurological condition. There is degeneration of the dorsal columns (loss of vibration and proprioception, e.g. positive Romberg's test), corticospinal tracts (pyramidal upper motor neuron pattern of weakness, e.g. extensor plantar response), spinocerebellar tracts (cerebellar syndrome, e.g. ataxia, intention tremor) and peripheral large myelinated nerve fibres (lower motor neuron pattern, e.g. absent distal reflexes). Other associated features include diabetes mellitus, optic atrophy, hypertrophic cardiomyopathy (ejection systolic murmur), sensorineural deafness, high-arched palate and pes cavus. Marfan's syndrome can also cause a high-arched palate and kyphoscoliosis. However, it is associated with primarily musculoskeletal rather than neurological dysfunction, as well as pes planus (flat foot arches) and aortic/mitral regurgitation.

Pes cavus is a high-arched foot that doesn't flatten on weight bearing, and can be unilateral or bilateral. There are many causes:

- Idiopathic
- Orthopaedic
    - Post-traumatic calcaneal/talar fracture malunion
    - Plantar fascia contraction
    - Achilles tendon shortening
- Neuromuscular
    - Friedreich's ataxia

- o Poliomyelitis
- o Spinal trauma/tumour
- o Syringomyelia
- o Muscular dystrophies (e.g. Duchenne/Becker muscular dystrophy)
- o Charcot–Marie–Tooth disease.

Charcot–Marie–Tooth disease represents a heterogenous group of chronic polyneuropathies, also referred to as hereditary motor and sensory neuropathy. The typical features are a predominantly motor peripheral neuropathy (sensory involvement is later) with distal lower motor neuron signs (e.g. weakness, absent reflexes), as well as palpable peripheral nerves (especially the common peroneal nerve over the head of the fibula) and absence of upper motor neuron signs.

In addition to Friedreich's ataxia, only a select group of conditions can cause mixed upper and lower motor neuron signs. Most commonly the cause is dual pathology, in which there are two heterogeneous conditions causing both upper (e.g. stroke, myelopathy, spondylosis) and lower (e.g. peripheral neuropathy) motor neuron features simultaneously. The examples of standalone unifying causes of the mixed motor pattern are as follows (the final three of these are also associated with dorsal column signs):

- Amyotrophic lateral sclerosis
- Conus medullaris lesions (the lower tapered end of the spinal cord)
- Friedreich's ataxia
- Taboparesis (tertiary syphilis; tabes dorsalis and general paresis of the insane)
- Subacute combined degeneration of the cord (vitamin B_{12} deficiency).

Of these, Friedreich's ataxia is the only one to present with this patient's constellation of symptoms and signs. The most likely differential diagnoses in the current scenario would be amyotrophic lateral sclerosis (the patient would be older and have purely motor signs, with no cerebellar or sensory involvement), tabes dorsalis (patient will likely have an Argyll Robertson pupil) and a lesion of the conus medullaris (would cause mixed upper and lower motor neuron signs of the legs alone).

5.60

B – Demeclocycline

This patient has developed the syndrome of inappropriate antidiuretic hormone, most likely as a result of his head injury. In the syndrome of inappropriate antidiuretic hormone there is dilute plasma that has an osmolality of less than 260 mmol/kg and concentrated urine that has an osmolality of greater than 500 mmol/kg.

The antidiuretic hormone is made in the hypothalamus and is usually secreted from the posterior pituitary in response to a high plasma osmolality or reduced circulating volume. It acts on the kidney, causing insertion of aquaporin II channels into the distal convoluted tubule and collecting ducts. The function of aquaporin II is to reabsorb water from the tubules back into the interstitium. Thus, there is a dilute plasma and concentrated urine in the syndrome of antidiuretic hormone.

Treatment for the syndrome of antidiuretic hormone is usually by fluid restriction to 0.5–1 L per day. In severe cases, demeclocycline (a tetracycline antibiotic) can be used to antagonise the effects of antidiuretic hormone on the collecting ducts. It acts by inhibiting the insertion of aquaporin II channels and causes nephrogenic diabetes insipidus. Tolvaptan is a vasopressin V2 receptor antagonist that can be used if fluid restriction and demeclocycline are ineffective.

Diabetes insipidus is the opposite of the syndrome of antidiuretic hormone. Patients have a concentrated plasma and produce dilute urine. Diabetes insipidus can be either craniogenic, where there is a failure to produce antidiuretic hormone, or nephrogenic, where there is insensitivity to the action of antidiuretic hormone. Treatment for craniogenic diabetes insipidus involves replacement of antidiuretic hormone using the synthetic analogue desmopressin.

Amiloride is a potassium-sparing diuretic that acts by inhibiting sodium reabsorption in the distal convoluted tubule. In theory, diuretics should increase free water excretion; however, they are not widely used in the treatment of the syndrome of antidiuretic hormone.

Addison's disease and hypothyroidism are also causes of hyponatraemia; however, there is nothing in this scenario to suggest these diagnoses and so treatment with hydrocortisone and thyroxine, respectively, is not indicated.

Index by Topic

Gastroenterology	1.9, 1.10, 1.32, 1.33, 1.48, 1.49, 1.50
	2.9, 2.44, 2.50, 2.53
	3.9, 3.28, 3.32, 3.46, 3.49, 3.50, 3.51, 3.57
	4.6, 4.42, 4.43, 4.46, 4.47, 4.48
	5.44, 5.49
Haematology	1.12, 1.36, 1.37, 1.53
	2.10, 2.11, 2.12, 2.15, 2.32, 2.33
	3.12, 3.13, 3.39, 3.52, 3.58
	4.7, 4.15, 4.30, 4.52
	5.6, 5.8, 5.25, 5.43, 5.46, 5.53, 5.58
Infectious diseases	1.4, 1.19, 1.13, 1.23, 1.24, 1.38, 1.57, 1.58
	2.4, 2.13, 2.22, 2.23, 2.28, 2.38
	3.20, 3.23, 2.24, 3.60
	4.19, 4.20, 4.24, 4.33, 4.36, 4.49, 4.51
	5.7, 5.18, 5.19, 5.28, 5.35, 5.37, 5.54
Nephrology	1.14, 1.15, 1.18, 1.39, 1.54, 1.56
	2.34, 2.48, 2.54
	3.2, 3.14, 3.15, 3.27, 3.55
	4.11, 4.31, 4.32, 4.58
	5.9, 5.10, 5.11, 5.48, 5.50
Neurology	1.16, 1.40, 1.41, 1.42, 1.60
	2.16, 2.25, 2.35, 2.36, 2.37,
	2.39, 2.49, 2.59
	3.16, 3.22, 3.37, 3.38,
	3.40, 3.41, 3.56
	4.13, 4.34, 4.35, 4.37, 4.40
	5.12, 5.22, 5.30, 5.36, 5.38, 5.39
Oncology	1.20, 1.25, 1.43, 1.55, 1.59
	2.5, 2.21, 2.24, 2.41
	3.25
	4.21
	5.20, 5.29, 5.31, 5.55, 5.56

Index by Keyword